Clinical and Experimental Restricted Environmental Stimulation

Arreed F. Barabasz
Marianne Barabasz
Editors

Clinical and Experimental Restricted Environmental Stimulation

New Developments and Perspectives

With an Introduction by
Ernest R. Hilgard

Springer-Verlag
New York Berlin Heidelberg London Paris
Tokyo Hong Kong Barcelona Budapest

Arreed F. Barabasz, Ed.D., Ph.D., A.B.P.P.
Professor, President, International REST Investigators Society, Director,
Attentional Processes Laboratory, Washington State University, Cleveland Hall,
Pullman,WA 99164-2131, USA

Marianne Barabasz, Ed.D.
Associate Professor, Attentional Processes Laboratory, Washington State University,
Cleveland Hall, Pullman, WA 99164-2131, USA

With 33 Illustrations.

Library of Congress Cataloging-in-Publication Data
Clinical and experimental restricted environmental stimulation : new
developments and perspectives / Arreed F. Barabasz, Marianne
Barabasz, editors : introduction by Ernest R. Hilgard.
p. cm.—
Includes bibliographical references

1. Restricted environmental stimulation—Congresses.
I. . Barabasz, Arreed F. II. Barabasz, Marianne.
[DNLM: 1. Psychotherapy—methods—congresses. 2. Sensory
Deprivation—congresses. WM 420 C641]
RC489.S44C6 1993
616.89'14—dc20
DNLM/DLC 92-48872
for Library of Congress

Printed on acid-free paper.

Softcover reprint of the hardcover 1st edition 1993

Production managed by Christin R. Ciresi; manufacturing supervised by Vincent Scelta.
Camera-ready copy prepared by the editors using WordPerfect.

9 8 7 6 5 4 3 2 1

ISBN 978-1-4684-8585-1 ISBN 978-1-4684-8583-7 (eBook)

DOI 10.1007/978-1-4684-8583-7

This is also the first volume to introduce the dry float, a new form of REST. This innovative approach combines features of the chamber method with those of the salt water wet float. Dry float and wet float effects are compared in a number of chapters emphasizing electroencephalographic, blood pressure, and plasma cortisol responses. New methodologies, such as continuous blood sampling during flotation REST, are elucidated in detail sufficient to facilitate use in laboratory and clinical situations.

The first experimentally controlled study of the immunological effects of REST is presented. Other studies report REST effects on physical dysfunctions and psychological disorders. These later studies emphasize a variety of foci including REST prescriptions for the treatment of premenstrual syndrome and extended REST sessions to treat children with autism. Finally, the clinical utility of REST in physical therapy and the treatment of physical disabilities is introduced.

We have tried to stress the presentation of information to make methodology amenable to replication, verification or disproof. It is hoped that these characteristics will stimulate further interest, study and application of what is already one of the most exciting and efficacious interventions available to the researcher and clinician.

The preparation of this volume was made possible by the supportive atmosphere provided by Washington State University. Special thanks are extended to Dennis Warner and Dean Bernard Oliver.

Special gratitude is expressed to Leigh Ann Matson and Cindy Sollinger, the recipients of many hours of dictation. Final preparation was made possible by Leigh Ann Matson and Christina Rulffes.

Arreed Barabasz
Marianne Barabasz

Washington State University
Pullman, Washington, USA

Contents

Part II: Sensory Restriction and Hypnotizability

Section III. Enhancement of Performance

Section IV. Stress Management

Section V. Treatment of Habit Disorders

Section VI. Psychophysiological Effects

Section VII. Biological Effects

Contributors

RICHARD ATKINSON — Fort Hays State University, Fort Hays, Kansas 67601-4099 USA

ELIZABETH BALLARD — Vancouver Community College, Langara Campus, Vancouver, British Columbia V5I 2Z6 CANADA

ARREED BARABASZ — Washington State University, Pullman, Washington 99164-2131 USA

MARIANNE BARABASZ — Washington State University, Pullman, Washington 99164-2131 USA

RODERICK BORRIE — Sensorium Institute, East Setauket, New York 11733 USA

CHARLES BROWNFIELD — Audubon, New Jersey 08106 USA

HELEN CRAWFORD — Virginia Polytechnic Institute and State University, Blacksburg, Virginia 24061 USA

JAMES DANA — Advanced Bio-Physical Care, East Setauket, New York 11733 USA

ANNA DELEON — Medical College of Ohio, Toledo, Ohio 43699 USA

DAVID DIRITO	Colorado Mental Health Institute, Pueblo, Colorado 81003 USA
CPT. REBECCA DYER	United States Army, Fort Drum, Community Mental Health Service, Watertown, New York 13601 USA
THOMAS FINE	Medical College of Ohio, Toledo, Ohio 43699 USA
MARTIN FRIEDMAN	Sensorium Institute, East Setauket, New York 11733 USA
WILLIAM GERARD	Medical College of Ohio, Toledo, Ohio 43699 USA
CATHY GIBSON	Medical College of Ohio, Toledo, Ohio 43699 USA
JOHN HARRISON	Community Medical Center, Missoula, Montana 59801 USA
ERNEST HILGARD	Stanford University, Stanford, California 94305 USA
JOHN HYLAND	Medical College of Ohio, Toledo, Ohio 43699 USA
WALTER JESSEN	Regeneration Institute, Los Gatos, California 95032 USA
PATRICK MCALENEY	Mercy Center for Health Services, Watertown, New York 13601 USA
SEAN MEE	Community Mental Health Center, Spokane, Washington 99202 USA
PETER MIGALY	Lafayette Clinic, Detroit, Michigan 48207 USA Formerly Semmelweis Medical University, Budapest, HUNGARY

DONNA MILLS	Medical College of Ohio, Toledo, Ohio 43699 USA
PAMELA NIELAND	Medical College of Ohio, Toledo, Ohio 43699 USA
SANDRA PERRY	Advanced Bio-Physical Care, East Setauket, New York 11733 USA
VLADIMIR RAIKOV	Center for Preventive Medicine, Petroverigski, DOM 10, Moscow, RUSSIA
NOEL RATHER	Texas A & M University, College Station, Texas 77843 USA
PATRICIA RUZYLA-SMITH	Center for Nursing Education, Spokane, Washington 99208 USA
HARMONY SHROEDER	Medical College of Ohio, Toledo, Ohio 43699 USA
GARY STEEL	University of British Columbia, Vancouver, British Columbia, V6T 1Z4 CANADA
PETER SUEDFELD	University of British Columbia, Vancouver, British Columbia, V6T 1Z4 CANADA
JOHN TURNER, JR.	Medical College of Ohio, Toledo, Ohio 43699 USA
CPT. JEFFREY WAGAMAN	United States Army, 130th Station Hospital, Heidelberg, AEO9102 GERMANY
IAN WICKRAMASEKERA	East Virginia Medical School, Norfolk, Virginia 23507 USA

Introduction

Ernest R. Hilgard

The chapters gathered together here serve as the selected proceedings of the 4th International Congress on Restricted Environmental Stimulation (REST) held in Washington, DC, in 1990. The congress was sponsored by the International REST Investigators Society (IRIS). Arreed Barabasz, President of IRIS, and his wife Marianne Barabasz, edited the volume. They have been very active researchers in this area, and authored or coauthored 11 of the 30 chapters. Altogether there are 34 different authors and coauthors represented.

The basic arrangements for isolating the subjects in experiments of this kind are two, the *chamber* method and the *flotation* method. The chamber method was introduced by Donald Hebb of McGill University, and the first account that appeared was published with his students and collaborators, Heron, Bexton, and Hebb (1953), followed by Bexton, Heron, and Scott (1954). Hebb (1949) had invented perceptual isolation as a method to test his theoretical proposal that behavior is centrally directed. A student could be isolated for two or three days in a soundproof compartment box with a bed in it. Patterned visual stimulation was reduced through the wearing of translucent goggles as the student lay quietly in bed, and special stimulation from self-induced movements was reduced by wearing cardboard sleeves over arms and hands. Communications between subject and experimenter were made through a headset. The occasional hallucinations induced served to attract interest to the method. Current methodology (Barabasz, 1980a; Suedfeld, 1980) typically limits exposure to a maximum of 24 hours. Arm sleeves and other anxiety producing props have been eliminated.

The flotation method had been introduced independently at the National Institute of Mental Health, under the general direction of

John C. Lilly, although his publications began later than those from Hebb's laboratory. In his first publication (Lilly, 1956), while he referred to his flotation experiments, a good deal of emphasis was placed upon the consequences of isolation in life experiences as reported in autobiographical accounts such as those of isolated sailors or those enduring the polar night. In a later publication he gave in detail what he considered the desiderata for an isolation tank (Lilly & Shurley, 1961). These earlier accounts and his subsequent experiments appeared in book form after a lapse of several more years (Lilly, 1975). In it he gives a full account of his specifications for the flotation tank and gives numerous memory protocols of the experience as recounted by named persons who had experienced spending from one to several hours in the tank, then written out what they recalled, with permission for him to publish what they wrote.

The water is somewhat below body temperature, at which it feels neither warm or cold (93.5° F) and comfortable flotation is achieved by dissolving ordinary commercial Epsom salt in the water to raise the specific gravity to 1.3. The body is submerged except for the head and neck, resting on the hands held behind the head.

The range of topics covered in the eight sections into which the present book is divided point clearly to the relevance of the restricted environmental stimulation data to many topical fields that are of interest to various specialties within psychology and education.

Because of my own special interest in research on hypnotic phenomena and dissociation, I was pleased to see that the testing for changes in hypnotic responsiveness, along with electrophysiological indicators, had led to efforts to find some common theoretical ground, especially in Sections I, II, and VI, all of which indicated a new type of integration in REST findings. Those with interests in many other fields will find occasions to celebrate the findings relevant to their own interests. The headings of the eight sections are good guides to the findings of greatest pertinence.

This rich account should reach many readers who may as a result correct their beliefs that the restricted environmental stimulation investigations lie only as a specialty outside the domain of their own interests.

1

Stimulus and Theoretical Reductionism: What Underlies REST Effects?

Peter Suedfeld

One of the interesting aspects of being a REST researcher is being frequently asked, "Why does REST have all these effects?" The question is asked by reporters, actual or prospective participants, and professional colleagues. Unfortunately, no one so far has given a totally satisfactory answer. One attractive kind of answer tries to ally the supposedly more "scientific" biological sciences with our work by proposing theories of REST phenomena that focus on how stimulus reduction affects the functioning of the central nervous system (CNS). Because these explanations approach the understanding of behavioural and psychological phenomena from a neural viewpoint, they can be called reductionistic.

One distinction to be borne in mind is the one between neurophysiological effects of REST and neurophysiological explanations for REST effects. Even a well-established demonstration that REST brings about a particular change in CNS functioning does not establish that the change is responsible for the psychological changes exhibited by REST subjects on measures of perception, cognition, mood, and the like (for an interesting recent discussion of this issue, see Cacioppo &

Tassinary, 1990). Correlation is not evidence of causation. The common tendency to ignore that point is exacerbated by the fact that there are seductive metaphors across levels of explanation in the language that we use: arousal (neurological/physiological or cognitive/emotional), dominance (of a mode of thought, of a cerebral hemisphere). With that warning, let us look at the theories.

From the very infancy of the field, stimulus reduction has been accompanied by such theoretical reductionism. The theory that led to the invention of "perceptual isolation" was Hebb's (1949) neuropsychological speculation that behaviour is centrally, not peripherally, directed. His theory stressed the complexity of behaviour-environment interactions, and the holistic aspects of brain activity: neuronal networks, reverberating circuits and feedback mechanisms, all working in a probabilistic rather than a deterministic fashion. This was a far cry from the simple primary drive models of motivation and telephone-switchboard models of brain functioning that had been in vogue only a few years earlier.

Monotonous stimulation should, according to this approach, interfere with the functioning of phase sequences, which would lose their organization and persistence. As a result, environments in which stimulation was monotonous or meaningless should result in disorganization of both brain and behavioural processes. The direct CNS results consisted primarily of progressive increased density of alpha activity (later replicated in many studies, although more recently identified as possibly confounded--see Barabasz & Barabasz, 1985; Zubek, 1973) and high delta wave activity.

The McGill REST data, as well as evidence from research with animals reared under deprived conditions, were compatible with the hypothesis of psychological/behavioural disorganization. But as we know, the preponderance of more recent REST research has shown drastically different and even opposite results, leading to general disavowal of the first group of studies (Suedfeld, 1980). We tend to forget that the original theory, and the original research, emphasized monotony and lack of meaningful patterning in the experimental environment. In contrast, later and current research, using drastically reduced absolute levels of stimulation, may have switched without notice to a completely new paradigm, irrelevant to Hebb's hypotheses. Comparisons of monotonous and reduced stimulation do not always show significant differential effects, so that we cannot definitively conclude whether Hebb's theorizing was wrong or whether it was right but not given an adequate empirical test.

Another ignored problem was that of using exclusively psychological data to test a neuropsychological theory. There was no alternative, as the fairly rough and global EEG measures then available were inadequate to test Hebb's sophisticated model of brain functioning; but any behavioural test was necessarily inferential and open to other explanations. Shortly after this period, I suggested (Suedfeld, 1969b) that it was not useful to explain a set of mysterious facts (REST effects) by invoking an equally mysterious set of constructs (brain processes). Although both sets of variables have become much less mysterious in the ensuing 20 years, I still maintain the basic principle of that criticism.

The next interesting neuropsychological hypothesis was that of Lindsley (e.g., 1961), who first implicated the Ascending Reticular Activating System (ARAS) in REST effects. Because the ARAS appeared to coordinate and control arousal, alerting and attention, its responses to stimuli in turn affect both general cortical activation and specific processes such as perception. When there is a gross change from the ARAS's accustomed stimulation level, it is not completely able to adapt; in consequence, cortical functioning and psychological processes are disrupted. This was the first time that arousal and adaptation level were brought in as major hypothetical constructs. Hebb referred to this line of work as having "knocked the props out from under [his] theoretical position" (1961, p. 7). Once again, however, the theory seems to stand without a clear guidepost to empirical testing, whether at the psychological or the neurological level.

Schultz (1965) proposed the first integrative theoretical framework. To the role of the ARAS, he added that of the hypothalamus, which also appears to be responsive to both sensory and cortical stimulation. Furthermore, sensory variation is not only needed to maintain an optimal arousal level in the brain, but also serves to reinforce behaviour. Most importantly, Schultz hypothesized a drive for sensory variation, which he called "sensoristasis", analogous to homeostasis. This is a drive state of cortical arousal that leads the waking organism to maintain an optimal level of sensory variation which, in turn, maintains optimal arousal in the cortex. Sensoristasis is, however, a "fluctuating constant" (Schultz, 1965, p. 31), a shifting optimal range rather than a setpoint. Neurologically, it is the ARAS that monitors and regulates sensoristatic balance.

This theory is closely akin to Zuckerman's Optimal Level of Stimulation idea (1969a), except that the latter downplayed the CNS aspects of the optimal or sensoristatic level. A number of other theories focusing on information processing could also be incorporated into the general category of explanations based on departures from and attempts to restore some accustomed level and/or quality of input. During the 1960s, these theories were probably the most widely accepted. Their central constructs--stimulus hunger, stimulus/action hunger, the postulated drives for information, exploration, meaningfulness, novelty, structure--are compatible variants of the basic hypothesis (Jones, 1969; Suedfeld, 1969b).

One major difficulty with these propositions is that the drive construct seems to be transferred from physiology without adequate thought. The generally accepted primary drives, such as hunger and thirst (sex being an anomalous and perhaps inappropriate drive in this category), are associated with measurable tissue deficits, motivate a narrow range of consummatory behaviours, and are reduced by a similarly limited number of substances from the environment. There are no verifiable analogues to any of these factors in the case of the information-based drives. Nor, once again, is there neurological evidence that either the ARAS or the hypothalamus shows major functional changes during or after REST. Last, with the now well-established relaxing and reinforcing nature of REST (especially, but not exclusively, short-term flotation), the postulate that stimulus-related "hunger" is activated in REST is contrary to observations. Many subjects complain about information and stimulation that disrupts states of serenity or euphoria reached during the session.

The 1970s and early 1980s saw a gap in the chronology of theory-development, which coincided with a notable decrease in the volume of experimentation with REST. The research that did take place tended to explore practical and generally atheoretical applications in clinical treatment, health maintenance, skill and cognitive improvement, etc.

Fortunately, that phase now appears to have passed. The new wave of brain-centred theories reflects both an altered paradigm, much more open to grappling with such amorphous concepts as states of consciousness, and increased technological power for the investigation of brain functioning.

One major advance was the two-part theory advanced by Budzynski (1990). One of these parts was the hypothesis that REST is similar to various consciousness-altering manipulations that induce a "twilight state" characterized by a preponderance of EEG theta wave activity, associated with creativity, insight, intuition, and serenity. Barabasz (1990b) demonstrated significant theta power increases for subjects in flotation REST but not for control subjects in conditions of normal stimulation. Some research from the Medical College of Ohio has confirmed increased theta during flotation as opposed to a control condition, although replication is needed. However, while self-reports assert that REST is associated with the kinds of mental states described by Budzynski, quantitative objective measurements have had inconsistent results at best.

The second component of the Budzynski hypothesis is that the normally dominant cerebral hemisphere, which monitors and responds to the constant flow of ambient events, becomes deactivated by an environment in which that flow is seriously reduced. In consequence, the normally nondominant hemisphere assumes a greater role, and psychological processes shift toward the mode characteristic of that hemisphere: again, nonlinear thinking, imagery, free flow of ideas, and novelty. This aspect of the theory should be easy to test with bilateral EEGs, but the attempts to do so in my own laboratory, and elsehwere (Barabasz & Londsale, 1983), have not obtained supportive data. And, again, the behavioural data are both mixed and--as in the case of Hebb's and other early theories--equally well explained by theories that do not invoke such, or even any, changes in how the brain is affected by REST.

Last, we have the possibility of neurochemical explanations. Most of this work has been done by Turner and Fine (1983, 1985b, 1990b;

Turner, Fine, McGrady, & Higgins, 1987; but see also Zubek, 1969a), and most of it demonstrates consistent decreases in the secretion of stress- or arousal-related hormones. Early findings indicated that the adrenal cortex was not activated to any substantial degree during REST, and that noradrenaline production among REST subjects was no different from that of recumbent controls. Both it and adrenaline production decreased, possibly because of the supine position. However, output did increase among subjects who terminated the experimental session early, and also in a group that underwent a more rigorous REST and physical restriction procedure (Zubek, 1973). Another set of early studies showed no effects of 24-hr. REST on 17-ketogenic steroids, 17-ketosteroids, pituitary thyroid stimulating hormone, ACTH, and other activation or stress-related substances.

Recent studies in the flotation tank have tended to show reductions in the secretion of cortisol, ACTH, and other stress-related hormones, although the data are not uniformly consistent. But we must remember the distinction made previously between data and theories: the findings on how REST effects hormonal secretions do not mean that lower levels of hormonal productions explain psychological phenomena.

An even more recent set of studies, showing that naloxone injections have an impact on the psychological effects of REST, is more interesting theoretically. The possibility arises that REST evokes an increase in the production of endogenous opioids, which may indeed be used to understand emotional, cognitive and other REST-related changes. Even if this relationship is confirmed, however, it leads to the next question: why should REST lead to higher endorphin levels?

It should be apparent that in my opinion, it is still premature to draw even semi-firm conclusions about the CNS substrates of the great variety of established REST effects on psychological functioning. Theories that themselves are formulated on the psychological level, dealing with such factors as attention, information processing, interactions between cognition and emotion, introspection, and the like, may be more fruitful and more directly testable at this point.

This does not mean that neurological theories are inappropriate or unacceptable. In fact, I am sure that they will someday be better worked out conceptually and better supported empirically, and a recent paper (Crawford, 1990c) provides an example of how this can be done. New technologies--full spectral EEG analyses, PET and NMR scanning--also have the potential to contribute to this effort. But I want to emhasize that psychological events cannot now, and perhaps not fully ever, be completely reduced to neurophysiological ones if we are to understand them in any meaningful way.

2

A Neo-Dissociation Conceptualization of REST

Sean Mee

Restricted Environmental Stimulation Therapy (REST) research demonstrates a wide range of powerful effects but lacks a single compelling theoretical explanation. Sensory deprivation research, beginning in the 1950s explored how monotonous or reduced environmental stimulation affects various aspects of an individual's abilities, cognitions, attitudes and awareness. Since Hebb (1961) and his associates Bexton, Heron, and Scott began experimentally studying the effects of sensory deprivation on human subjects, numerous effects have been reported. Many of these findings appear to be conflicting. The diversified and contradictory nature of these results made it difficult to develop an underlying conceptual framework which would explain this wide range of data.

Early experimenters had difficulty differentiating the effects of stimulus reduction from expectancy effects and other non-REST factors. Suedfeld, Ballard, and Murphy (1983) suggested early research findings of increased stress and anxiety resulting from REST were actually associated with non-REST factors. Much of the observed stress and anxiety was a reaction to: 1) a psychosocial atmosphere emphasizing negative anecdotal reports (M. Barabasz, A. Barabasz, & O'Neill, 1991); 2) the lack of structure; 3) requiring subjects to remain in isolation until the situation became intolerable; and 4) utilizing elaborate breathing apparatus and total underwater immersion sensory deprivation (Suedfeld et al., 1983). As the experimental procedures have been refined by addressing the above confounds, the effects found in earlier studies, such as overall cognitive impairment, hallucinations and a strong aversion to REST are no longer prevalent. The refinement of REST experimentation engenders compatible findings of increased suggestibility, openness to new information, temporary impairment limited to complex cognitive abilities (Suedfeld, 1980) and increased hypnotizability (A. Barabasz, 1980, 1982; A. Barabasz, Baer, Sheehan, & M. Barabasz, 1986). These findings, free from the spurious effects associated with the early sensory deprivation studies, may provide a basis for understanding the mechanisms underlying REST.

A theory which explains the mechanisms underlying REST is needed. Because both REST and hypnosis seem to share common factors such as reducing external distractions, increasing internal focus and openness to suggestion, perhaps they also share a common underlying theory. One theory of hypnosis may be particularly relevant to REST. Barabasz implied (1982) and later (1984a,b) suggested that E. R. Hilgard's (1977) neo-dissociation interpretation of hypnosis might serve as a conceptualization of the process occurring in REST. If both hypnosis and REST involve a dissociative process, the two interventions might be expected to share common features such as induction of a dissociative state, characteristics of a dissociative state, and effects of a dissociative state. As Barabasz (1979) once mused "phenotypic commonalities may imply genotypic bases."

This preliminary attempt is intended to elucidate these commonalities in an effort to more comprehensively conceptualize REST within a neo-dissociation theory.

Both REST and hypnosis appear to induce comparably altered states of awareness in contrast to "normal awareness". Qualitatively, the focus of awareness shifts from what could be considered the dominant processing system in normal awareness to a subordinate processing system, as opposed to an overall diminished awareness. This shift is a dissociation of the subordinate cognitive processing system from the "normal" processing system (E. R. Hilgard, 1989). This alternative experience arises because awareness is being processed through a subordinate system dissociated from the usually more dominant "normal" awareness system. E. R. Hilgard's use of the term "subordinate" system implies the processing system is not completely inactive, rather, it is lower in the hierarchy of processing systems and as such is less active, yet utilizable.

Both REST and hypnosis must induce a change in the dominant processing system for dissociation to occur. This is accomplished by decreasing the information or stimulation being received by the dominant cognitive processing system (Barabasz, 1990a). E. R. Hilgard (1989) theorized that each processing system has its own input and output channels. Therefore, one way to decrease the dominance of a particular system is to decrease stimulation in the environment that would be received by the processing system through its input channels; this is how REST could bring about a decrease in the dominant system. Hypnosis on the other hand appears to bring about a decrease in the dominant system by narrowing the focus of the input channels so that stimuli reaching the system is greatly reduced. Both interventions, therefore, reduce the stimulation or information being received by the dominant system, one by reducing the available stimulation in the environment (REST) and the other by restricting the amount of stimulation "flowing" through the input channels (hypnosis). The similarity of hypnosis and REST in this regard was recognized by J. R. Hilgard and Lebaron (1984, p. 32). They noted:

> Thus, seeing and hearing, two of the most important channels for making contact with a variety of experiences in the environment begin to narrow the focus. The voice keeps suggesting comfort and contentment, as well as mental and physical relaxation to the point where the eyelids become tired and may feel like closing. When the eyes close a major device for orientation toward outer reality disappears.

Quoting Barabasz, Hilgard and Lebaron (1984, p. 32) went on to point out more directly the analogous relationship between hypnosis and REST:

> This general relaxation and withdrawal from external stimulation other than the voice of the hypnotist produces responses that have much in common with the more extreme experiences reported in sensory deprivation; for example, Barabasz (1982) suggests sensory restriction forces the organism to focus, perhaps as seldom before, on internally generated imaginal activity.

Both techniques appear to decrease the activity of the dominant processing system, thereby, allowing a less dominant system to become more active. One main difference may be the manner in which this decrease occurs. The individual being hypnotized must actively strive to effect a change on the dominant processing system, whereas, it is the environment in REST that modifies the dominant processing system of the individual.

Both techniques reduce the information coming into the usually dominant system and thereby set up a situation in which the individual must turn to internal stimulation. The experiences of reminiscing, fantasizing and daydreaming reported in *The Deep Self* (Lilly, 1977) could be examples of this increased focus on internal stimuli or what J. R. Hilgard considered imaginal involvement. Imaginal involvement appears to be dissociative in nature (A. Barabasz, 1982; M. Barabasz, A. Barabasz, & Mullin, 1983; A. Barabasz, 1984a; J. R. Hilgard, 1974). For example, J. R. Hilgard (1974) noted that imaginal involvement serves as a dissociative coping mechanism utilized by children to block the physical pain of punishment or to combat the boredom of being sent to their rooms. Consistent with A. Barabasz's (1982) hypothesis, this suggests to the present author that a tendency towards an internal stimuli focus and, thus, a dissociative experience can be fostered by reducing environmental stimulation. The isolation experiences of adults in Antarctica, as reported by Barabasz (1984), appear to involve a similar process. In his conceptualization of experimental laboratory REST results, Barabasz (1982, 1990) emphasized that reducing the amount of stimulation reaching the dominant processing system sets up a situation in which an individual will become imaginally involved, a defensive maneuver to cope with the environment. As suggested by J. R. Hilgard (1974) these individuals thereby dissociate.

For the REST subject, focusing on internal stimuli and using a less dominant processing system may or may not be a completely new experience. For REST subjects who have used this dissociative mechanism in the past, it may enhance their imaginative involvement since their is no distracting "outside" stimuli which might tend to get processed through the usually dominant non-dissociated or stimulus driven cognitive processing mechanism. For REST subjects who have minimal experience with imaginative involvement, REST might be viewed as relaxing but they will have no prior experience with which to make a comparison. Due to this lack of previous experience these subjects may in fact be "learning" quite a bit about the experience of dissociation and their capacity to dissociate. Barabasz (1990c) studied the spontaneous occurrence of hypnosis upon exposure to flotation REST. The post-experimental inquiry showed both high and low hypnotizables viewed REST as relaxing and pleasant but only the high hypnotizables added descriptions consistent with E. R. Hilgard's (1977) neo-dissociation conceptualization of hypnosis. The high hypnotizables' descriptions involved comparisons of REST with the experience of hypnosis. The low hypnotizables did not because they probably had no previous experiences involving hypnotic dissociation with which to make the comparison.

J. R. Hilgard (1974) suggested that previous experience with imaginal involvement may in fact relate causally to an individual's ability in hypnosis. This implies that the low hypnotizables' experience of dissociation in the form of increased focus on internal stimulation and imaginative involvement in REST could be their first such experience. This is consistent with A. Barabasz's (1982) demonstration of increased hypnotizability after six hours of chamber REST. However, Barabasz (1990e) and Barabasz and Kaplan (1989) found that one hour of flotation REST is not adequate to produce imaginal involvements in subjects without previous experience. The failure of one hour of flotation REST to produce increased hypnotizability test scores was a devastating finding for those who once viewed REST as producing apparent effects merely because of the experimental demand characteristics of the apparatus. Orne and Scheibe (1964) believed that effects could be produced by experimental cues without actual REST. However, Orne and Scheibe's study failed replication (M. Barabasz, A. Barabasz, & O'Neill, 1991).

Hypnosis appears to incorporate a similar shift from a dominant processing unit to a more internal processing unit. Since hypnosis involves an active relinquishing of the dominant processing unit, it is up to the individual choosing to experience hypnosis whether or not they will switch to the more internal subordinate processing unit. The difference between high hypnotizables and low hypnotizables involves not only a willingness but, as Barabasz (1982) implies, an ability to utilize the subordinate processing system. The low hypnotizable subject's inability to switch to an unused or infrequently used processing system seems consistent with J. R. Hilgard's (1974) suggestion that high hypnotizables have an ability to switch to a subordinate processing system and that they use this ability more frequently. The low hypnotizables relative inexperience with the subordinate processing unit connected with imaginative involvement might, in terms of E. R. Hilgard's neo-dissociation theory, allow the processing system to remain farther down in the hierarchy of available systems. It might be expected for individuals who have made use of this processing system that it will be higher up in the hierarchy and as such easier to "switch" to in hypnosis.

If both REST and hypnosis involve dissociation then individuals in REST should show characteristics of a dissociative state. Reports of individuals in REST experiencing blank periods (Woodburn, 1961), feelings of detachment from their usual experience (Lilly, 1977) and increases in imaginal involvement (Barabasz, 1984) appear to be consistent with a dissociative state.

If both REST and hypnosis bring about a dissociative state then both techniques should show similar effects. Suggestion is one effect that is an integral part of hypnosis (Sheehan & McConkey, 1982). Independent of the hypnosis literature, there is evidence that REST increases suggestibility. This is supported by reports of subjects being more easily persuaded to accept an attitude contrary to their own (Heron, 1961; Suedfeld & Kristeller, 1982), and increases in suggestibility (Barabasz & Gregson, 1979) following periods of restricted environmental stimulation.

Both hypnosis and REST appear to create a situation in which the individual is more open to suggestion. Suedfeld (1985) suggested that in REST, complex cognitive functions needed in order to counter argue suggestions, are impaired. Therefore, the ability to resist suggestions or educational information is somewhat lost to the REST subject. Individuals in REST might find themselves in a dissociated state using a subordinate cognitive processing system more attuned to internal stimuli and imaginative involvement. Then suddenly they have to deal with a message more appropriate for the dominant cognitive processing system and the related complex cognitive abilities. It is not difficult to argue that in this situation the individual would be less able to logically combat the message, or possibly unwilling to bother.

Suggestion in hypnosis might involve a similar process. E. R. Hilgard and J. R. Hilgard (1975, p. 18) stated in regards to hypnosis: "Reality testing is set aside, so that the imagined experience is accepted as real". Suggestibility in both hypnosis and REST seems to involve a lack of reality testing and tolerance of conflicting ideation.

There appears to be evidence that both hypnosis and REST involve a process of dissociation. If this is the case, then why would REST increase an individual's hypnotic ability? Previous experience with dissociation as a mechanism for coping with isolation or punishment, is associated with higher levels of hypnotizabilty (J. R. Hilgard, 1974). This suggests that previous experience with dissociation enables one to more easily dissociate in another situation. As a possible explanation of increased imaginative involvement in Antarctica, Barabasz (1984) points out, that imaginative activity might be learned through practice of a dissociative reaction initiated in an attempt to cope with reduced external stimulation. The conceptualizations of J. R. Hilgard and A. Barabasz suggest to the present author that individuals will be more likely to enter a dissociative state if they have used dissociation as a coping strategy in the past. This is supported by the finding that one hour of flotation REST produced significantly higher hypnosis responsivity scores for high hypnotizables compared to low hypnotizables in the absence of a hypnotic induction (Barabasz, 1990e).

If REST provides the opportunity for the individual to enter into a dissociative state it would explain why an individual who has not been plateaued would be more highly hypnotizable after REST; but if an individual has already been plateaued to produce maximal hypnotizability more experience with dissociation should not increase their hypnotizability. Barabasz (1982) found an increase in plateaued subject's hypnotizability scores following six hours of chamber REST, while Barabasz and Kaplan (1989) found no significant change in hypnotizability after one hour of flotation REST.

This increase in hypnotizability following long-term exposure to chamber REST beyond that of the plateaued hypnotizability level might be explained in two ways. Perhaps the sheer amount of time spent in a dissociative state, while in a restricted stimulation environment, would be very difficult to replicate through repeated comparably brief hypnotic sessions.

The second more plausible explanation is eluded to by Barabasz (1982) where he stated: "Sensory restriction forces the organism to focus as seldom before, on internally generated imaginal activity." Barabasz's hypothesis raises two main points. The first is that the individual may for the first time be focusing on internally generated imaginal activity. If this is the case then prior to REST the individual would have little if any hypnotic talent and, thereby, little or no previous experience with dissociation. An individual who has no previous experience with dissociation would continue using their dominant cognitive processing system as they have limited or no awareness of an alternative system. The second point he brings to light is the fact that the organism is "forced" to dissociate. This allows for a change over basal plateau hypnotizability. If an individual strives to utilize a less dominant processing unit but is unable to because of lack of experience, then no dissociative experience will occur. On the other hand if the individual in REST does not need to labor but is forced into a dissociative state in order to cope with the reduced environmental stimulation, then when this experience is over he/she will have access to a subordinate cognitive processing system and the experience associated with it. If long term chamber REST creates a situation in which one can enter a dissociative state, without previous experience, then the experience will enable them to actively reproduce the dissociative state in hypnosis.

This paper has attempted to conceptualize both REST and hypnosis within Hilgard's neo-dissociation theory by drawing from the hypotheses and findings of Barabasz. Both REST and hypnosis appear to involve similar "induction" strategies of decreasing the information and other potentially activating stimuli reaching the dominant cognitive processing system. Both REST and hypnosis involve similar characteristics of a dissociative state (e.g., ceasing to make plans, increased focus on inner stimuli, feelings of detachment, etc.). Both REST and hypnosis appear to increase the individuals' suggestibility by reducing reality testing capacity. Finally, the view that REST and hypnosis both involve dissociative states can account for the increases in subjects' hypnotizability level following long term chamber REST (Barabasz, 1982; Barabasz & Kaplan, 1989) and spontaneous hypnosis for high hypnotizables in brief flotation REST (Barabasz, 1990c,d,e).

3

Bridging the Gap

Roderick Borrie

Nine years ago the first International Conference on Restricted Environmental Stimulation (REST) was held. The mood was one of excitement and anticipation of growth, fueled considerably by the publicity and popularity produced by John Lilly's creation, the flotation tank. Commercial centers sprouted everywhere as people looked for new ways to feel better, find themselves (and God), and make money. REST researchers who had been around for years were joined by a new generation of researchers and practitioners seduced by the undeniable effects of Flotation REST. Conferences two, three, and four attest to the creativity, industriousness, and tenacity of these people, particularly commendable in view of the scarcity of research funding for their work.

In the meantime, the flotation fad died. A recent *Time* magazine article reviewing an electronic relaxation device warned that it may be "another fleeting relaxation craze that attracts the curious and eventually bores them, like the flotation-tank phenomenon of the early 1980s". Those involved with the commercial flotation industry know that business has been off for a long time. Many centers have closed, several tank manufacturers have folded. REST research, however, continues because efficacy has little to do with popularity.

REST has many consistent, striking effects. It facilitates relaxation and pain relief. This is consistently supported by physiological data coming out of the Medical College of Ohio and the University of

British Columbia, and the symptom reduction data from Lawrence University, SUNY/Stony Brook, and elsewhere. REST fosters a state of mind that can enhance an individual's inner explorations *and* increase receptivity to therapeutic interventions. This has been demonstrated by the work with hypnosis and REST at Washington State University and by the work with biofeedback and REST at the Medical College of Ohio to name just a few of many research programs.

If the effects of REST could be dispensed in the form of a pill, it would be more prescribed than Valium. Why not? REST produces relaxation without drowsiness, gradual natural pain relief, lowering of blood pressure, decreased muscle tonus, increased range of motion, enhanced learning, a feeling of well-being, and increased introspection, and all without side-effects. Or, main effects could be decided according to the needs of the patient. The other effects would then be side-effects. Imagine the physician prescribing this REST pill to the patient suffering from rheumatoid arthritis along with the side-effect precaution, "This may give you a feeling of inner peace or lead to unusual introspection". Or to the patient taking the REST pill for essential hypertension, "Be careful when operating machinery, it may become much more enjoyable."

The idea of a REST pill touches on some of the major problems Restricted Environmental Stimulation Therapy faces in attempting to fit into our society. Our society is materialistic and, for the most part, externally oriented. Time is a commodity to be used, to be filled. To not fill each minute with some externally-bound activity is to be wasteful of time. Keeping busy is equated with success and health. Being alone is to be avoided; it is a sign of unpopularity, lack of involvement, sickness, and even failure. Being alone and overtly inactive is also to risk serious boredom. Asking people in our culture to voluntarily shut themselves off from the outside world even for an hour is to touch on some of their greatest fears.

And what exactly is REST? A term for a variety of ways to remove a person from the external world, to allow a person to be totally with and within self, doing nothing (at least overtly) for a given period of time. In other words, REST is diametrically opposed to the ways of our culture. At least it would seem so at first glance. This is one of the gaps that members of the International REST Investigators Society (IRIS) face today.

The theme of our fourth conference is "Bridging the Gap". The conference flyer referenced closing the gap between REST and a variety of other treatment modalities: psychotherapy, hypnosis, biofeedback, physical therapy, and performance enhancement. The gap is actually one of REST's credibility and acceptance as a viable treatment modality compared to other therapies. We would like to see greater acceptance for REST as a therapy. With greater acceptance of what we do, perhaps we could get on to closing other gaps, like the financial gap to fund our research. This would allow us to get on with the job of answering the myriad questions we still have about REST, the information gap.

At our second conference, in New Orleans, Peter Suedfeld commented on a distinction between his own work with REST and that of John Lilly. "John", he said, "is an explorer and I am a map-maker". Extending the analogy to my own work as a clinician, I would add that I am an engineer. The explorer probes the unknown to experience and know it for himself, and then informs others of the extension of known boundaries. The map-maker watches the expanding frontier and doggedly tries to fill in the gaps of what is known and disseminate his map to all who travel. The engineer takes the map and builds roads and bridges making these new areas accessible and useful to greater numbers. Each of these roles - explorer, map-maker, and engineer - represents a different focus, a different approach, and different goals. Each role also has a different set of critical questions and a different way of contributing to bridging the gap in REST's credibility and acceptability as a treatment. IRIS is composed of all three roles.

For the engineers, the "T" in REST is for Therapy and some of the critical questions are, "How can REST be used?", "What disorders can REST treat?", "With which therapeutic modalities can REST be most effectively interfaced?", and "What are the contraindications for its use?". The past decade has seen the emergence of REST as a therapy and the expansion of its applications. It has been used to treat stress and stress-related disorders, headache, chronic pain, arthritis and other pain. It has been used to modify addictive behaviors, to treat phobias, and to treat compulsive behaviors. Recently it has been applied to the treatment of a variety of physical disabilities, such as, cerebral palsy, stroke, and Parkinson's Disease. REST is showing itself to be quite beneficial.

Still, some of us find ourselves nervously giving elaborate justification and explanation to our clinical colleagues as to why we use REST in treating our patients. While more research is crucial to impress the medical community about the advantages of REST as a treatment, more data will not make it legitimate. REST already is a legitimate treatment, because it produces desired effects with specific disorders. It works. This is our biggest asset. It is also safe. Reported negative effects are minimal and trivial. Some have reported temporary physical or mental discomfort and a small percentage leave REST before their scheduled time. Some people do not care for REST but they are not harmed by it.

Although I speak of a gap in REST's acceptability, it has been my experience that the medical community is increasingly open, if somewhat skeptical, to its possibilities. As some of you have probably found, a few doctors will even refer their most difficult patients for REST treatment. Positive results with these patients will lead to additional referrals, one key to our acceptance into the mainstream of medicine.

Two other keys are education and standardization. If we want REST to be taken seriously, we must view it as the powerful tool it is. It is not too early to offer training to professionals interested in incorporating REST into their practices. Educating practitioners from different disciplines about applications of REST will accelerate its dissemination and present new opportunities for interfacing REST with other therapies. We can also begin the process of setting standards for the therapeutic use of REST and establishing certification procedures. If REST has the power to affect patients so profoundly, it certainly has a potential for misuse. Therapeutic standards for the use of REST and eventual certification for practitioners are the responsibility of IRIS. It is better that we regulate the clinical use of REST ourselves than wait until someone else does it for us.

An IRIS committee on standards and certification should be formed to at least begin this process. The questions of cautions and contraindications need to be formally addressed. We need to understand and predict which patients may react poorly and how personality may dictate the manner in which REST is presented. We need to be pooling and examining our data on adverse reactions. Are there personality variables we should screen for? Early psychiatric applications of chamber REST reported that obsessive-compulsive patients responded poorly. My own experience with obsessive patients is that they need more intervention in the early stages of treatment. Initially, they need some external focus to distract them from their obsessing. Gradually, their tolerance for more complete REST can be shaped over repeated sessions. This increased tolerance of REST may even lessen their obsessiveness in other situations. Another cautionary question concerns the possible absorption of magnesium during flotation REST. If magnesium is absorbed is there an optimum amount? Are there some patients for whom magnesium absorption would be a problem?

Realistically, part of REST's acceptability as a treatment modality lies in its profitability. Ultimately this means having an insurance code for Restricted Environmental Stimulation Therapy. At present, practitioners around the country are getting insurance reimbursement for REST but it is coded as psychotherapy by psychologists and as hydrotherapy by physicians or physical therapists. Neither of these accurately describes the treatment. The establishment of a separate code is probably the most important factor in the acceptance of REST as a treatment modality.

Research remains a mainstay in bridging the credibility gap. While clinicians, the engineers, are providing valuable information from their clinical studies, most systematically controlled research comes from the map-makers. For the map-makers the critical questions are not restricted to REST as a therapy. Questions about REST effects, what produces them, and individual differences in reactions to REST are posed with the general view of REST as a technique. It is interesting at this conference that the majority of research focuses on the issues of applicability. As our numbers are small, the shared focus on the potential of REST's clinical application is important, both to the acceptance of REST as a treatment and to the procurement of research funds.

The focus on applications is making us much more interdisciplinary. Demonstrating that REST can increase the effectiveness of certain existing treatment procedures will insure a place for REST as a supplement to, rather than as a competitor with other treatments. As this happens, our colleagues from these other disciplines will see advantages to incorporating REST, pick up the proverbial research ball and run with it in their own directions. This is what has happened at the REST lab at SUNY/Stony Brook with the research push into physical disabilities.

The map-maker also keeps in mind the question "How does REST, as a unique set of conditions affecting the human organism, fit into the broader picture of human functioning?" In Peter Suedfeld's 1985 IRIS Presidential Address he appealed to us to bring our theories up-to-date and to guide our research with theory-derived hypotheses. These are tall orders. As we interface REST with techniques like hypnosis or biofeedback, or fields like psychotherapy or psychoneuroimmunology, new questions arise, as do new theories. Scientists are making remarkable progress in the understanding of brain functioning, mind-body interaction, and consciousness, largely due to enormous advances in technology. Naturally, theoretical advances follow and we see a whole new generation of theoretical models, like quantum physics or chaos theory, used to further understanding of human functioning. We have a tremendous opportunity and challenge, as we expand the horizons of REST's applicability, to broaden the theoretical context in which we view REST and its effects.

Let us finally consider the "explorer" of REST, who is actually an explorer of self. The explorer poses the questions "Who am I, particularly in the absence of external definers?", "What realities are available to me?", "What are the potentials of the human mind?" and, of course, questions of spirituality. Those of us who see the potential of REST as a path toward inner awareness are, perhaps, painfully aware of a personal gap between where we are and where we want to be. This we must resolve individually. However, reports from the explorers and map-makers ahead of us, do help to assuage our frustrations and encourage our personal struggles. But these remain solitary pursuits.

As we begin to treat patients with specific disorders and symptoms, we should stay aware of REST's ability to evoke their own inner Lewis and Clark. As we use REST to help a patient suffering from TMJ, or arthritis, or cerebral palsy we need to be aware of the "side-effects" they may experience in their treatment. These patients enter REST to find relief from their suffering and may be surprised to find themselves developing a new perspective toward their lives. The refocusing of attention that occurs during REST often contributes to a new self-awareness. New insights and awareness contribute to real changes in the patient's thoughts and behaviors that could benefit from a helpful and understanding professional hand. We must remain sensitive to the powerful personal nature of REST and the fears that many patients bring with them. Used with compassion, Restricted Environmental Stimulation Therapy has the potential to provide far more than alleviation of symptoms; it has the potential to foster self-awareness and empower the patient to mobilize his or her own inner resources.

As the clinical use of REST becomes more commonplace, it could begin to impact on both the medical mainstream and society itself by making us more aware of abilities within the mind and ways of accessing those abilities. In the film *Flashback* Dennis Hopper makes the prediction that the 90s are going to make the 60s look like the 50s. I don't know exactly what *he* meant but to me it means a society that is less materialistic and more conscious of human potential and powers of mind. The 90s is the time for REST.

4

Temporal Patterns of Affect in an Isolated Group

Gary Steel and Peter Suedfeld

This study is part of an on-going series of investigations into psychological adaptation to the challenges of polar living. The focus of this particular study was the temporal patterning of mood during isolation in a high Arctic location. We were interested in investigating three aspects of such isolation. First, it has been suggested that an isolate's mood and morale drop to a low point shortly after the midpoint of the duration. This drop has been labelled the "third-quarter phenomenon" (Bechtel, 1987); however, up to this time, no empirical research has been conducted to verify the existence of this pattern. Second, intuition would lead us to believe that significant events in an isolate's day-to-day existence could have a profound effect on his or her mood state, due mainly to the relative monotony of the environment. Third, it has been shown that an isolate's emotional stability contributes positively to the social and functional well-being of the group (Gunderson, 1973). This study investigated the existence and correlates of such stability in a group of subjects who had never before been isolated together.

Method

Subjects

All subjects (n = 8) were personally recruited by the project head. Each individual was required to supply their own personal equipment and to pay their own way to the base camp at Resolute, N.W.T.; food, lodging, transportation, and camp equipment were supplied from that point on.

Three subjects left prior to the scheduled end of the isolation period (Subjects 6 and 8: Day 8; Subject 2: Day 20). These departures were planned at the beginning of the project; however, this left the researchers with relatively few data points for these people. The data presented, therefore, is based on the remaining subjects. A description of these subjects follows:

Subject 1: 28-year-old female, single. She was a physician in practice for two years. Prior to Isachsen, she had been to the Arctic twice, both times as a medical officer in an isolated community.

Subject 3: 29-year-old male, married. This subject was a graduate student pursuing his doctorate in psychology. He had no Arctic experience prior to Isachsen.

Subject 4: 36-year-old male, married. Subject 4 was serving in the Canadian Armed Forces. He was, at that time, holding the rank of captain, and had been attached to the forces for 15 years. His only Arctic experience had been a training exercise 10 years ago; this exercise lasted two weeks.

Subject 5: 37-year-old male, single. This subject holds a Masters in geography and was employed as a geographic technician in an Ontario university. He had been to the high Arctic six times prior to this study, serving each time as a project coordinator for a glaciology camp on Axel Heiberg Island.

Subject 7: 41-year-old male, married. Subject 7 holds the equivalent of a Masters in human biology. He was unique in that, where the other subjects were all Canadian citizens, Subject 7 was Argentinean. He had been to the Antarctic many times in his capacity as a researcher for the Argentine Antarctic Institute; this was the first time he had been to the high Arctic.

It is noteworthy that these five people had had minimal interaction with each other prior to isolation. In essence, they were strangers to one another.

Procedure

When it came time to choose a methodology for this study, we faced a number of problems. Unlike the majority of studies in psychology, we were going to have access to very few people; regular parametric methods would be unsuitable with just five subjects. Second, the phenomenon we wished to study, namely the interplay between isolation, significant events and temporal patterning of mood, does not lend itself well to standard quantitative methods. Third, and perhaps most important, the thrust of the study was exploratory. When all of these factors were taken into account, it became obvious that a quasi-experimental field study methodology would be best suited to this project.

Time Frame: Entry, Exit, and Significant Events

The group met at the base station at Resolute, N.W.T., during the last week of June, 1989. Entry into Isachsen, some 500 kilometers northwest of Resolute, occurred over a period of three days, from June 30 to July 1. Because of several logistical difficulties that had to be overcome in making the quarters habitable, the mood scales were not begun until July 2 ("Day 1" in all tables and figures that follow). Physical contact with anyone from the "outside" occurred at four different times during the on-site period: July 9 (Day 8), July 21 (Day 20), July 31 (Day 30), and August 20 (Day 50). The isolation segment of the study ended with the last contact; at this time, the first of the "long-timers" was taken out. All subjects were out of isolation by August 23 (Day 53); however, all daily measures were continued for a two week period after isolation. In summary, Weeks 1 to 7 represent the time spent in isolation; Weeks 8 and 9 are the period immediately following isolation.

Measures

The primary measure used in this study was a modified version of the Russell Mood Scale (Russell, 1980; Russell & Snodgrass, 1986), which was completed each evening by all subjects. This scale consists of 12 bipolar mood descriptors, six of which represent the arousal dimension and six of which represent the pleasure dimension. It has been shown elsewhere (Russell, 1980) that an individual's mood state can be expressed as a function of these two orthogonal dimensions. Dimensional scores, arrived at by averaging across the appropriate descriptors, range from 0 (low) to 8 (high).

Other measures taken at Isachsen were diaries, interviews, and on-site observations made by two subjects who served as observers. One of these observers was fortuitously blind to the phenomena being examined; as it turned out, he had undertaken to write up a set of case notes on the group as a summer project. He graciously allowed us access to these notes at the end of the isolation.

Due to safety demands, total cut-off from the outside was not possible. These limitations were similar to those of the first polar studies of REST effects (Barabasz, 1980a, 1984a). The group was physically isolated; in addition, mail and personal messages originating externally were not allowed. However, with the exception of a seven day radio blackout caused by solar flare activity (Week 7), radio contact was made twice daily with the base station, at which time a weather report and operational messages were passed along.

Results

The final analyses were based on the five subjects who remained for the entire isolation period. Such a low number of subjects precludes parametric statistical techniques; therefore, a purely descriptive approach will be adopted in this section. With regard to the third quarter phenomenon, it was felt that weekly means would give a clear picture of major trends in mood. Table 4-1 gives the means for each subject, as well as the group means for each week. It can be seen that, for the isolation period (Weeks 1 to 7), neither the lowest point in pleasure nor that of arousal showed much of a common pattern among the subjects.

Table 4-1

Mean Dimensional Scores (0 - 8) per Week

Week	Pleasure	Arousal	Week	Pleasure	Arousal
Subject 1			*Subject 5*		
1	5.14	4.59	1	5.30	3.54
2	5.19	4.16	2	4.90	3.69
3	5.11	4.07	3	4.85*	3.30*
4	6.50	4.92	4	5.23	3.66
5	6.11	4.73	5	5.38	3.69
6	4.80	3.76*	6	5.16	3.73
7	4.78*	4.42	7	5.52	3.88
		Post-	isolation		
8	5.61	6.00	8	4.61	3.42
9	4.02	5.69	9	5.92	4.23
Subject 3			*Subject 7*		
1	4.90	3.40	1	6.07	4.95
2	4.73	3.90	2	6.23	5.00
3	4.83	3.88	3	6.42	4.02
4	4.95	3.92	4	6.80	3.71*
5	6.02	3.97	5	6.85	4.45
6	4.57*	3.50*	6	6.33	3.47
7	5.21	3.57	7	5.78*	4.19
		Post	isolation		
8	5.54	4.88	8	6.69	4.40
9	5.33	3.80	9	6.40	4.16
Subject 4			*Group Means*		
1	5.52	4.02	1	5.09	4.10
2	4.97	4.04	2	5.04	4.16
3	3.85*	3.90*	3	4.82*	3.83
4	5.09	4.16	4	5.51	4.07
5	4.69	4.33	5	5.40	4.23
6	5.64	4.64	6	5.09	3.82*
7	5.28	5.45	7	4.99	4.30
		Post-	isolation		
8	5.69	5.19	8	5.50	4.78
9	6.09	4.80	9	5.25	4.52

* minimum during isolation period

Examining the group means, we see that the lowest general point of pleasure occurred in the third week, while the lowest point in arousal came about in the sixth week.

As isolation was the primary manipulation in this study, it seemed appropriate to examine interruptions in the isolation for the effect that these events had on mood. The four times such contact occurred were, of course, coincidental with airplane arrivals. At this time, all members of the group had some form of interaction with the pilots of the aircraft. The fact that these contacts were of some significance to the members is supported by both participant observers' notes and the group members' respective diary entries: All members commented on the aircraft's arrival and the impact, logistical and/or affective, that it seemed to have on the group.

Group arousal and pleasure means before and after each of these events can be found in the data tables accompanying each event chart (Figures 4-1 to 4-4).

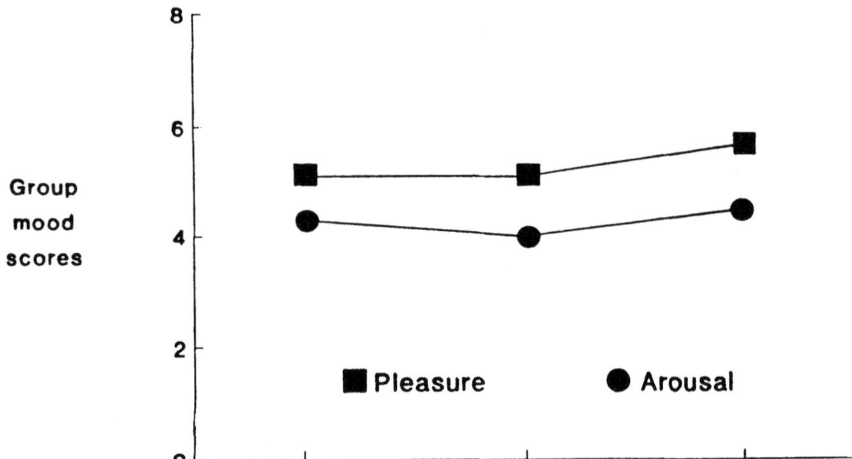

Pre-event	Day of event	Post-event
5.1	5.1	5.7
4.3	4	4.5

Figure 4-1. Mood change before and after Event 1 (short-timers out; supplies in). Pre-event and post-event data points represent the average over four days before and after the event.

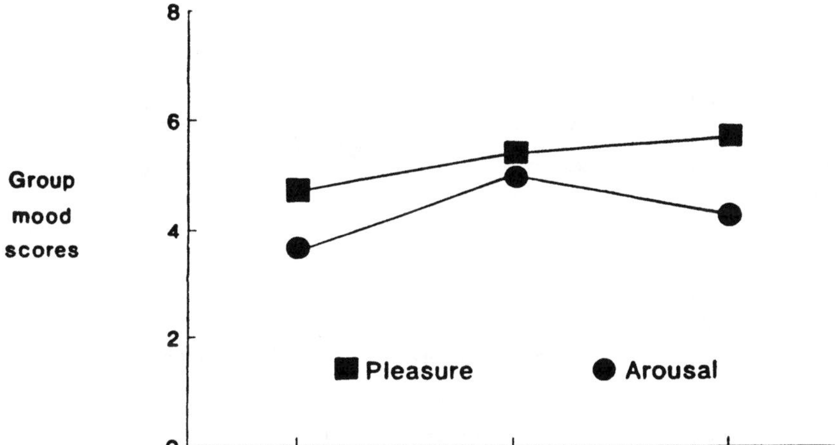

Pre-event	Day of event	Post-event
4.7	5.4	5.7
3.6	5	4.3

Figure 4-2. Mood change before and after Event 2 (Subject 2 leaves; supplies in). Pre-event and post-event data points represent the average over four days before and after the event.

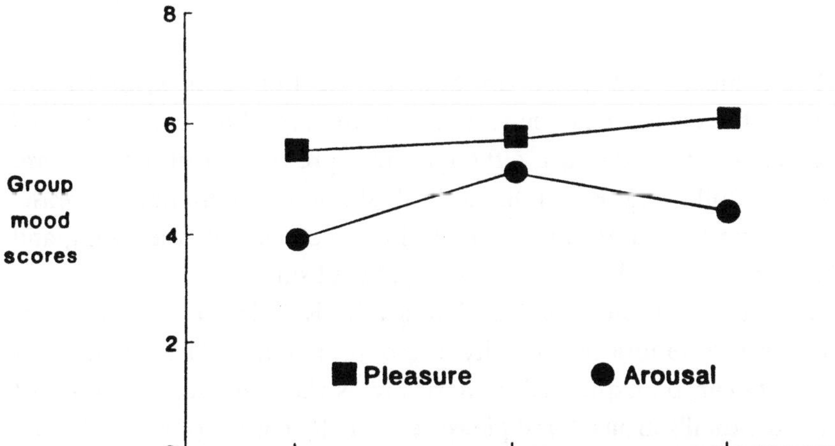

Pre-event	Day of event	Post-event
5.5	5.7	6.1
3.9	5.1	4.4

Figure 4-3. Mood change before and after Event 3 (Pilots to dinner; supplies in). Pre-event and post-event data points represent the average over four days before and after the event.

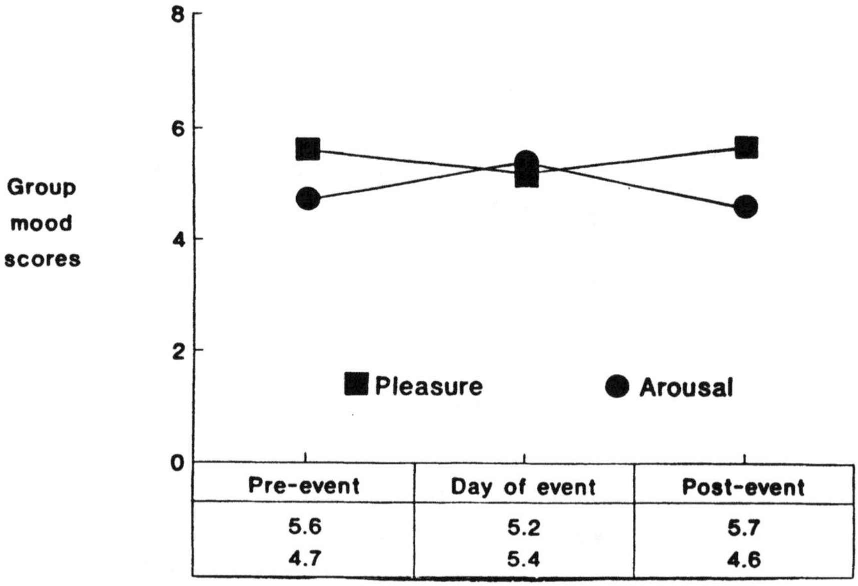

Figure 4-4. Mood change before and after Event 4 (Subject 5 leaves; mail arrives). Pre-event and post-event data points represent the average over four days before and after the event.

These means are based on data for the four days prior to and following the event. It can be seen that, in the first three events, arousal increased after the contact, although these pre-to-post differences are minimal. Following Event 4, arousal showed a minimal decrease. Pleasure, on the other hand, increased in all cases after the event, and in Events 2 and 3, this increase was quite substantial.

One of the more reliable findings in isolation research is the importance of emotional stability in group members. This stability (or lack of it) can be expressed numerically as the standard deviation of each individual's arousal and pleasure over the course of the isolation; when considered in conjunction with the means for each of these dimensions, a rough picture emerges of the affective quality of the members' stay. As can be seen in Table 4-2, the subjects did not vary a great amount in their moods during isolation. As well, means for each subject indicate that they were all generally calm, pleased, and happy during the field portion of the study. This pattern is repeated in their post-isolation means and standard deviations, with one exception: Subject 1 seemed less pleased upon re-entry into southern civilization, and the pleasure component of her mood varied considerably.

Table 4-2

Subjects' Grand Means and Standard Deviations

	Mean		SD	
Isolation:	During	After	During	After
Subject 1				
Pleasure	5.38	4.82	1.47	2.08
Arousal	4.38	5.83	1.40	1.13
Subject 3				
Pleasure	5.03	5.45	1.02	1.15
Arousal	3.72	4.36	.85	.92
Subject 4				
Pleasure	4.98	5.86	1.13	1.35
Arousal	4.34	4.98	1.16	1.22
Subject 5				
Pleasure	5.20	5.27	.61	.77
Arousal	3.64	3.82	.54	.61
Subject 7				
Pleasure	6.36	6.54	.93	.75
Arousal	4.26	4.24	.95	.92
Group				
Pleasure	5.40	5.59	.70	.65
Arousal	4.01	4.66	.77	.52

Discussion

Although there is anecdotal evidence for the existence of a "third quarter phenomenon", this mood pattern only showed up in our data as a result of averaging across all subjects. Even then, the pattern held only for the arousal component of behavior and not for the pleasure component. As a caveat, however, we would like to underscore the fact that the results of this study are based on relatively few subjects. Having noted this, we can suggest that it may be that arousal is indeed tied to length of isolation; more specifically, it is likely that arousal is a function of the subject's expectations regarding the duration of their stay. The pleasure component, on the other hand, seems to vary as a function of specific day-to-day events.

With regard to such events, our data indicate that short-term contact with "outsiders" has a positive impact on both dimensions of mood. This finding is confounded, however, with the fact that fair to good weather conditions were required before an aircraft could be sent to Isachsen. Thus, a quite plausible alternative explanation of the significant events analysis is that good weather induced good mood; this is made even more likely as Isachsen is rather infamous among Arctic veterans as a place for extremely poor weather conditions. We are currently exploring this hypothesis in a reanalysis of the data. Nevertheless, both participant observations and diaries strongly indicated that personal contact with people outside the immediate group had a pronounced effect on the mood of the subjects.

The lack of variability in each subject's mood ratings was quite interesting. With all the rigors of Arctic living, including such features as prolonged inclement weather, difficulties with the diesel heaters, unheated sleeping quarters, primitive bathing and toilet facilities, and all the joys of cooking in a kitchen equipped with a three-burner iosol stove and no running water, the group members showed a pronounced lack of fluctuation in their mood, maintaining a generally positive affective state through the entire isolation period. Of equal interest is the fact that the most stable members of the group were Subjects 5 and 7, the two who had extensive polar experience prior to their taking part in this study. Perhaps Arctic experience attracts the affectively stable individual; perhaps the Arctic experience enables one to achieve a sense of stability. The field methodology employed in this study does not allow us to make causal inferences, but the findings have led to some interesting hypotheses for future work.

5

Neo-Dissociation Accounts For Pain Relief and Hypnotic Susceptibility Findings: Flotation REST Elicits Hypnosis

Arreed Barabasz

Chamber REST has been demonstrated to dramatically enhance hypnotizability in both experimental (A. Barabasz, 1982) and clinical (A. Barabasz & M. Barabasz, 1989) settings. Both studies demonstrated REST to be effective in significantly raising test scores on a standardized test of hypnotizability. Furthermore, these apparent score increases were found to generalize to significantly increased responsiveness to hypnotic suggestions for the relief of both experimental and chronic clinical pains. These results (A. Barabasz, 1982) were conceptualized within E. R. Hilgard's (1977a) neo-dissociation theory in combination with J. R. Hilgard's (1974, 1979) findings regarding the role of imaginative involvement. It was hypothesized (A. Barabasz, 1982, p. 162) that "REST forces the subject to focus, perhaps as seldom before, on internally generated imaginal activity." It appeared that subjects developed imaginative involvements in REST as a mechanism for coping with reduced stimulation. These skills, once learned, were viewed as accounting for the enhanced hypnotizability and the maintenance of this newly developed talent following exposure to chamber REST.

Despite Suedfeld and Ballard's (1984) emphasis on the need for procedural specificity and the obvious differences in methodologies, the literature frequently fails to discriminate between chamber and flotation REST. Kaplan and Barabasz (1989) replicated the hypnosis enhancement effects for chamber REST but showed no significant effects for the flotation method. However, these findings do not preclude the possibility that flotation REST might serve to facilitate the production of spontaneous hypnosis in subjects who have already demonstrated high levels of hypnotic talent.

Independent of the hypnosis research, Suedfeld (1980, 1985, 1987) reviewed several recent investigations showing REST, in combination with educational messages aimed at behavior change, to be dramatically efficacious in the treatment of a number of severe habit disorders. The data showing increases in hypnotizability (A. Barabasz, 1982) and the behavioral responsiveness to messages given to subjects during REST suggest the possibility of the spontaneous occurrence of hypnosis in REST. This possibility seems all the more likely given the anecdotal reports of pain relief (Lilly, 1985; Perry, 1985) and other experiences consonant with the neo-dissociation explanation of hypnosis.

In a preliminary study, high (n=5) and low (n=5) hypnotizables spent 45 minutes in flotation REST and in a non-REST control condition. Left arm ischemic pain was induced, without a hypnotic induction, while subjects were asked to think of their left arms as detached from their bodies. Both groups reported significantly less pain in the REST condition. High hypnotizables reported significantly less pain than lows in the flotation REST condition and reported REST as "just like hypnosis."

The purpose of the two investigations reported here was to further explore the possible occurrence of spontaneous hypnosis in flotation REST.

Method: Study Number 1

Subjects

Ss (n=20) consisted of student volunteers enrolled at a large rural university. Ss were drawn from high and low hypnotizability subject pools and had participated in one or two hypnosis experiments within the preceding 12 months. All Ss had been exposed to a minimum of 15 hypnotic inductions aimed at plateauing maximal hypnotic responsiveness. High hypnotizables (n=10) had Stanford Hypnotic Susceptibility Scale: Form C (SHSS:C) scores of 10-12 while lows (n=10) had SHSS:C scores of 1-4.

Apparatus

The REST tank (Floatarium Model SWS) (2.4 meters long X 1.4 meters high X 1.3 meters wide) is an enclosed, sound insulated, fiberglass tub that contains a 25 cm. deep dense solution (D=1.30 g/cc) of tap water and epsom salts (20% solution). The solution is maintained at 34.5° C (±.2°). A feature of the Floatarium brand tank is the provision of special tank floor contours which facilitate Ss' ability to sit upright. The tank is sound attenuated and light free once the S or experimenter activated door is closed. Ss float supine with ears submerged (Ss wore 20 db wax earplugs). Ss' vocalizations are monitored by a built-in microphone. Messages can be transmitted to Ss from the monitoring room via underwater transducers. The tank is ventilated by a silent positive pressure system. Between float sessions, the water is filtered and purified by an ultraviolet irradiation system. A shower is immediately adjacent to the tank for hygienic purposes immediately before and after each float experience.

The cold pressor pain apparatus consisted of a picnic cooler filled with ice and tap water. The water was maintained at 5° C (±1°). Cold pressor pain was reported by standard methodology (E. R. Hilgard & J. R. Hilgard, 1975). Briefly, Ss immersed their left hand and arm in the ice water just over the elbow. Ss were asked to report, on command, every five seconds by assigning a numerical value to their experience using 1 as no pain and 10 as an anchoring value - the point at which Ss "would very much like to remove the arm from the water." Upon reaching the anchoring value Ss were asked to continue reporting. Ss were reminded at the beginning of each session that they were free to terminate cold pressor pain at anytime simply by removing their arm from the cooler. All Ss kept their arms immersed for at least one minute. All Ss were asked to remove their arms at the 1 1/2 minute point.

Procedure

All Ss were exposed to three conditions in random order. Condition A consisted of flotation REST. After 45 minutes in the tank, Ss were asked to sit upright and to extend their left (non-dominant for all Ss) arm out of the tank porthole. Without any hypnotic induction, Ss were then instructed to place the arm into the picnic cooler and to think of this arm as detached from their body. Ss left the tank after cold pressor data were obtained. Condition B was conducted outside of the tank room with Ss comfortably seated. In this condition Ss were exposed to the hypnotic induction instructions from the Stanford Hypnotic Clinical Scale (Morgan & J. R. Hilgard, 1975) and a hypnotic suggestion to think of their arms as detached from their bodies. Cold pressor data were then obtained as in condition A. Condition C was conducted in the same manner as condition B but no hypnotic induction was used.

The sequential progression of the three conditions was randomized for each subject. E was blind with respect to Ss hypnotizability level in an attempt to assure that all Ss would be treated in an equivalent manner. Low hypnotizables were instructed to simulate hypnosis; their instructions were taken from Orne's (1979) real-simulator design procedure. The low hypnotizable subjects simulated hypnosis in all respects, except that their cold pressor pain report scores, obtained in the last minute of the experiment, were real. Subjects were told not to simulate their pain reports but rather to give accurate reports (A.

Barabasz & M. Barabasz, 1992). An independent post-experimental inquiry was conducted to assess Ss' experiences in each of the three conditions.

Results: Study Number 1

All Ss kept their arms in the ice water for a minimum of one minute in each condition. Each S provided at least 12 numerical pain reports for REST, hypnosis and control conditions.

Since all possible between conditions and between groups contrasts were of interest, appropriate t-tests were calculated by the Dunn Method of multiple comparisons (Dunn, 1961). Dunn's method was chosen because it protects alpha error by distributing type I error risk over each series of within or between comparisons. The effect is similar to Scheffé and Tukey post-hoc comparisons but without the need for analysis of previous calculations or loss of statistical power. Omega square was calculated for each comparison to estimate the degree of statistical association from the data. The results of the within groups comparisons appear in Table 5-1.

The results presented in Table 5-1 demonstrate significant effects for REST in contrast to the control condition for both high ($p < .01$) and low hypnotizables ($p < .05$). Lows showed no significant ($p > .05$) effects in either the control versus hypnosis comparison or the REST versus hypnosis comparison. Hypnosis was significantly more effective in reducing reported pain than either the control condition ($p < .001$) or the REST condition ($p < .01$) for high hypnotizables. Results of the between group comparisons appear in Table 5-2.

The results presented in Table 5-2 show equivalence between high and low hypnotizables for control condition pain reports ($p > .05$). High hypnotizables demonstrated significantly lower pain reports than lows in response to either hypnosis ($p < .001$) or REST ($p < .05$) conditions.

Table 5-1

Within Groups Cold Pressor Pain Comparisons
for Low and High Hypnotizability Ss

Treatment Condition	N	Mean	S.D.	D.F.	T	Omega Square
Control Lo	10	7.65	1.58			
vs.				9	2.4*	.30
REST Lo	10	6.70	1.49			
Control Lo	10	7.65	1.58			
vs.				9	1.0	.01
Hypnosis Lo	10	7.35	1.68			
REST Lo	10	6.70	1.49			
vs.				9	1.18	.03
Hypnosis Lo	10	7.35	1.68			
Control Hi	10	8.65	4.24			
vs.				9	3.0**	.42
REST Hi	10	4.30	1.87			
Control Hi	10	8.65	4.24			
vs.				9	4.2***	.60
Hypnosis Hi	10	1.70	1.05			
REST Hi	10	4.30	1.87			
vs.				9	4.0*	.57
Hypnosis Hi	10	1.70	1.05			

*$p < .05$
**$p < .01$
***$p < .002$

Table 5-2

<u>Between Groups Cold Pressor Pain Results for Low and High Hypnotizability Ss</u>

Hypnotizability Group	Treatment Condition	N	Mean	S.D.	D.F.	T	Omega Square
Lows		10	7.65	1.58			
vs.	Control				18	.7	.07
Highs		10	8.65	4.24			
Lows		10	6.70	1.49			
vs.	REST				18	3.2*	.31
Highs		10	4.30	1.87			
Lows		10	7.35	1.68			
vs.	Hypnosis				18	8.9**	.80
Highs		10	1.70	1.05			

*p < .05
**p < .001

Discussion: Study Number 1

The results of the study show both low hypnotizables, simulating hypnosis, and high hypnotizables demonstrated significantly lower cold pressor pain scores in flotation REST than in the control condition. However, highs reported significantly lower pain scores than lows. The post experimental inquiry showed that both highs and lows viewed the flotation REST session as relaxing and pleasant but only the highs added descriptions consistent with Hilgard's (1977a) neo-dissociation conceptualization of hypnosis. High hypnotizables reported "...like in hypnosis I could imagine myself anywhere like (it was) real," "...my arm was just floating out there when he asked me to put it in the ice water," "...being in the tank was about as close to hypnosis without actually doing it (hypnotic induction)."

These findings, supported by the relatively high levels of statistical association as indicated by Omega Square calculations, suggest that the pain reductions may be the result of a combination of two mechanisms of action. Flotation REST has been shown to produce substantial relaxation effects (Turner & Fine, 1983) and relaxation reduces pain perception (McGlashen, Evans, & Orne, 1969). McGlashen, Evans, and Orne (1969) found hypnosis effects on pain reduction to be much more than that associated only with relaxation. Analogous to this data the present study's results suggest pain reduction for low hypnotizables may be due to relaxation while the greatly enhanced pain reduction for highs may be due to the combination of relaxation and hypnosis. These findings raise the question as to whether flotation REST produces spontaneous hypnosis in subjects known to have hypnotic talent.

Despite the fascinating data, Study Number 1 was limited. It was intriguing to see that both REST and hypnosis produced similar pain scores in high hypnotizables. However, it was not clear as to whether or not hypnosis was the active mechanism in both conditions because measures of hypnotic responsiveness could not be directly obtained in REST without confounding the cold pressor pain procedure. Furthermore, the post experimental inquiry did not determine whether high hypnotizable Ss in REST may have merely been engaged in self-hypnosis entirely independent of REST. Study Number 2 was intended to build upon the findings of Study Number 1 by providing a direct measure of hypnotic responsiveness and information on the potential use of self-hypnosis.

Method: Study Number 2

Subjects

Ss (n=28) consisted of student volunteers enrolled at a large rural university who had not participated in Study Number 1. High and low hypnotizability Ss met the same hypnosis experience criteria and test score ranges as Ss in Study Number 1.

Apparatus

The same REST tank (Floatarium Model SWS) and flotation procedure used in Study Number 1 was employed for Study Number 2.

Procedure

The high and low hypnotizable groups were each randomly divided into two subgroups (highs - groups A [n=7] & B [n=7] and lows - groups C [n=7] & D [n=7]). After 45 minutes in flotation REST Ss in groups A and C were then exposed to a prerecorded hypnotic induction from the Stanford Hypnotic Clinical Scale (SHCS) (Morgan & Hilgard, 1975). Ss in groups B and D were not exposed to an induction. As in Study Number 1, pre-experimental hypnosis testing and administration of induction/non-induction conditions were completed by experienced assistants. E was blind with respect to hypnotizability group or induction condition. Therefore, the possibility of bias in the administration of hypnosis responsiveness testing was precluded.

To assess hypnotic responsiveness, in the flotation REST environment, eight items were drawn from the SHCS and the SHSS:C. The items were given by this investigator in the following order: 1) mosquito hallucination (SHSS:C); 2) taste hallucination (SHSS:C); 3) dream (SHCS); 4) age regression (SHCS); 5) anosmia to ammonia (SHSS:C); 6) hallucinated voice (SHSS:C); 7) post-hypnotic suggestion (SHCS); 8) post hypnotic amnesia (SHCS). To suit administration in the tank environment some modifications were necessary. For example, scoring of the mosquito hallucination did not allow observation of grimacing but movement (to chase the mosquito away) was easily scored by the sound of Ss hand moving in the tank solution. The anosmia to ammonia item involved exposure to ammonia via the positive pressure tank ventilation inlet with the filter element removed and an instructional modification reflecting this procedure.

Results: Study Number 2

Hypnosis responses were scored on the basis of the criteria established for the scales from which they were drawn with the exception of the visual observation of overt signs. The data were analyzed by a 2 (hypnotizability) by 2 (induction condition) analysis of variance. Significant effects emerged for hypnotizability $F(1,24) = 258.5$, $p < .001$. Means and standard deviations are shown in Figure 5-1.

Separate analyses determined that the hypnosis response scores for high or low hypnotizable Ss were not significantly influenced by the absence or presence of the SHCS hypnotic induction [highs $F(1,12) = 2.8$, $p > .11$, lows $F(1.12) = 1.8$, $p > .20$.]

Results of the post experimental inquiry showed marked differences between high and low hypnotizable Ss. Both groups consistently reported flotation REST to be relaxing. However, high hypnotizables engaged in deep imaginal activity with one to three themes while lows reported a variety of distraction oriented activities (e.g., pushing off the tank wall with a toe), multiple brief imaginal attempts and simple boredom. Five of the 14 high hypnotizables reported engaging in self-hypnosis. The hypnosis response scores of these five Ss were, however, not significantly different from the nine Ss who did not report hypnosis activity ($p > .05$).

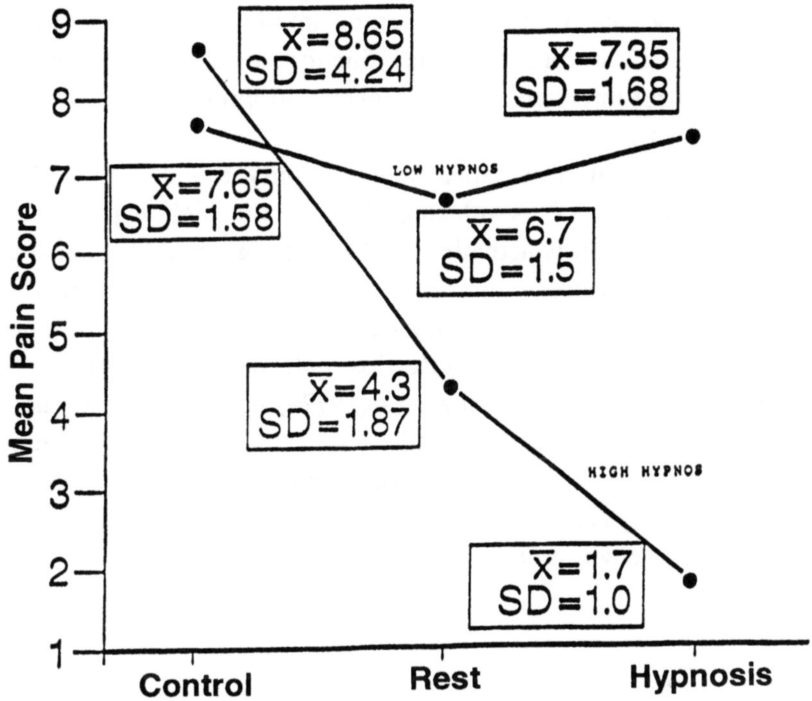

Figure 5-1. Cold pressor pain results.

Discussion: Study Number 2

The results of the study which show significantly higher hypnosis responsivity scores for high hypnotizables contrasted with lows, regardless of the presence or absence of a hypnotic induction, lend further support for the hypothesis that flotation REST can elicit spontaneous hypnosis in Ss known to have hypnotic talent. These general findings support Study Number 1 which used cold pressor pain scores as a criterion measure. However, contrary to Study Number 1 which showed significantly lower pain scores for the induction versus non-induction condition, the present investigation showed no significant differences between the hypnotic induction condition and the flotation REST without a formal hypnotic induction condition. This finding, if replicated, may have rather far reaching implications for the use of REST, as a substitute for a hypnotic induction, for patients whose fears of loss of control interfere with the normal attentional shifts required to enter hypnosis.

The independent post experimental inquiry revealed that all Ss viewed flotation REST as relaxing. Five of the high hypnotizables engaged in self hypnosis activities but the hypnosis responses of these Ss were not significantly different from the other nine highs. The inquiry also showed prolonged dissociative deep imaginal involvement for the high hypnotizables. The effortless nature of this activity for the highs seems consistent with Hilgard's (1977a) neo-dissociation theory of hypnosis and previous data (Miller, A. Barabasz, & M. Barabasz, 1991). In sharp contrast to these effortless automatic responses, the low hypnotizables engaged in a variety of alternative effortful strategies in response to the environment.

6

REST and Hypnotic Phenomena: Some Similarities Observed in European Case Studies

Peter Migály

More than a decade before the original McGill studies of sensory deprivation, psychoanalytic authors dealt with the potential role of sensory-motor manipulation, and with the progressive elimination of stimuli in hypnotic inductions (Kubie & Margolin, 1944; cit. Chertok, 1966, p. 33). The enhancement of hypnotic susceptibility by sensory restriction procedures was also predicted by a psychoanalytic model (Gill & Brenman, 1959; cit. Chertok, 1966, p. 33; cit. Wickramasekera, 1977a, p. 144).

Several studies in this field have presented sufficient evidence of increased hypnotizability due to Restricted Environmental Stimulation (REST) (Barabasz, 1979, 1980c; Barabasz & Barabasz, 1989; Barabasz & Kaplan, 1987; Pena, 1963; Sanders & Rehyer, 1969; Wickramasekera, 1969, 1970, 1977a).

In 1987 at the 4th European Congress of Hypnosis, Oxford University, evidence was presented that hallucinatory states, including REST and hypnosis, share not only psychological, but electrophysiological and neurochemical similarities as well (Migály, 1987a,b,c). In that paper, a comparison was made of the hypnotic hallucinations and hallucinations which occur in dreams, in isolation (REST), in psychotic (schizophrenic) states, and in states induced by psychomimetic drugs. Electrophysiologically, the investigations of cerebral hemispheric asymmetry were found important (Migály, 1987a). During REST, similarly to hypnotic and other hallucinations, a shift in the left and right hemispheric dominance was observed (Goldstein, Sugarman, Marjerrison, & Stoltzfus, 1973; Migály, 1987a; Macleod-Morgan, 1985; Lynn, 1985). Neurochemically, the neurotransmitter imbalance model of hallucination was pointed out, and the interaction of hypnosis with other hallucinatory states was also discussed (Blanc, Hervé, Simon, Lisoprawski, Glowinski, & Tassin, 1980; Glowinski, Tassin, & Thierry, 1984; Migály, 1987a,b,c, 1988, 1991; Migály & Jakab, 1986; Migály, Jakab, & Károvits, 1987). Psychological, electrophysiological and neurochemical data support the idea of a close connection between these altered states of consciousness.

The following European case studies permit a further psychological comparison of hypnosis and REST. The use of hypnosis to reproduce the sensory restriction experience is also analyzed.

Cases

In *Case 1*, a male subject experienced REST by immersing in a tank of salt water kept at body temperature in a Scandinavian Yoga and Meditation Center. He described his experience to me more than a year after he returned from his Scandinavian trip. In the pyramid shaped tank his vision and hearing were blocked and the feedback from the muscles was reduced because he remained motionless. Some time later, while he was floating in this water, he lost his orientation and his first feeling was similar to that of being in outer space. He also mentioned during his report that for a time he felt as if he could see his head or mind from the outside. Most of the time he had a floating feeling or the feeling that his body had disappeared. Some time later he experienced hallucinations. He "saw" a wonderful Indian hand in color with the little finger and thumb gently touching.

His second spontaneous picture was quite unpleasant. He saw his own heart from the outside as the talon of an eagle grasped it. He did not see the eagle, only its talon, which deeply pierced his heart. This heart was not dark and it was beaded with blood tinged sweat. However, he had a feeling that he was more powerful than the grasp of the eagle and that he would survive.

His next vision was that of a trip on a riverboat. The boat went under a bridge, which was like an old bridge in Florence. Then he arrived at a wonderful house which was like a castle and he knew that he had arrived home. He was very optimistic afterward.

During his experience of REST he had an increasing time distortion. He reported that he did not know the time, and it seemed as if it had stopped. He also mentioned that at first he did not hear when someone knocked and said that his session was over. He did not know where this voice came from and did not want to end his experience. He knew from being told that the time he spent in the pyramid was about 45 minutes.

In *Case 2*, a female subject participated in REST in a similar way, but in London. She said that she was told she would have about one hour for her experience. Then she would hear music, which would be a sign that the time for her experience had ended. After observing everything and immersing in the tank of water, she stopped moving and waited, but nothing happened. However, she did not feel that everything remained the same. First she felt as if she were floating, then she did not feel her body at all. Then she paid attention to the falling drops of the condensing vapor. Some time later this sound changed in nature to resemble the murmur of the sea. Then, it, too, disappeared. She had no thoughts and felt nothing. She waited. She reported that she did not see anything, only the face of her friend, which was quite large. Some time later--she did not know when--she suddenly heard music. She became angry that nothing had happened yet and that she already had to end her experience. She started to go out from the tank of water and due to her movement the music seemed to be discontinued. She also noticed that she was not used to listening to this kind of music. She later realized that it was an inner music. Then she returned to the previous state, but not as deeply, as the sensations of her body had been restored. She waited and fidgeted, and only later did she hear the real music signaling the end of her time for this experience.

The Hypnotic Phenomena Compared with REST

The above case studies are comparable to the experience of hypnosis. The experience of REST or hypnosis might be influenced by expectations. One of the major differences, however, is that the psychodynamic and imaginative process are not controlled by a therapist under REST. In spite of this, there are some interesting similarities between sensory restriction and the hypnotic phenomena.

Time distortion, for example was experienced in both of the above cases (see also Suedfeld, 1980, p. 45), and is also frequently reported in hypnosis. This might develop in a trance spontaneously or by specific suggestions (Kroger & Fezler, 1976; Cooper & Erickson, 1954). Proprioceptive changes by specific hypnotic suggestions are sometimes utilized therapeutically, for example to enhance age regression or anesthesia (Kroger & Fezler, 1976). In other cases--like in the above reports on REST--spontaneous proprioceptive changes, the feeling of the disappearance of the body, developed. Similar changes might develop spontaneously under hypnosis too. Two of my hypnosis patients reported that kind of feeling during the induction phase. It should be noted however, that on both of these occasions, under hypnosis, the therapeutic goal was to develop anesthesia. One of these patients interpreted this spontaneous hypnotic phenomenon--the feeling of the disappearance of her body--as disturbing, and the other as neutral.

Another, perhaps the most important phenomena to be compared, is hallucination. About 80% of the McGill subjects reported some form of hallucination (cit. Burns & Dobson, 1984, p. 107). Spontaneous visual hallucination was an important part of both of the above case reports on REST. In the second case, auditory hallucination was also reported. As is well known, all kinds of hallucinations can be elicited under hypnosis. This is used in standardized scales to measure hypnotic susceptibility, and it also has a major importance in the therapeutic process of clinical hypnosis (Kroger & Fezler, 1976; Leuner, 1969).

The above case reports might focus our attention on some other psychological similarities between REST and hypnosis. The floating feeling, the feeling of being in outer space and the feeling of seeing oneself from the outside are worth mentioning. The unwillingness to end the experience or the reducive attitude (as if nothing particular had happened) can also be found under both hypnosis and REST.

Reproduction of Sensory Restriction Experience by Hypnosis

It has been reported in the literature that it was possible to simulate some of the hallucinatory states through hypnosis. This is well demonstrated for night dreams in the standardized items of some hypnotic susceptibility scales. The hypnotic dreams of deep trance subjects were reported to be very similar to their nocturnal dreams (Barrett, 1979; Tart, 1966).

The hypnotic simulation of schizophrenia and psychotic hallucination are also possible (Erickson, 1980, Vol. I. p. 267). What is more, success in increasing and later eliminating psychotic hallucination was also reported (Zeig, 1974). In one case, Fogel and Hoffer (1962) demonstrated that it was possible to reproduce an LSD psychedelic experience by hypnosis alone. The hypnotic subject felt as if she had been drugged and she reported a similar experience to LSD, which she had had three weeks previously (Fogel & Hoffer, 1962).

Therefore, it seemed challenging to try to reproduce by hypnosis the sensory restriction experience in Case 1. Similar hallucination and perception changes developed during the two experiences. After the induction of hypnosis, the subject, however, reported a new imaginative scene. Then he was guided to relive his previous REST experiences, which he reported he did successfully. However, in the previous month he had some cardiac symptoms. He suspected a possible connection between his psychosomatic symptoms and his prior vision under REST (see also Haberman, 1987). Therefore, a careful change was initiated in his imagery, for therapeutic reasons, when he imagined his second scene and saw his heart as the talon of an eagle grasped it. First, the imagined talon was changed to his own hand, which was strong and helped his heart to beat rhythmically. Then it was suggested that he could take his hand off of his heart as the continuum would remain between his hand and heart through his arm and body, even if he did not think about it. Additional therapeutic suggestions were also used at this point. He had no difficulty in reliving under hypnosis the other hallucinatory and perception changes of his previous REST experience.

Conclusion

Psychosomatic problems might develop in spontaneous trance during REST. Therefore, psychological counseling should be available with this method. Therapists must be prepared to solve any potential psychological problem arising from spontaneous hallucination during REST. Hypnosis can be the method of choice in such problematic cases.

The above case studies on REST permitted a comparison with hypnosis. Time distortion, spontaneous proprioceptive changes, the feeling of the disappearance of the body, spontaneous or suggested hallucination, and other similarities were pointed out. It was also demonstrated that the sensory restriction experience can be reproduced by hypnosis. These data support a close relationship between these altered states of consciousness.

7

A Model of the Common "Active Ingredient" in Stress Reduction Techniques

Ian Wickramasekera

Psychophysiological Stress, Short Term Memory and Negative Affect

Psychological stress (Lazarus, 1966; Appley & Trumball, 1967) has been implicated in the exacerbation or etiology of several medical symptoms (e.g., headaches, peptic ulcers, essential hypertension) and behavioral symptoms (alcohol, drug and tobacco abuse). Analyses of psychological stress emphasize the critical role of cognition (e.g., threat appraisal and labelling) in the sequence of events that comprise psychological stress (Lazarus & Folkman, 1984) and suggest that it is unlikely that physiological arousal alone, without aversive cognitive labelling of the arousal, is a sufficient condition for the acquisition and maintenance of chronic stress related clinical symptoms.

The stressors that impinge on these patients seldom involve tissue damage or the threat of tissue damage. Frequently, they present in intermittent ambiguous forms of threat to well-being or conflicts that elicit cumulative physiological arousal and/or intense ambivalent emotions in these people. These "psycho-social" conscious or unconscious perceptions of threat and conflict may include an unhappy marriage, a problem child, the care of a sick or aging parent, a hypercritical boss, an unrealistic performance standard, rejection, or loneliness. These complex psycho-social problems elicit sympathetic activation that cannot be adequately remediated by primitive "fight or flight" methods of coping, or alternatively by modern drugs and surgery, as the somatizing patient (Wickramasekera, 1989) attempts to do.

The importance of conscious or unconscious (Kihlstrom, 1987) cognitive activity lies in the simple fact that most psychological stress is initiated and maintained not by tissue damage, but by rigid and developmentally primitive cognitive appraisals of threat to well-being, and the fixed emotional meanings we assign to psycho-social and environmental events over which we have little or no direct control. Rigid and irrational habits of cognitive appraisal (Ellis, 1962; Beck, 1976) can generate catastrophizing verbalizations which can transduce into "stressors," the inevitable psycho-social events (failure, delays, loss, uncertainty, rejection, etc.) of life. When cognitively appraised rigidly and simplistically as "threatening" or "intolerable", these events can lead to excessive and chronic psychophysiological arousal through the hypothalamic-pituitary-adrenal axis (H.P.A.A.) and other physiological mechanisms. Causing immunosuppression (Ader, 1981; Geiser, 1989), muscular or vascular pain, negative cognitive ruminations (e.g., anxiety, depression), neurotic avoidance (phobias) or self-medication (e.g., substance abuse).

The ability to transcend irrational cognitive constrictions and to see fresh solutions to perceived "threats" is the essence of creativity and insight. High negative (Watson & Clark, 1984; Watson & Tellegen, 1985) affect (fear, anger) and high levels of cognitive catastrophizing (Ellis, 1962; Wickramasekera, 1979, 1983, 1986, 1988) can keep the hypothalamic-pituitary-adrenal axis (H.P.A.A.) on "red alert," constricting cognitive resources. Consciousness or short term memory has a maximum attentional capacity limited to seven items, plus or minus two (Miller, 1956). If high chronic sympathetic activation (e.g., tachycardia) is cognitively appraised as a "threat" to well-being, then the bulk of limited conscious cognitive resources can be seized and dedicated reliably and exclusively to internal cognitive monitoring and cognitive coping with the cognitive system's own inner subjective processes of threat perception and threat management. Cognitive resources may be chronically devoted to security operations like maladaptive cognitive scanning (repetitious scanning of internal cognitive threat perceptions) and maladaptive behavioral coping (avoidance). This may leave little or no conscious cognitive resources available for objective scanning and appraisal of the external environment or for creative cognitive coping with the problematic situation. Thus, the present perceptual representation of a "stressor" can be dominated by internally generated cognitive fantasies and memories and relatively devoid of externally generated sensory and environmental informational input. So that the perception of a given threat may be largely a constructed cognitive fantasy rather than a perceived sensory event. It is likely that the bulk of the cognitive resources of both the 1) conscious cognitive system and perhaps also the 2) unconscious cognitive system (Kihlstrom, 1987; Wickramasekera, 1991) are preempted whenever a threat is perceived, sympathetic activation occurs, and strong negative affect (e.g., fear or anger) is evoked. Hence, no cognitive resources may be available to appraise objectively and to cope creatively with the actual external problem. Threatening cognitive labels sustain sympathetic activation which can 1) inhibit objective perception of the "sensory" world and 2) block creative cognitive coping with real environmental threats. All the above factors increase the probability that the everyday perceptions, the emotions and the coping methods of the present and future will be similar to those of the past.

Creativity, the Perception of Threat, and Hypnotic Ability

Alterations in the perception of everyday events have been psychologically described by Kris (1951), Schachtel (1959), and others. Perception is altered in a way that increases the probability that events and problems in living (Szasz, 1960) will be looked at freshly. Schactel (1959) called this the "allocentric mode of perception" and described it thus. "This openness means that the sensibilities of the person, his mind, and his senses, are more freely receptive, less tied to fixed anticipations and sets, and that the object is approached in different ways, from different angles, and not with any fixed purpose to use it for the satisfaction of a particular need, or the testing of a particular expectation or possibility". Reducing sympathetic activation, as in sleep, may indirectly reduce threat perception and disinhibit cognitive creativity. This disengagement of limited cognitive resources from chronic threat appraisal and coping and their availability for fresh or objective cognitive appraisal of the environment and creative coping can liberate present and future perceptions from the domination of the past maladaptive emotions and coping methods. Stressors may be recognized as the fantasies of a mind preoccupied with scanning its own inner workings and insulated from the objective environment by this cognitive preoccupation. Stressors can be perceived as stepping stones rather than as obstacles to well-being.

There is empirical evidence of a modest (r=.55) relationship between hypnotic ability and creativity (Bowers & Bowers, 1979). Hypnotic ability is an empirically well established construct and tools to measure its magnitude have high and known reliability and validity (Hilgard, 1965). There is evidence that two common procedural components in stress reduction techniques can at least temporarily increase hypnotic ability. The common procedural components that potentiate hypnotic ability are sensory restriction and muscular relaxation.

Stress Reduction Techniques

Five techniques have been proposed to combat psychophysiological stress. The best known of these methods are 1) Transcendental Meditation (TM), 2) Autogenic Training, 3) Progressive Relaxation, 4) Symbolic Desensitization, and 5) Frontal EMG and Thermal Biofeedback. There is some evidence for the clinical utility of these techniques with some patients with certain stress related problems (Blanchard et al., 1986, 1988; Wolpe, 1973; Schultz & Luthe, 1959;

Jacobson, 1970; Wallace & Benson, 1972). Where data is available, careful study demonstrates that: 1) there are individual differences in response to these stress reduction methods, 2) the "active ingredients" are not clear in these superficially very different procedures, and 3) the mechanism of change in clinical status and psycho-physiological response is not clear in these studies.

Similarities Among Stress Reduction Techniques

In spite of many historical, cultural, and philosophical differences between these stress reduction methods, it appears that they share at least three similarities at a procedural level. 1) All five techniques require the trainee to explicitly or implicitly restrict sensory stimulation during the exercises. For example, subjects are asked to close their eyes, lay or sit still, and concentrate attention on a repetitive stimulus or phrase. Hence, at least in this respect they are like Restricted Environmental Stimulation Therapy (REST). 2) All five procedures instruct the patient to relax, let go, and to reduce his level of psychophysiological arousal. Hence, all five techniques try to reduce sympathetic activation and threat perception. 3) All five techniques explicitly or implicitly seek to impact the patient's belief systems and structure positive therapeutic expectations. Their credibility is boosted by their association with systems (e.g., science, medicine, etc.) that already have high credibility (Wickramasekera, 1977b, 1985). For example, TM training is introduced with a display of charts and graphs and a lecture on the scientific basis of TM. Progressive relaxation (Jacobson, 1970) stresses its roots in the muscle physiology laboratory and EMG measurement. Desensitization (Wolpe, 1973) is introduced to a patient in clinical practice with reference to its roots in the conditioning laboratory and its presumed origins in scientific psychology. Clinical biofeedback uses impressive scientific-medical instruments and in fact, appears to have such high face validity that it requires no explicit statement of credentials. Autogenic training is preceded by a serious ritualistic measurement of vital functions (pulse, blood pressure, etc.), which can create the impression that grave and healing events are at hand. The scientific and medical packaging of these five procedures may inhibit critical analytic skeptical brain functions. Their claims of clinical effectiveness are supported by empirical data and at least plausible and logical rationales. Hence, there is a deliberate structuring of positive therapeutic expectations.

1. Sensory Restriction and Potentiated Hypnotizability

Sensory restriction (REST) is one common procedural component of the five stress reduction techniques. It appears that sensory restriction procedures can be used to increase human secondary suggestibility (persuasibility) and to potentiate therapeutic expectations (Azima et al., 1961; Adams et al., 1963; Suedfeld, 1969a; Lilly, 1956; Hebb, 1966; Zukerman & Cohen, 1964; Orne & Scheibe, 1964; Lindsley, 1957). These reports have been critically and exhaustively reviewed in at least two authoritative texts (Zubek, 1969b; Rasmussen, 1973) and will not be elaborated on further. The studies to be reviewed here, however, constitute the first controlled empirical demonstrations that sensory restriction procedures also reliably increase primary suggestibility (Eysenck & Furneaux, 1945; Evans, 1967) or hypnotizability. Previous studies focused on secondary suggestibility and did not incorporate pre-post measures of secondary suggestibility of known reliability and validity.

Increased patient sensitivity to cognitive expectational manipulations can also be indexed by changes in primary suggestibility. Primary suggestibility or hypnotizability can be operationally defined by standardized pre-post scales, such as the Stanford Hypnotic Susceptibility Scales (1959) or the Barber Suggestibility Scale (1969) which have been designed to measure these behaviors. Hypnotizability is a variable whose parameters have been well established through careful laboratory studies (Hilgard, 1965; Barber, 1969).

In the last 25 years, several independently replicated studies with progressively tighter controls demonstrate that sensory restriction procedures increase hypnotizability (Pena, 1963; Wickramasekera, 1969,

1970, 1977; Sanders & Rehyer, 1969; Barabasz, 1982; Barabasz & Barabasz, 1989). Superior hypnotic ability appears to be associated with potentiated cognitive control of physiological functions (Barabasz & Lonsdale, 1983; Speigel & Barabasz, 1989; Spiegel et al., 1985; Spiegel el al., 1988; Ewer & Stewart, 1986; Murphy et al., 1989; Klein & Spiegel, 1989; DeBenedittis et al., 1989; DePascalis et al., 1988). Hence, the REST component common to all five stress reduction techniques may potentiate through hypnotic mechanisms the cognitive reduction of 1) sympathetic activation, 2) negative affect (N.A.), and 3) threat perception at least temporarily. Reduced threat perception (indexed indirectly by reduced sympathetic activation) may liberate cognitive resources for more 4) objective cognitive appraisal of the environment, and 5) creative cognitive coping with challenges in living.

An early study (Wickramasekera, 1969) supported the hypothesis that 30 minutes of sensory restriction enhanced hypnotizability as measured by Forms A & B of the Stanford Hypnotic Susceptibility Scale (SHSS). Experimental subjects were subjected to REST Experimental subjects wore padded earphones providing white noise, light attenuating goggles and wore cotton gloves. They were instructed to be silent and motionless for 30 minutes while seated in a recliner. Control subjects were simply told to come back after 30 minutes for post-testing. This study showed a significant increase ($p < .007$) in hypnotizability in the sensory restriction group and no change in the control group.

The second study (Wickramasekera, 1970) was a replication and extension of the previous study using 45 white male prisoners randomly assigned to one of three groups of 15 subjects each. Subjects in both experimental groups (one and two), received 60 minutes of sensory restriction (auditory-visual-tactile) delivered by a procedure identical to that described above. But subjects in experimental one were additionally read before exposure to REST, a set of verbal instructions intended to arouse anxiety about the effects of REST. Controls simply sat on the same chair in which experimental subjects had sat and listened to music and read magazines for sixty minutes. The results of this study confirmed the observations of the first study. Subjects in the two experimental groups (REST) increased significantly ($p<.005$) in hypnotizability, but controls did not. Analysis revealed that the three groups were equated on initial susceptibility. When this second study was being prepared for publication, Professor Ernest Hilgard brought to my attention an unpublished dissertation by Pena (1963), which also used male prisoners. Pena used a control group plus two experimental groups receiving, respectively, one and one-half and three hours of sensory restriction. He found that the enhancement scores of the three groups were ordered in a direction that was consistent with the enhancement hypothesis. The group receiving three hours of sensory restriction obtained the greatest enhancement of hypnotic ability, and the control group the least.

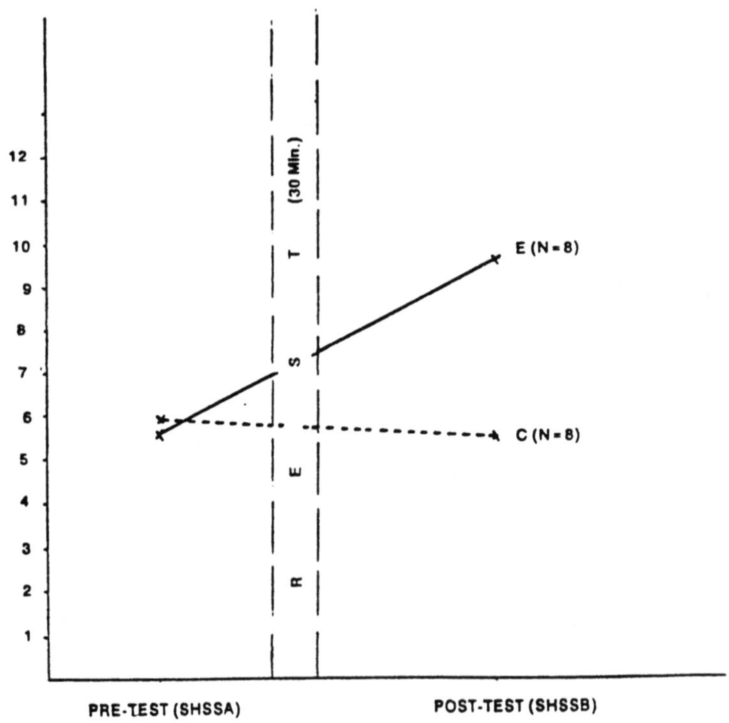

Figure 7-1. Hypnotic ability and sensory restriction (REST). Wickramasekera, 1969

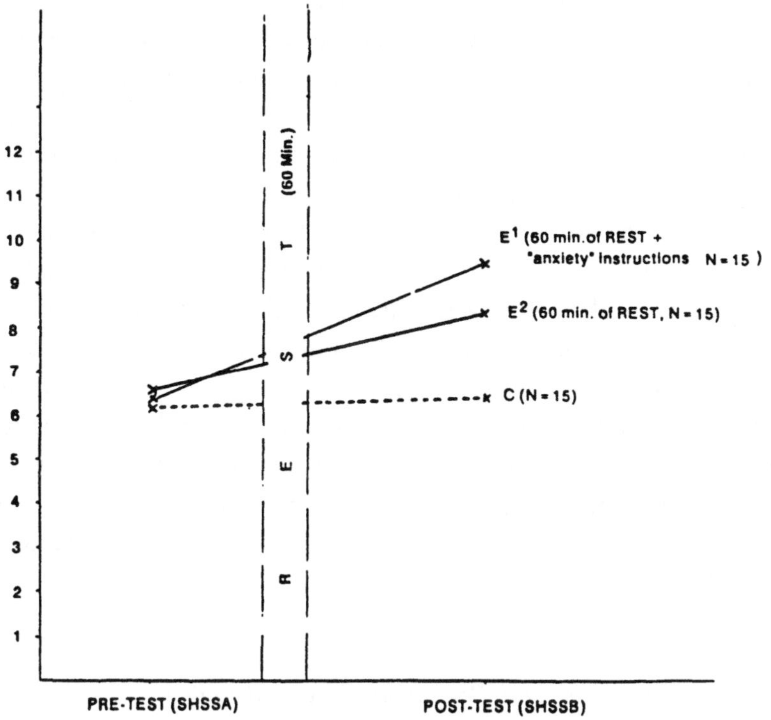

Figure 7-2. Hypnotic ability and sensory restriction (REST). Wickramasekera, 1970

A study by Sanders and Rehyer (1969) which used previously "resistant" subjects, also found that four to six hours of sensory restriction significantly increased hypnotizability at least temporarily. There is only one study (Levitt et al., 1962) involving hypnotizability that failed to replicate the above observations. The Levitt study involved three "resistant" student nurses. It appears that sensory restriction in a laboratory situation may enhance hypnotizability or primary suggestibility at least temporarily.

More recently, a series of very tightly controlled studies (Barabasz, 1982; Barabasz & Barabasz, 1989) used the most stringent measure of hypnotic ability, the Stanford Form C. Clever and careful controls for generalization, follow-up testing, plateau hypnotizability, experimental demand characteristics, and motivational instructions were used. The Barabasz studies clearly show that chamber REST (six hours) enhances hypnotic ability. Reviews (Adams, 1964; Suedfeld, 1977) support the hypothesis that in a clinical situation, subjects show a positive therapeutic response to even a single session of mild to moderate sensory restriction. But these studies did not illuminate the mechanism of change elucidated by Barabasz (1982). The therapeutic regimens of autogenic training, progressive muscular relaxation, transcendental meditation, clinical biofeedback, and systematic desensitization increase the probability of numerous brief consecutive periods of sensory restriction which may have cumulative therapeutic effects through potentiated hypnotic ability. Potentiated hypnotic ability may be used through cognitive procedures to reduce sympathetic activation, reduce negative affect, indirectly reduce threat perception, and increase the cognitive resources available to access the "allocentric mode of perception".

2. Muscle Relaxation and Potentiated Hypnotizability

Relaxation instructions are a second common procedural component of the five stress reduction techniques. Relaxation instructions are one of the independent variables that increase suggestibility (Barber, 1969). It would seem that increasing the precision of relaxation training, and reducing sympathetic activation with EMG feedback may increase suggestibility even more significantly. In a preliminary study (Wickramasekera, 1971), contingent EMG feedback training temporarily but significantly increased hypnotic ability ($p < .001$). In the control group there was no change in hypnotic ability.

Encouraged by these preliminary observations, we attempted replication. The only differences were that in the present (Wickramasekera, 1973) study, 1) there were 10 30-minute feedback training sessions; 2) the post-testing for hypnotic susceptibility was done by a research assistant who was blind to the nature (contingent or non-contingent) of the feedback training the subjects received. We again found that response contingent (true) feedback training increased hypnotic susceptibility significantly ($p = .001$) if only temporarily. There was no change in the control group which got false or non-contingent EMG feedback. Radtke et al., (1983), using procedures unlike mine, has reported a failure to replicate the above results.

But within the constraints of both our experimental situation and our clinical procedures with tension headache patients, we have often observed that those who succeed in learning to voluntarily and reliably drop frontal (to approximately 2 uV.p-p) EMG levels, appear more responsive to hypnosis on post-testing on the SHSS:B (Wickramasekera, 1976, 1977a). These observations are also consistent with the systematic EEG studies of Engstrom (1976) and the clinical EEG study of Melzack and Perry (1975) who used EEG feedback to potentiate relaxation induction.

The muscle relaxation training component common to these five stress reduction techniques may be another mechanism (in addition to REST) through which hypnotic ability is temporarily increased. Relaxation potentiated hypnotic ability may be a mechanism through which 1) sympathetic activation is reduced, 2) cognitive threat perception is indirectly reduced, 3) the probability of access to the "allocentric mode of perception" is increased.

3. Potentiated Placebo Effects and Positive Therapeutic Expectations

Structuring positive therapeutic expectations is another common component in the five stress reduction techniques under review. There is good consensus in both the psychotherapy and the medical literatures, that patient expectations can powerfully influence clinical outcome with both psychological and biological disorders (Frank, 1965; Shapiro, 1971; Beecher, 1959; Kaxdin & Wilcoxin, 1976; Strupp & Bergin, 1972; Goldstein, 1962). The medical literature shows that the effects of an active drug can be attenuated, potentiated, or reversed by expectational manipulations. The literature on the placebo effect (Shapiro, 1971) has shown that placebos can be more powerful than potent active drugs for placebo responders and that they can reverse the action of such drugs. Placebos can have therapeutic effects on organic illness and malignancies. Studies have shown the dose-response, time-effect curves and the side effects of an active drug and a placebo to be similar (Evans, 1974). Beecher (1959) and Evans (1974) reviewed 36 double blind studies and found that a placebo reduced surgical pain by half its original intensity in 36 percent of patients.

There are currently at least three explanatory models of the placebo effect. The suggestion hypothesis (Shapiro, 1971; Barber, 1969) and the anxiety reduction hypothesis (Evans, 1974a,b) are the best known. Recently, I have proposed (Wickramasekera, 1977b, 1980, 1985) a conditioned response model of the placebo effect that operates through acquired expectations and Pavlovian conditioning. This third model (Wickramasekera, 1977b, 1980, 1985) explains and predicts the observed clinical outcomes of the present five stress reduction procedures.

It appears that people of high hypnotic ability condition more rapidly in both operant and respondent learning situations (Edmonston, 1979; Wickramasekera, 1980, 1985). The REST and relaxation training procedures in the five stress reduction techniques appear to potentiate hypnotic ability. Hence, people with increased hypnotic ability should condition more reliably and powerfully and will therefore be better placebo responders than people of low hypnotic ability. The five stress reduction techniques may also potentiate the conditioned response mechanism of the placebo effect.

Hypnotizability as a Factor in Risk, and Therapy of Stress Reactions

High and low hypnotic ability people are especially at risk for stress related disorders, because they are respectively hyper- and hyposensitive (Wickramasekera 1979, 1983, 1986, 1988). Therefore, enhanced hypnotic ability may be both a liability (hyper- and hyposensitivity) and an asset (because it can be used to reduce sympathetic activation, reduce threat perception and to increase creativity) in the management of stress related disorders.

The enhanced hypnotizability associated with REST and/or muscular relaxation (e.g., low frontal EMG) potentiates the verbal-cognitive control of behavior and physiology (Wickramasekera, 1976, 1977a) bringing even temporarily, psychological and physiological systems closer together in a functional sense.

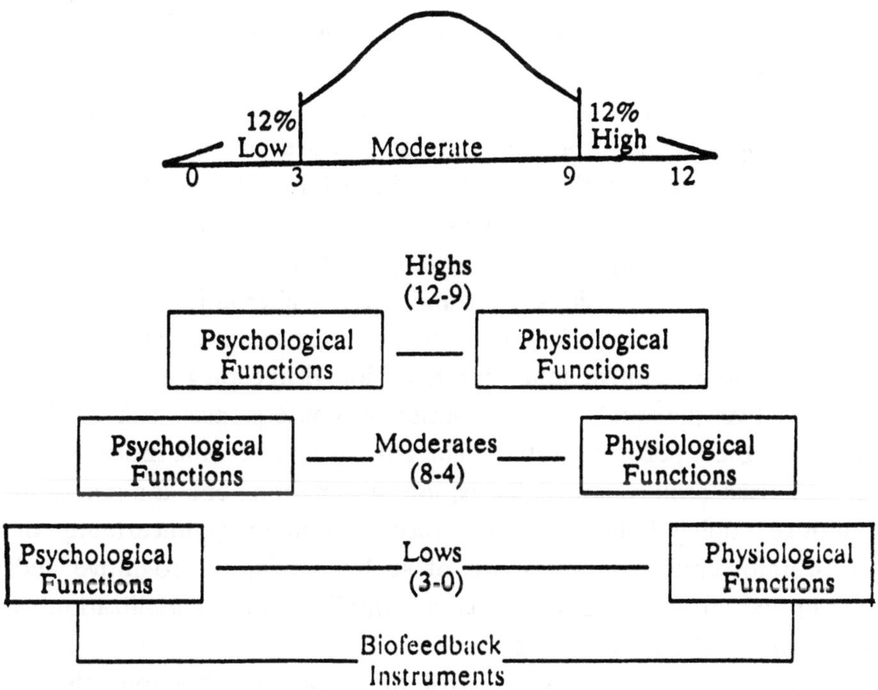

Figure 7-3. Degrees of proximity between psychological and physiological functions.

Hence, verbal relaxation instructions (a psychological function) can be used to induce a state of low physiological arousal (inhibition of the H.P.A.A.) which is very often an indirect index of reduced threat perception in the cognitive system. Limited cognitive resources (seven, plus or minus two) may be liberated from chronic dedication to security operations. This cognitive state (inhibition of chronic preoccupation with the perception of threat) will be indexed in the cognitive system by 1) reduced conscious catastrophizing, 2) reduced conscious negative affect (neuroticism), and 3) reduced unconscious negative affect (reduced sympathetic reactivity) (Wickramasekera, 1979, 1983, 1986, 1988, 1991). In this low threat perception mode ("allocentric" mode of perception), larger portions of the cognitive system are available to freshly appraise old problems and for creative coping and problem solving as described by Kris (1951) and Schactel (1959). The "allocentric mode of perception" increases the probability of creatively approaching old problems in living, finding "meaning" in what seemed meaningless, looking freshly at everyday events, and noticing alternatives where none seemed to exist before. These cognitive and perceptual changes can generate more adaptive behavioral and biological coping methods, and the positive personal or environmental consequences can further reinforce these perceptual shifts. The patient may become more willing to take risks, acquire new skills, explore his environment, and persist in adaptive coping behavior in the face of temporary uncertainty or non-reinforcement. The absence of such an adaptive cognitive and perceptual attitude can be at least as crippling to self actualization as the absence of an arm or leg.

The increased cognitive control of autonomic functions that a patient often experiences, with repeated practice of the five stress reduction techniques (all of which may unintentionally increase hypnotic ability) can add considerably to the patients conviction of "self efficacy" (Bandura, 1977), apart from actually reducing the frequency or intensity of a specific symptom (e.g., tension or migraine headache pain). "An efficacy expectation is the conviction that one can successfully execute the behavior required to produce an outcome" (Bandura, 1977). Self efficacy is postulated by Bandura (1977) to be the primary determinant of the intensity and duration of coping behaviors, assuming the patient has the relevant skills and incentives.

Conclusion

Sensory restriction and muscular relaxation potentiate hypnotic ability and the placebo effect. Potentiated hypnotic ability can cognitively reduce sympathetic activation and enhance creativity (Bowers & Bowers, 1979). It is a major hypothesis of this paper that an alteration in physiology alone is not a sufficient condition to induce durable positive clinical outcomes, particularly if there is little or no long term change in the aversive features of the patient's environment. Low physiological arousal may indirectly index temporarily reduced cognitive threat perception, and increased availability of cognitive resources for objective appraisal of the situation and creative cognitive coping. But an additional essential condition, for durable positive clinical outcome is a stable change in the way the patient cognitively appraises, and creatively copes with, "threatening" information, so that new coping skills are learned and social support systems acquired to elevate the patient's general level of positive affect (Watson & Tellegen, 1985).

The disengagement of constrained cognitive resources from preoccupation with threat perception and their availability for engagement in fresh and creative cognitive coping may enable obstacles to be seen as stepping stones. Reducing negative affect (threat perception) enables the patient in stress reduction therapy to risk experimenting with new cognitive and behavioral coping skills that are essential for dealing adaptively with the inevitable major and minor changes in life. It is predicted that: 1) Pre-post tests of hypnotic ability, before and after systematic and extended training in the five stress reduction techniques will show significant increases in hypnotic ability; 2) The delivery of a) pure forms of REST and b) generalized muscle relaxation will be more effective in increasing hypnotic ability than either condition alone.

8

Age Regression Phenomena

Vladimir Raikov and Marianne Barabasz

There is an obvious consistency between restricted environmental stimulation (REST) and hypnosis. While subjects can enter a state of hypnosis by active alert methods (Miller, A. Barabasz & M. Barabasz, 1991), typical hypnotic inductions involve relaxation. Subjects enter the state by means of a form of REST. Visual stimuli are eliminated when eyes are closed and outside annoyances are eliminated by the subjects' precisely focused attention on the hypnotist's voice. Sensory perception, due to movement, is markedly reduced by the subject's calm position in a comfortable chair or on a bed. Recently, A. Barabasz (1990c,e) demonstrated that REST alone could elicit spontaneous hypnosis without dependence on a hypnotic induction. Interestingly, REST alone has also produced some regressive child like inversion perception responses in adults (Miller & Barabasz, 1985).

Raikov (1980) reported that adults who were highly hypnotizable could be age regressed to a point where they could exhibit neurological reflexes and behaviors consistent with infancy which were convincing to the trained neurologists who served as observers. The study, using 10 subjects, demonstrated uncoordinated eye movements and sucking reflexes characteristic of infancy in all cases. Six subjects showed the foot bending reflex, five showed the Babinski reflex, while four subjects showed the infant grasping reflex. There was a clear positive relationship between the degree of hypnotic involvement, age regression and the production of these neonatal behaviors. The Raikov (1980) study appeared to demonstrate that neonatal reflexes could be produced during age regression with subjects who were high in hypnotic capacity. However, the design of the study did not rule out the possibility of motivated role enactment.

Raikov (1982) focused on the role enactment issue and attempted to control for this potential confound by comparing the performance of two highly hypnotizable subjects, two professional actors, and two low hypnotizable subjects. The two highly hypnotizable university students had considerable experience in hypnosis including previous age regression ability and elements of reflex activity. The remaining subjects were inexperienced. All subjects were individually given instructions in hypnosis which were intended to induce age regression to the newborn state. These subjects were subsequently tested for special movements, grimaces, crying without tears, and uncontrolled reflexes. All behaviors were filmed for later evaluation. Observation of the films suggested that the highly hypnotizable subjects showed neonatal responses 90 percent of the time. Professional actors showed neonatal responses 15 percent of the time while the low hypnotizable subjects showed such responses only 10 percent of the time.

The present study was intended to extend previous research by comparing regressed high and low hypnotizable subjects who had comparable REST and hypnosis training experiences prior to data collection.

Method

Subjects

Eight university student volunteers served as subjects. All subjects had had several sessions of experience with hypnosis using the key elements of REST, as noted above, for the hypnotic induction. This particular sample of subjects was chosen from a larger pool because of the demonstration of high hypnotic capacity (n=4) or the demonstration of essentially non-hypnotizable or low hypnotizable capacities (n=4).

Procedure

Following an eyes closed rest period of several minutes and relaxation instructions intended to produce hypnosis, subjects were exposed to regression instructions as follows: "You are newborn. You are an infant..." the instructions to remain deeply hypnotized and to open their eyes were given. Subjects were tested for foot bending and Babinski reflexes. All data were collected in the identical setting at the All Union Center for Preventive Medicine, Moscow, Russia. Sessions were professionally recorded on 16mm film with a sound track.

Results

Observations of the video record clearly demonstrated responses similar to those reported by Raikov (1980, 1982) earlier. All of the high hypnotizable subjects showed uncoordinated eye swimming movements. None of the low hypnotizables demonstrated such behavior. Half of the high hypnotizables but none of the lows demonstrated the Babinski reflex or foot bending reflex. As in the earlier studies, it appeared that there was a relationship between involvement in age regression and the production of neonatal behaviors.

Discussion

The apparent findings provide further preliminary evidence that highly hypnotizable subjects who respond to suggestions for age regression can reproduce the reactions of a newborn including both behaviors and reflexes. Independent neurologists who viewed the video records found the responses to be strikingly similar to those found in infants. The study represents improvements in research methodology as compared to the earlier attempts (Raikov, 1980, 1982). In contrast to the earlier studies, both high and low hypnotizability subject groups had similar experiences with hypnosis before the experimental inductions which were designed to maximize hypnotic performance. The sample size, while still small, had double the subjects in both the high and low hypnotizability groups as studied earlier.

The findings are exciting. However, the methodology would benefit from further improvements (A. Barabasz & M. Barabasz, 1992). Research is currently planned for a cooperative project between Russia and the U.S.A. to test the observed phenomena more thoroughly. Orne's (1979) real-simulator design will be employed. As in the present study, both high and low hypnotizability subjects will be plateaued for maximal hypnotic responsiveness before commencement of the investigation. However, the hypnotists conducting the video tape recorded age regression procedures will be blind to subjects hypnotizability level. Low hypnotizable subjects will be instructed to simulate hypnosis in an attempt to assure that hypnotists will not treat high and low hypnotizability subjects differently during the regression sessions. A rigorous criteria for high and low hypnotizability groups will be established by individualized independent testing using the Stanford Hypnotic Susceptibility Scale: Form C of Weitzenhoffer and Hilgard (1962). An attempt will be made to assure equivalent hypnotic depth by asking subjects to assign a number on an open ended scale once hypnotized, and then to indicate, by raising a finger, when they have doubled this level and feel they are deeply hypnotized (Miller, A. Barabasz & M. Barabasz, 1991). Upon completion of the regression sessions, a clinician blind to the experimental focus of the study will conduct an independent interview with each subject. The interviews will be aimed at determining whether or not subjects were able to retrieve lost memories during the session and to determine whether or not extra experimental factors may have influenced subjects' responses.

9

Effects of Flotation REST and Visual Imagery on Athletic Performance: Tennis

Patrick McAleney and Arreed Barabasz

Flotation Restricted Environmental Stimulation (REST) has produced promising preliminary results in sports performance enhancement (Hutchison, 1984; Lee & Hewitt, 1987; Stanley, Mahoney, & Reppert, 1987; Suedfeld & Bruno, 1990; Wagaman & Barabasz, 1990). The technique involves floating on a dense magnesium sulfate solution in a sound-attenuated, light-free tank. Unfortunately, the studies to date are limited. Only three studies presented data beyond anecdotal or case study reports (Lee & Hewitt, 1987; Suedfeld & Bruno, 1990; Wagaman & Barabasz, 1990).

Lee and Hewitt (1987) examined the use of the flotation tank for the improvement of gymnastic performance and the reduction of physical symptoms. Female gymnasts of novice and intermediate skill were randomly assigned to one of three treatment conditions: REST and visualization, non-REST and visualization, or control. In each condition subjects were exposed to audio-taped messages which included initial relaxation, visualization of routines, and "wake-up." Subjects floated for 40 minutes once a week for six weeks. Subjects in the REST condition performed significantly better than subjects in the non-REST visualization only and control conditions.

The two other studies of flotation REST and athletic performance (Suedfeld & Bruno, 1990; Wagaman & Barabasz, 1990) examined effects of flotation REST on basketball performance. Suedfeld and Bruno (1990) examined the use of visual imagery combined with flotation REST, an "Alpha Chair," and a normal room and chair, on the free-throw performance of occasional or nonbasketball players. Free throw (foul shot) accuracy improved by 50% the day after a one-hour flotation REST session with guided imagery. The two non-REST imagery only groups showed no improvement. It was suggested that REST may induce an optimal arousal state for the task and/or it may enable subjects to return to such a level 24 hours after treatment. Also suggested was the notion that imagery may be more vivid or accurate in a REST environment, or that REST may make the imagery more accessible later. A synergistic interaction between imagery and optimal arousal was hypothesized to explain the results. Unfortunately, the study employed only a single REST session. The specificity of REST effects are in doubt since a single flotation session could be expected to be perceived as more novel than the control condition. Furthermore, the results produced by nonexpert occasional recreational players tell us nothing about the potency of the effects of REST on well trained, high ability, dedicated athletes.

During the 1988-89 season, Wagaman and Barabasz (1990) examined the effects of REST on the basketball performance of players of high ability from two large Northwestern university intercollegiate varsity basketball teams. Subjects were randomly assigned to treatment groups, including REST (six flotation sessions) with visual imagery and relaxation with visual imagery (six sessions). Subjects were tested on performance and self-report measures before and after treatments. Analyses showed that the two groups were equivalent at the pretest but differed after treatments on basic athletic performance measures. Wagaman and Barabasz's (1990) results were viewed as consistent with the concurrent findings of Suedfeld and Bruno (1990). The study also suggested that two REST sessions per week were the most effective for performance enhancement.

To date, no study has tested the effects of flotation REST and visual imagery with comprehensive performance measures in a competitive environment, and no study has focused on tennis. The purpose of the present study was to test the effects of REST and visual imagery on the competitive performance of expert intercollegiate tennis players. Indeed, little can be said about the effectiveness of REST on athletic performance if data are not obtained in actual competition.

Method

Subjects

Members of a varsity tennis team (10 men, 10 women) (ages 18 to 22 years) from a Pacific Athletic Conference university volunteered for this study. To control for possible confounds due to sex differences, groups were balanced according to sex. Within the sex constraint, subjects were randomly assigned to one of two treatment groups, 1) flotation REST with imagery messages and 2) an imagery message only condition. Subjects in both groups understood that imagery training was widely used and had been shown to be an effective technique for enhancement of performance.

Apparatus

A Floatarium brand flotation tank was employed for the REST treatment. It is constructed of fiberglass, is lightproof and sound-attenuated. Intercommunication and ventilation systems are integral to the construction of the Floatarium tank. Subjects floated supine on a solution of water and Epsom salts (magnesium sulfate) at a density of 1.30 grams per cubic centimeter (Lilly, 1977). The solution was maintained at approximately 34.5° C (±.2° C) (Lilly, 1977).

Subjects in the imagery only condition were exposed to their treatment in a REST chamber, a sound-attenuated room (3 m x 1.7 m x 2.4 m). Entry to the chamber is provided by an elaborate double door. The experimental demand characteristics of the chamber are at least as great as those of the flotation tank. To eliminate potential REST effects for the imagery-only control condition, the room was fully lighted and normal sounds were provided by an open intercom hidden in a ceiling vent. Subjects moved about the room or sat in a comfortable chair. In other words, the experimental demands and situational cues were maintained to equate with the elaborateness of the tank environment but the potential REST effects of the chamber were entirely defeated.

Materials

The performance enhancement/visual-imagery message was similar to that used in the Wagaman and Barabasz (1990) study. It was devised under the guidance of a professional tennis instructor and was eight minutes in length. It included images of five or six alternative skills in which the subjects visualized themselves making optimal shots (Feltz & Landers, 1983). This relatively short message length was selected so that subjects would have adequate time to process the content of the message in the REST environment. In the Wagaman and Barabasz (1990) study, the message was approximately 20 minutes in length and was delivered at the 30-minute point of the 50-minute session. As a consequence, the subjects complained that they had no uninterrupted message processing time in the REST environment.

Measures

To obtain accurate performance data, subjects' tennis matches were videotaped before treatment and after completion of the six treatment package. Players' opponents were matched for ability by the coaches at the pre-treatment tournament. At posttreatment, opponents were determined by draw. At pretreatment, two of the study's players competed against each other; at posttreatment none did. Videotapes were scored by raters blind to subjects' treatment condition on three separate performance measures: first service, key shot, and points won/lost. The possible scores for service variables were: winner, in-play, or error. The key shot, that shot which produced or resulted in winning or losing the game point, had possible scores of winner, forced error, or unforced error. Frequency counts were kept for each subject (e.g., first service winners) precluding the need to attempt to assign equal interval scale values for the scores on the dependent measures. Length of time for scoring the videotapes was not standardized due to the variability in actual playing time. The number of points to be scored per player was set at the first 50 points per match. Interrater reliability for all performance scores was .88.

Procedure

To familiarize subjects with the experimental procedures (Suedfeld, 1980), those in the REST condition received an introduction to the tank and flotation procedures, including a 20-minute introductory float prior to their initial treatment session. Experience in our lab has shown that the introductory float may be important because subjects enjoy a non-experimental period which allows exploration of the environment. Novelty effects are greatly reduced. Subjects in the imagery-only condition received a similar orientation to their treatment condition.

Each group was exposed to six treatment sessions in the three-week period prior to the posttest (two sessions per week). Treatment periods were of 50 minutes duration. At the half-way point in each session, subjects were exposed to the tape recorded imagery message.

Results

Independent samples t-tests were computed for each of the three separate videotaped performance variables. At pretreatment no significant differences were found between groups on the performance variables. At posttreatment, a significant difference was found between groups on first service winners ($t = 2.11$, $p < .05$). In the REST treatment group (mean = 2.55, SD = 2.5), there were significantly more service winners than in the control group (mean = .67, SD = 1.4). An Omega squared showed that 15% of the variance was accounted for between the independent and dependent variables. Analyses of key shots and points won/lost data were not significant ($p > .05$).

Since first service data consisted of frequency counts of winners, which were not normally distributed, it was felt that complete reliance on the robustness of the sensitive parametric analysis might be inappropriate. To provide additional stringency non-parametric analyses were also calculated.

A Kruskall-Wallis analysis of variance showed no significant difference between REST and control groups at pre-treatment (He = 1.4, df = 1, $p > .05$). At posttreatment the REST group showed significantly better first service results than the control group (He = 4.3, df = 1, $p < .05$).

Pretreatment to posttreatment data were analyzed using the Wilcoxon Signed-Ranks test. Controls showed no significant change in performance (Ns-R = 5, T = 5, $P > .05$) while the REST group showed a significant improvement in first service winners after exposure to the six REST sessions (Ns-R = 8, T = 3, $p < .05$).

Discussion

This is the first study of the effects of REST with visual imagery on tennis performance. Data was obtained in actual competition. Both expert male and female athletes were employed and performance data were obtained on comprehensive competitive performance indicants. The results show that flotation REST combined with a visual-imagery message enhanced the performance of one previously well-learned key athletic skill among players of high ability. The significant first-service winner results indicate that players who are already at a high level of performance ability can improve the execution of this frequently repeated task.

The nonsignificant findings for the key shot analyses are not surprising. For this variable, a variety of skills or types of shots were scored, including forehands, backhands, forehand and backhand vollies, drop shots, and overhead smashes. These shots, although highly practiced and repeated often, are inherently more variable in a game or match environment. A player has less control of the direction, speed or spin of a ball returned by an opposing player. Therefore, these shots might be expected to be less responsive to imagery practice, no matter how favorable the learning environment. In contrast to this variability, the automatic nature of the service motion is under direct control of the server.

Also, the nonsignifcance of the point won/lost measure is not surprising, since it is affected by the performance of both players, subjects and opponents alike. In varsity athletics, there tends to be high similarity among the players, with the less skillful players not being selected for the teams so a convergence of over-all points scored is not unexpected. Despite this constraint, this measure was added to the study to provide over-all performance data. Perhaps increases in over-all points won might be observed for less highly skilled players.

It appears that REST was effective in enhancing the highly controlled skill of the service motion and was less effective for the more variable demands of the key shot. It also may be that the imagery message, which was generic in description, might be more effective if it were individually tailored to the needs of each player. Further research should assess the effect of individualized messages on enhancement of athletic performance.

Acknowledgment

The authors thank Marianne Barabasz, Rebecca Dyer, Dan Peterson, Ken Azbill, Dennis Warner, and REST Technologies Corporation.

10

Flotation REST and Imagery in the Improvement of Collegiate Athletic Performance: Basketball

Jeffrey Wagaman and Arreed Barabasz

Several psychological techniques have been used in an effort to enhance sports performance, including pre-game rehearsal, psycho-physiological arousal (psyching-up), biofeedback, and anxiety reduction by relaxation. Procedures such as visuo-motor behavioral rehearsal, hypnosis and guided imagery, have been either developed or adapted specifically for performance improvement (Garver, 1977; Hall & Erffmeyer, 1983; Lee & Hewitt, 1987; Suinn, 1986; Wojcikiewicz & Orlick, 1987). The findings favor mental practice as effective in performance enhancement but all of these interventions have been disappointing in terms of the magnitude of positive change produced.

Restricted Environmental Stimulation Technique (REST) (Suedfeld, 1980), has been shown to greatly enhance mental imagery (A. Barabasz, 1982). REST has been found to produce deep relaxation as shown by psychological test data (A. Barabasz, M. Barabasz, Dyer, & Rather, 1990) and psychophysiological measures (A. Barabasz & M. Barabasz, 1985; Jacobs, Heilbronner, & Stanley, 1984; Turner & Fine, 1983). In contrast to the mediocre athletic performance enhancement effects of non-REST interventions, flotation restricted environmental stimulation has produced remarkably promising preliminary results in both anecdotal (Daniel, 1985; Hutchison, 1984a,b; Stanley, Mahoney & Reppert, 1987) and recent controlled studies (McAleney & A. Barabasz, 1990; Suedfeld & Bruno, 1990; Wagaman & A. Barabasz, 1990; Lee & Hewitt, 1987).

Lee and Hewitt (1987) employed multiple REST sessions for novice/intermediate competitive gymnasts and found performance improvement on the basis of judges' subjective ratings. Suedfeld and Bruno's (1990) preliminary study exposed recreational basketball players to a single REST session with imagery and found improvement on the objective measure of foul shooting scores obtained in a non-game session. Only one controlled investigation of athletic performance enhancement by REST has been completed using expert players. McAleney and Barabasz (1990) demonstrated significant tennis performance enhancement in actual intercollegiate competition on a variety of objective measures.

The present study was designed to provide a comprehensive objective and subjective measures test of the effects of REST on athletic performance using expert collegiate basketball players.

Method

Subjects

Male collegiate basketball players (n=22) from two major university varsity teams volunteered for a "mental imagery and sports performance study." Coaches for each team agreed to allow requests for participation in the study on the basis of a group meeting with each team and informed consent. Subjects were randomly assigned to either REST or control conditions. The study was conducted in conjunction with the 1988-89 basketball season.

Measures

Performance "PERF" scores (Sonstroem & Bernardo, 1982) are objective performance measures based on several different skills performed during a basketball game. This standardized measure has consistently demonstrated concurrent validity coefficients of .73 to .83 (Sonstroem & Bernardo, 1982). PERF scores were calculated for each player on the eleven games played prior to the beginning of the study and on the five games immediately after completion of treatments.

The Performance Evaluation Questionnaire (PEQ) consists of a standardized coaches' report form (AAHPERD, 1984). The PEQ was filled out, pre- and post-treatment for a standardized non-game situation, by coaches who were blind to subjects' treatment group.

The Performance Questionnaire (PQ) (Stanley et al., 1987) is a short self report measure that assesses subjects' perceptions of treatment effects on basketball performance. PQ data was obtained within five days after completion of all treatment sessions.

Imagery Training

The Lee and Hewitt (1987) athletic performance enhancement tape was adapted for use with basketball players. The audio tape emphasized relaxation and visualization of skills in competition. Game performance shooting, dribbling, defense, and passing skills were emphasized. For example, Ss were asked to visualize themselves shooting successfully from various locations on the court, visualize the ball as an extension of their arm, visualize themselves being able to stop any opponents drive.

Treatment Environments

REST subjects floated supine on a solution of water and epsom salts at a density of 1.30 grams per cubic centimeter. The solution was maintained at approximately 34.5° C (±.2° C). The light proof, sound attenuating Floatarium brand SWS flotation tank was employed. Intercommunication and ventilation systems are integral to the tank which resembles an enclosed oversized bathtub. Subjects showered before and after flotation.

Control subjects sat in a comfortable chair in a lighted office. No attempt was made to attenuate normal ambient sound levels. Controls were free to study or simply sit comfortably during, before, and after the tape was played in their sessions.

Procedure

After completion of all pre-treatment performance measures, subjects were exposed to the above environments for six sessions of approximately 50 minutes each over a five week period. The performance enhancement tape was played at the mid-point of each session.

Results

A repeated measures ANOVA on PERF scores showed a significant interaction $F(2,49) = 3.69$, $p < .05$. A Scheffé test showed significant differences on the post test where the REST group (mean = 15.75, S.D. = 3.6) scored significantly ($p < .01$) higher than the imagery only control group (mean = 11.20, S.D. = 2.7). A Scheffé test contrasting subjects who completed two REST sessions between games with subjects completing only one session between games was also significant ($p < .05$). Subjects exposed to two REST sessions between games showed higher PERF scores (mean = 25.95, S.D. = 13.0) than subjects who experienced REST only once between games (mean = 15.75, S.D. = 3.6).

A Kruskal-Wallis one way analysis of variance was calculated on coaches blind PEQ post-treatment ratings of players. The REST subjects were rated as significantly better on passing and shooting but not on dribbling, defense or overall skill. The results appear in Table 10-1.

Table 10-1

Kruskal-Wallis Analysis of Post-treatment PEO Scores

Source	M Rank	Cases	Chi-Square
Passing			
REST	4.85	11	3.31*
Control	6.82	11	
Dribbling			
REST	5.00	11	2.34
Control	6.68	11	
Shooting			
REST	4.95	11	4.21*
Control	7.00	11	
Defense			
REST	5.68	11	0.64
Control	6.41	11	
Overall			
REST	5.64	11	0.60
Control	6.41	11	

* $p < .05$

A one way ANOVA of subjects' subjective ratings of treatment effectiveness (PQ scores) showed no significant ($p > .05$) difference between treatment the REST (mean = 29.72, S.D. = 4.2) and the taped imagery only control groups (mean = 30.7, S.D. = 3.9).

Discussion

The findings demonstrate that flotation REST, with performance enhancement imagery, produces greatly improved athletic skill. The REST-imagery group demonstrated superior performance compared to the imagery only control group on both objective game performance scores and coaches blind ratings of passing and shooting. The potential contribution of expectancy to these results appears to be negligible since subjects ratings of treatment effectiveness showed they perceived only neutral to slight effect with no significant difference between REST and the imagery only control group. Consistent with laboratory (A. Barabasz, 1982) and field (A. Barabasz, 1984) REST experiments, imagery seemed to be greatly enhanced by the state of arousal induced by REST. REST may function to increase the potency of imagery training or, as suggested by Suedfeld and Bruno (1990, p. 84), REST may make imagery more accessible later.

Unlike the preliminary studies which used novice-intermediate gymnasts and judges ratings (Lee & Hewitt, 1987) or recreational basketball players and a single REST session with only a single simple non-game measure (Suedfeld & Bruno, 1990), the present study demonstrated significant REST effects with expert intercollegiate players on objective game and non-game measures. Consistent with the concurrent findings of Suedfeld and Bruno (1990) it would seem that the use of REST is clearly justified in the training of high performance athletes especially when its speed, economy and freedom from known side effects is considered.

11

Short-Term Exposure to REST: Enhanced Performance on a Signal-Detection Task

Richard Atkinson

Past reports of long-term exposure to the restricted environmental stimulation technique (REST) have focused on its deleterious effects on perceptual/cognitive functioning. Attempts to precisely determine the visual functions disrupted by long-term exposure to REST indicate that Ss experience difficulty in focusing, objects appear fuzzy and not clearly distinct from their background, the environment appears to be two dimensional, colors are bright and highly saturated, shapes are distorted, contrast is increased, positive and negative after images are pronounced, and distortions occur in size constancy (Batten, 1961; Bexton, Heron, & Scott, 1954; Doane, Mahatoo, Heron, & Scott, 1956; Freedman & Greenblatt, 1959; Freedman & Held, 1960; Heron, Doane, & Scott, 1956; MacNeill & Zubek, 1967; Scott, Bexton, Heron, & Doane, 1959; Zubek, 1969b).

Long-term exposure to REST appears to produce additional deficits in cognitive performance. Ss undergoing the experience of REST report a rapid decline in the ability to maintain focused attention upon ideational content, difficulty in following a particular line of logical thought, inability to think logically, and disruptions in the organization of their thoughts (Courtney, Davis, & Solomon, 1961; Davis, McCourt, & Solomon, 1960; Goldberger & Holt, 1958; Scott et al., 1959; Smith & Lewty, 1959; Wexler, Mendelson, Leiderman, & Solomon, 1958).

Despite these apparent negative effects of long-term exposure to REST, the anecdotal accounts of short-term exposure are generally positive. For instance, corporate attempts to merchandise sensory-isolation flotation tanks report a plethora of benefits from their use, extolling such virtues as their ability to enhance perceptual skills, to generate clarity in thought, and to produce intense episodes of solitude and relaxation (Lilly, 1981).

A discrepancy also exists between the empirical evidence and the reports of various esoteric disciplines that utilize techniques similar to REST. The parallels between REST and concentrative meditation in Zen Buddhism are often striking (Naranjo & Ornstein, 1977). Concentrative meditation includes exercises that involve a restriction of awareness from distracting sensory stimulation (Ornstein, 1977, p. 160), which is similar to the impoverished perceptual environment of REST. According to the Zen tradition, the primary advantage of concentrative meditation is that through the process of "turning off" input processing for a period of time, an aftereffect of "opening up" or enhanced awareness is achieved. Gurdjieff (1973) has provided a clue as to the way in which perception may be enhanced through meditation by comparing that experience to a child who has not yet developed many of the automatic ways of tuning out the external world; hence, the child may perceive a repeatedly-viewed stimulus in the same manner as when perceived the first time. Deikman (1966) referred to this phenomenon as "deautomatization" or "dishabituation." In support of this concept, Kasamatsu and Hirai (1966) found that advanced masters of Zen were able to dishabituate to a repeated clicking sound, while control Ss were unable to perform the same task.

Based on the similarities between REST and concentrative meditation, it would seem reasonable to expect some positive perceptual/cognitive effects of REST. In support of this assertion, Lilly (1981) reported that levels of awareness, feelings of relaxation, and vividness of mental imagery increased in the verbal reports of 500 Ss during short-term exposure to REST. These case studies support the hypothesis that short-term exposure to REST may be a positive experience.

Barabasz and his colleagues (Melchiori & Barabasz, 1990) completed the first and only experimental study of the effects of brief flotation REST on the complex cognitive/perceptual task of instrument flight performance using commercial pilots as subjects. Only those exposed to REST, but not controls, showed significant improvements on the instrument flight task.

To assess the cognitive/perceptual effects of REST, the current study contrasted the performance of subjects on a signal-detection task (SDT), consisting of "strong," "weak," and "no signal trials, before and after one hour of exposure to one of the following conditions: REST, sensory alertness, and sensory relaxation. The purpose behind the brief one hour period of exposure was to compare the results of this study with those that involved long-term exposure to REST. It was anticipated that short-term exposure to REST would enhance cognitive/perceptual performance on the SDT.

Since performance on a SDT may vary partly as a function of arousal level, a related concern was the level of sensory arousal in each of the conditions. The relationship between performance and arousal is usually represented as an inverted U-shaped function. According to this function, information-processing activities will be poor or nonexistent during sleep, but will improve in waking, reaching some optimal level as cortical arousal increases. It is possible the brief exposure to REST may minimize distracting sensory input found in normal alert/aroused states without significantly reducing levels of sensory arousal. Therefore, it was anticipated that exposure to REST would produce greater enhancement on the SDT than exposure to sensory alertness or sensory relaxation.

Method

Subjects

A total of 45 Ss (27 women, 18 men) from Eastern Montana College participated in the study, with 15 Ss assigned to each experimental condition via a block randomization procedure.

Materials

A plywood sensory-isolation flotation tank (4' high X 4' wide X 10' long) was utilized to restrict sensory stimulation. The tank was filled to a depth of 15" with a 94° F solution of epsom salts in water to create a density of 1.30 gms/100 gms. An Apple IIe microcomputer was used to present an Apple Basic "Signal Detection Task" program to the Ss.

Procedure

There was one experimental session involving pre-exposure performance on 36 SDT trials, an exposure period of one hour (REST, relaxation, or arousal), and post-exposure performance on 36 SDT trials. For a given trial, a sequence of "F's" was presented at random positions one at a time on the screen until there was a total of 60 letters. Each trial lasted for an interval of 30 seconds. On 24 trials, one of the letters was an "E" instead of an "F." The Ss task was to detect the presence of the "E." Signal strength was manipulated by the timing of the target letter to be identified. On 12 trials, the "E" was presented within the first 15 seconds. These were classified as the "strong signal" trials, since at least 15 seconds was allowed to locate the target. On another 12 trials, the "E" was presented in the last three seconds of the trial. These were classified as the "weak signal" trials, since the time allotted to identify and locate the target was so brief. On the remaining

12 trials, the "E" was not presented. These were classified as the "no signal" trials.

For REST Ss, exposure lasted for one hour in the sensory-isolation flotation tank. In sensory alertness, Ss were instructed to read preselected passages from the book, "Personality and Hypnosis: A Study of Imaginative Involvement" by Hilgard (1979) for one hour. In sensory relaxation, Ss were told to relax on a large air mattress in a sound- and light-attenuated room, where they listened to a cassette tape of contemporary classical music combined with sounds of the ocean for one hour.

Results

The mean number of hits and false alarms for REST, alertness, and relaxation groups on pre- and post-test trials appear in Table 11-1.

A Groups (REST, Arousal, Relaxation) X Trials (Pre-test, Post-test) X Signal Strength (Strong, Weak, No Signal) analysis of variance (ANOVA) was performed on these data. A significant interaction was present for these three variables ($F(4, 84) = 3.40, p < .025$). Post hoc comparisons yielded a significant increase in "strong" and "weak signal" hits from pre-test ($M = 8.27, 5.07$) to post-test ($M = 9.27, 7.67$) for the REST group ($F(1, 43) = 17.15, p < .001$; $F(1, 43) = 18.42$; $p < .001$). A significantly greater number of "weak signal" hits was also observed for the REST group ($M = 7.67$) on the post-test trials as compared with the relaxation ($M = 5.47$) and alertness ($M = 5.47$) groups ($F(1,43) = 3.33, p < .05$; $F(1, 43) = 3.56, p < .05$). Within and between group comparisons did not yield significant differences in false alarm rates on the pre- and post-test "no signal" trials.

The number and percentage of REST, relaxation, and alertness Ss who increased, remained constant, or decreased in hits from the pre- to the post-test on "strong" and "weak signal" trials can be found in Table 11-2.

Table 11-1

Mean Number of Hits and False Alarms From Pre-Test to Post-Test Across Experimental Conditions

Signal Strength	Pre-Test		Post-Test	
	M	SD	M	SD
Strong Signal Hits				
REST	8.27	1.29	9.27	1.62
Sensory Alertness	8.40	1.50	8.73	1.79
Sensory Relaxation	8.87	1.46	9.13	1.73
Weak Signal Hits				
REST	5.07	2.17	7.67	2.07
Sensory Alertness	5.20	1.14	5.47	2.33
Sensory Relaxation	5.13	1.69	5.47	1.69
No Signal False Alarms				
REST	.07	.00	.20	.41
Sensory Alertness	.20	.41	.00	.00
Sensory Relaxation	.13	.35	.20	.41

Discussion

The results of this study indicate that exposure to REST is capable of enhancing visual perception as measured by a SDT. This conclusion is evident from the significant improvement in the performance of Ss from the pre-test to the post-test on "strong" and "weak signal" trials. The findings support those of Melchiori and Barabasz (1990). Moreover, the

Table 11-2

Individual Variations in Ss Performance from the Pre-Test to the Post-Test as a Function of Signal Strength and Condition

Signal Strength	Decrease		Same		Increase	
	N	%	N	%	N	%
Strong Signal Hits						
REST	1	7	0	0	14	93
Sensory Alertness	5	33	4	27	6	40
Sensory Relaxation	6	40	2	13	7	47
Weak Signal Hits						
REST	1	7	0	0	14	93
Sensory Alertness	6	40	3	20	6	40
Sensory Relaxation	6	40	3	20	6	40

results suggest that exposure to REST may contribute to enhancement of visual perception in Ss more than does relaxation and alertness, a conclusion supported by the significantly greater number of hits scored by the Ss in the REST condition on the post-test trials as compared with Ss in the relaxation and alertness conditions. Possible evidence has also been garnered to support the anecdotal (Lilly, 1981) and experimental (Melchiori & Barabasz, 1990) reports that show that exposure to REST enhances awareness. Finally, it is clear that high levels of perceptual vigilance are required to perform competently on a SDT. Perceptual vigilance, in turn, demands increased skill at focusing and maintaining visual attention. In the present study, greater perceptual vigilance was required on "weak signal" trials than on "strong signal" trials. Since the differences between the REST condition and the other two conditions were more pronounced on "weak signal" trials, short-term exposure to REST likely increases the ability to focus and maintain attention. The ability to continue to perceive monotonous visual stimulation in this way is comparable to the deautomatization or dishabituation that occurs with Zen masters using concentrative meditation techniques (Kasamatsu & Hirai, 1966). Those abilities are also highly similar to the skills engendered by repeated exposure to various esoteric disciplines in which a fresh perception is "awakened," allowing the practitioner to perceive more and from a new vantage point (Ornstein, 1977).

Obviously, a discrepancy exists between the results of this investigation and those of previous REST studies (e.g., see Bexton et al., 1954; Courtney et al., 1961; Doane et al., 1959; Davis et al., 1960). A partial explanation for this discrepancy may be found in the variable of exposure duration. Most early studies of REST were long-term in nature, sometimes lasting for several days (e.g., see Bexton et al., 1954). In contrast, the present experiment utilized an exposure duration of only one hour consistent with Melchiori and Barabasz (1990). Too little or no stimulus change may become an aversive state to be avoided only after long-term exposure to REST. The average subject has not been trained to focus attention inward during long episodes of exposure to REST, resulting in less than optimal functioning in the central nervous system. In contrast, short-term exposure to REST may reduce the number of irrelevant stimulus details without reducing optimal levels of arousal.

Another finding that requires additional comment is the evidence for enhanced performance among REST Ss on the post-test trials as contrasted with Ss in the relaxation and alertness conditions. One possible explanation for this disparity may be that Ss in the relaxation condition experienced sensory arousal comparable to the alertness condition as a result of listening to the musical selection. Certainly the tape was producing sensory stimulation that may have resulted in some increase in sensory arousal.

12

Slow REST or Fast Drugs: Meditation or Medication?

Charles Brownfield

Change in Viewpoint

Serendipity is credited with playing a ubiquitous role in the discovery of neuroleptic drugs in the 1950s, followed by antidepressants and anxiolytics in the 1960s. With little foresight about the consequences of long term use of these new medications, or their adverse effects, and encouraged by the dramatic control they exerted on behavior, the excitement, intellectual vigor, and prestige of psychiatry changed from humanistic to predominantly chemical conceptions of treatment (cf., Ayd & Blackwell, 1970; Lickey & Gordon, 1983; Schowalter, 1989).

Yet, there are still some of us in the mental health community who are deeply concerned about the efficacy (and safety) of these psychotropic drugs versus psychotherapy. Most textbooks suggest both are used, in concert, for maximum benefit to the patient. But we know from our own direct clinical experience that, usually, only one is used (or, at least, emphasized) to the exclusion of the other. For psychiatrists trained in the past 35 years, the pendulum has swung away from the dynamic, and toward the organic treatment of both major and minor mental disorders. Psychiatry's prevailing view, now, is that an organic cause underlies (nearly) all disturbances of thought, emotion, and behavior. The image of the psychiatrist as an astute listener interested in patients' histories and intrapsychic processes now belongs to a bygone era. The unconscious is irrelevant and the conscious is only an epiphenomenon of neurochemistry. Those who espouse the "you-are-what-you-synapse" approach to human understanding are the dominant force today; those holding to more dynamic, elegant, holistic theories are the dinosaurs of the profession (and sometimes even persecuted). Treating symptoms is the acceptable standard now.

Profit-oriented insurance companies pay for psychotropic therapy, and cost-conscious government agencies fund drug-based treatment programs. Drugs seem to be a fast, time-limited, practical, less complicated, easily coded, cost-effective means of "managing" mental illness within the perfunctory, but consensually accepted, "standard of care". Psychiatrists can "treat" more patients per hour, and sometimes do invite "ancillary" workers (like psychologists, social workers, nurses, and mental health counselors) to do the talking. If patients are better off now than they were 35 years ago because of these advances, why should there be any controversy?

Some Problems with Drugs

Complicating matters, now, is the fact that even busy non-psychiatric physicians routinely prescribe a variety of psychoactive drugs for a wide range of physical and mental complaints without adequate psychodiagnosis, management, or follow-up. Consequently, there is considerable minimization of, insensitivity to, and defensiveness about, the adverse effects these substances have been reported to produce in patients (Abramowicz, 1975; 1981a; Melville & Johnson, 1983; Siler, 1979; Wolfe et al., 1988).

For example, the most frequently prescribed class of anxiolytic "minor" tranquilizers, the benzodiazepines, including Valium (diazepam), Ativan (lorazepam), Centrax (prazapam), Halcion (triazolam), Dalmane (flurazepam), Paxipam (halazepam), Restoril (temazepam), Serax (oxazepam), Tranxene (clorazepate), Xanax (alprazolam), Versed (midazolam), etc., are reportedly associated with impairment of concentration, memory, learning, motor coordination, reaction time, and driving skills. They are addictive and can induce increased confusion, restlessness, hallucinations, withdrawal seizures, drowsiness, fatigue, rebound insomnia, speech defects, nightmares, hostility, paradoxical rages, panic attacks, and increases in suicidal and homicidal ideas and acts (Abramowicz, 1981b; Associated Press, 1989a,b; Bargmann et al., 1982; Bowen, 1978; Edwards & Medlicott, 1980; Feldman, 1986; Greenblatt et al., 1984; Mills & Eth, 1987; Ryan et al., 1968; Soldatos et al., 1985, 1986; Wolfe, 1985, 1987, 1988; Woods, Katz, & Winger, 1987; Zisook & DeVaul, 1977).

The usual retort is that these adverse effects are "rare" and, on balance, they help more people than they harm. Large collections of small N studies covering relatively brief periods of administration and follow-up, and attending to minor (and non-lethal) side effects seem to support this (c.f., Woods, Katz, & Winger, 1987). There are reasons, however, to suspect that the really serious adverse effects are more widespread than the profession generally acknowledges. Adverse reactions are only voluntarily reported to the FDA. These constitute only a small fraction of the actual number of cases which are never reported because the connection is overlooked, the process is too troublesome, or there is fear of legal liability. Large scale studies that look at benzodiazepine use as causing suicide, homicide, or violence simply do not get funded for fairly obvious reasons. Studies, done mostly in western Europe, have resulted in greater restrictions on benzodiazepine prescribing there. Some recent legal actions based on studies there, and in the United States, are establishing that just such a relationship probably does exist (Associated Press, 1989a; Raphael, 1989; Sigelman, 1989).

Zisook (1990), a psychiatrist at the University of California (San Diego), offered that at the time he published his warnings about adverse behavioral effects (c.f., Zisook & DeVaul, 1977), "these medications were overused and overprescribed without a full appreciation of their potential adverse effects". He goes on to state, "Over the past decade, however, the benzodiazepines have assumed a more realistic place in medical therapeutics and more prescribing physicians are aware of their limitations". He now feels that "these medications are relatively safe, have an important role, but need to be prescribed with constraint and realistic caution". In my clinical practice, at least half the patients I have been seeing in the past 10 years were placed on addictive benzodiazepines by their family physicians with very infrequent monitoring (if at all) for months and years at a time. I have seen psychiatrists treat outpatients with such drugs, almost exclusively, ignoring caretaking families' attempts to provide information that was prodromal for suicide. Does this suggest "constraint" or "realistic caution?"

Benzodiazepines seem relatively "safe" only because it is very difficult to commit suicide by overdosing with them. Interacting with alcohol or other drugs at the same time, the safety margin diminishes. Since "serendipity" played such a ubiquitous role in the discovery of psychoactive drugs in the first place, it could now be prompting us to suspect that, in some cases, they exacerbate problems more than we might want to recognize. Since physicians and drug companies are not likely to admit fallibility or wrongdoing, we would do well to question their practices and products more closely.

Benzodiazepines are effective for the treatment of symptoms of anxiety and insomnia. The major differences between them are their lengths of action. Calling some "anti-anxiety" drugs and others "hypnotics" has more to do with marketing than with pharmacology. They seem to be prescribed frequently, by general practitioners, without adequate history-taking, monitoring, or concurrent psychotherapy, for everything from anxiety to work stress, dermatitis, sleeplessness, and depression associated with bereavement, separation, and divorce. Nor is it below the standard of care for psychiatrists to prescribe them for patients diagnosed with "primary depression or psychosis", contrary to recommendations by drug manufacturers in the Physicians Desk Reference (Barnard, 1987).

Zisook (1990) also suggests that the literature on Xanax, originally marketed as an anti-anxiety drug, hints at its potential for the treatment of some types of depression. A recent news article in the *Philadelphia Inquirer* (Sifford, 1990) suggests that current psychiatric thinking supports the notion that a single drug (unnamed) can be effective in the treatment of multiple psychiatric illnesses, including depression, anxiety, bulimia, smoking, alcohol abuse, eating, and panic disorders! The director of the Philadelphia Medical Institute, Dr. Joseph Mendels, is quoted as saying, "non-psychiatric doctors - mainly general practitioners - are very much in favor of the concept of one drug for many illnesses. Using the same drug to treat four or five conditions simplifies life for them. They don't have to call in a psychiatric consultant. They can just give a drug."

Consumer Concerns

The growing mistrust and disaffection with mainstream psychiatry and psychology is reflected in the development of a consumer movement, questioning the mystique of the mental health professions, objecting to the style with which patients are treated (and their families ignored or even blamed), noticing the exacerbation of mental problems in adverse drug reactions, and counter-reacting to the "one-size-fits-all" neurobiochemical bias. Contemporary psychiatrists seem to see mental patients getting better and better under their regimen, while others see them getting worse and worse (cf., Fisher & Greenberg, 1989; Greenberg & Fisher, 1990).

The users of psychiatric and psychological services, and the advocacy organizations that now represent them, such as the National Alliance for the Mentally Ill, Public Citizens' Health Research Group, the Citizens' Commission on Human Rights, Activists for Alternatives, and the Alliance on Human Rights and Psychiatric Oppression, to name a few, are doing their homework and raising relevant issues that deserve attention. No matter how well-intentioned the biological treatment perspective is meant to be the mere consensus of authoritative opinion has become less credible to more people. Even groups as unlikely as the National Rifle Association and The Firearms Coalition lobby, in furthering their own special interests have documented firearms-related mass murders correlated with the concurrent use of prescribed neuroleptics, antidepressants, and benzodiazepine anxiolytics (Knox, 1989). Should all this be ignored or dismissed as irrelevant and-inconsequential?

The Psychotropic Promise of the Fifties

When neuroleptics were first introduced in the early 1950s, it was a time of "Cold War" hostilities and "Iron Curtain" intrigues, Communist-baiting "McCarthyism" and the Korean War confessions to atrocities by "brainwashed" American P.O.W.s in camps north of the 38th Parallel, stalemated peace talks at Panmunjam, and images of awesome mushroom clouds rising over Bikini Atoll and Yucca Flats. It was a pivotal era when the treatment of psychoses with the first major tranquilizer, Thorazine (chlorpromazine), rapidly impacted on mental hospital populations, quieting the agitation, and minimizing overtly bizarre and regressed behaviors.

It also caused heavy-footed shuffling, restlessness, and thickly slurred speech (and, we later learned, involuntary tongue thrusting and permanently impaired motor coordination, i.e., tardive dyskinesia). But it rapidly made patients far more "manageable". This was "success". It laid the foundation for conceiving that "mind-altering" drugs and community-based care might replace long term hospitalization. The ramifications of a "drug culture", or deinstitutionalization, or homelessness when the community faltered, had not yet been realized. It was only just beginning to be hinted at in those days (Huxley, 1954, 1958; Meerloo, 1955, 1956; Rolin, 1956; Szasz, 1960, 1961).

The Development of RES Research and Therapy

With this background of both uncertainty and optimism, published reports of experiments at McGill University on human responses to a restricted stimulus environment (originally "perceptual isolation") captured the attention of the psychological community (Bexton, 1953; Bexton, Heron, & Scott, 1954; Doane, 1955; Doane, Mahatoo, Heron, & Scott, 1959; Hebb, 1955b, 1958; Hebb, Heath, & Stuart, 1954; Heron, 1957, 1961; Heron, Bexton, & Hebb, 1953; Heron, Doane, & Scott, 1956; Melzack, 1954; Melzack & Scott, 1957; Scott, 1954; Scott, Bexton, Heron, & Doane, 1959). "Sensory deprivation", a term favored more by psychiatric, rather than psychological, writers quickly came into vogue. A spate of books and articles followed during this period chronicling the growth of scientific knowledge about what we, now call "restricted environmental stimulation" (Biderman & Zimmer, 1961; Brownfield, 1965; Burns, Chambers, & Hendler, 1963; Fiske & Maddi, 1961; Schultz, 1965; Solomon et al., 1961; Vernon, 1963; West, 1962; Zubek, 1969b).

Also in the 1950s, other RES researchers in Montreal were reporting positive therapeutic effects in psychiatric patients exposed to "partial perceptual isolation" (Azima & Cramer, 1956; Azima & Cramer-Azima, 1957; Azima, Vispo, & Azima, 1961; Azima & Wittkower, 1956; Azima, Wittkower, & Latendresse, 1958). Soon, similar findings were being published by other investigators. Suedfeld's monumental book, Restricted Environmental Stimulation (1980), summarizes and documents, in historical perspective, reports of effective remission of drug-induced psychotic reactions with RES; enhancement of receptivity to conventional forms of verbal psychotherapy; amelioration of substance addictions; and lasting positive therapeutic outcomes, using RES alone, with mental patients. Relatively briefer RES procedures evolved, with longer-lasting remission of symptoms and more profound water tank immersion techniques were added to room isolation (Lilly, 1956, Lilly & Shurley, 1958). Individual responses to RES became more predictable as awareness of the relevant variables grew (c.f., Brownfield, 1964a,b; Kammerman, 1977; Suedfeld, 1980; Zuckerman, 1979).

By contrast with the initial positive reception enjoyed by psychiatric drugs in the 1950s and 1960s the climate of those times nurtured misconceptions about RES. It was suggested, early on, that environmental restriction of sensory experience usually produced aversive, stressful, and mentally disruptive effects. This appeared to have some support in the literature which, in turn, created further misconceptions in both the popular and scientific media. Quite often, these had the effect of equating "sensory deprivation" with "brainwashing" and, therefore, by implication, suggesting it was a form of torture capable of producing hallucinations and zombie-like obedience. This confusion eventually found its way into novels that were made into movie screenplays that fueled fantasy and nurtured unwarranted generalizations.

Introductory psychology texts either ignored the research altogether, or associated it with forcible indoctrination, vigilance, or boredom. More kindly disposed writers pointed to similarities between RES phenomena and the benefits of Eastern mysticism, Zen, Transcendental Meditation, and yoga (c.f., Carrington, 1977). A sense of both mystery and danger pervaded the field which, in turn, tended to impede (though not to halt) the progress of RES research in understanding the etiology of, and successfully treating, a wide variety of mental and behavioral disturbances - even biologically based ones - without drugs.

Ergot, Mushrooms, Buttons, and Seeds: The Psychedelic "Turn-on"

The 60s massive social unrest, precipitated by increasing U.S. involvement in Vietnam, the development of an active Civil Rights Movement, anti-war protests, the jolting assassinations of charismatic leaders like the Kennedys and Martin Luther King, Jr., and the emergence of a strong "counter-culture" movement, heir to the pharmaceutical promises of the 50s emphasizing personal freedom and spiritual enlightenment, harbingered a dramatic increase in the manufacture, cultivation, and use of illicit drugs such as marijuana, heroin, and hallucinogenics like LSD (lysergic acid diethylamide-25), mescaline and peyote buttons, mushrooms, and morning glory seeds. The idea that personal liberation could be attained by "turning on, tuning in, and dropping out" with the aid of psychoactive substances derived from flowering plants was hardly alien in the context of those times.

LSD-25, for example, was synthesized from the ergot on rye, and initially touted by psychiatrists as a cure for alcoholism and a panacea for understanding and treating personality disorders and schizophrenia before it was made illegal in the early 60s (Crocket et al., 1963; Hoffer, 1965; Mogar, 1969); it rapidly evolved into the drug of choice for the "trip" to enlightment, and became the model for personal experimentation. It also portended the nightmare of chemical abuse which has persisted to this time.

Restricted Environmental Stimulation Therapy: The High Road Back?

By the mid-70s it had become possible to use RES environments and RES therapy (REST) procedures as a safe and effective non-pharmaceutically dependent addition to psychotherapy's repertoire. It had been successfully used with a wide range of mental and behavioral disorders subsuming dysfunctions of eating behavior (including anorexia nervosa and obesity), phobias, smoking, drug, and alcohol abuse, stuttering, hypertension, depression, schizophrenia, autism, intellectual retardation, hyperactivity and conduct disorders in children, as well as PCP and LSD psychoses. Researchers who continued to explore the early clinical applications of reduced sensory environments produced highly significant and positive results which are detailed in Suedfeld's (1980) book.

As an environmental therapy, designed to optimize external sensory stimulation for individuals with different needs in the context of treatment, REST carried none of the risks of adverse reactions which characterize psychotropic drugs. It also worked best with patients thought to be least accessible to verbal psychotherapy (Adams, Cooper, & Carrera, 1972; Brownfield, 1981) and who were thus most likely to be seen as candidates for psychotropics. Relatively few psychotherapists were aware of these findings. Moreover, few knew how, or dared risk being called "quack", to use REST in clinical contexts like private practice because it was so poorly understood as a therapy technique, negatively associated with "brainwashing" and, with some already noted exceptions, largely neglected in the clinical literature. It seemed cumbersome and impractical for insurance reimbursement purposes and less than optimally appealing for high sensation-seeking psychotherapists. For psychiatrists, drugs were quicker and satisfied their criteria for an "acceptable" standard of care that produced maximum cost-effective returns on their investments of time and effort.

The deinstitutionalization movement of the 60s was made possible, in part, by the development of psychotropic drugs. Politics and economics created a need for briefer therapies and quicker "fixes". This need was ostensibly filled over the past two decades by managed health care plans, community mental health centers, employee assistance programs, health maintenance organizations, preferred provider groups, private psychiatric hospitals, transitional living facilities, substance abuse treatment programs, group homes, nursing care facilities, and an even greater variety of newer, more potent antipsychotic, antidepressant, and antianxiety drugs which, we are now told, are evolving toward the "one-size-fits-all" model.

The Future

REST is a "psychological" approach to what may be, in all likelihood, biochemically mediated disturbances of the brain/psyche/behavior. Whether this always is a "disease entity" (such as a genetic abnormality, or lesion, or toxin, or virus) or an acquired disorder (such as in social learning, or modeling, or in response to environmental stress), the living organism does not usually exist in an environmental vacuum. It responds and adapts to external sensory stimulation. The evidence of RES research is that the nature of that stimulation, when carefully controlled, is able, by itself or in conjunction with other forms of psychotherapy, to produce improvements in the person which are, at least, quantitatively equal to, and probably qualitatively better than, the improvements attributed to psychotropic drugs. Interest in RES has been preserved and advanced by those persistent few who were responsible for the formation and development of the International

REST Investigators Society (IRIS) and who, in turn, have taught, published, and inspired their students to persevere and to extend the frontiers of RES research, technology, and therapy.

REST requires more time, effort, careful structuring, and close monitoring than psychotropic medication (or verbal psychotherapy), but it has the advantages of greater safety, freedom from adverse (and serious) mental effects, recognition of the patient's most salient individual personality characteristics, and the opportunity to facilitate natural homeostatic/sensoristatic processes. To become viable as a better alternative, REST must demonstrate its superiority over psychotropics in efficacy and outcome, as well as cost-effectiveness. It needs to come out of the laboratory and into clinical practice at every level of service delivery.

13

Effects of Chamber REST, Flotation REST and Relaxation on Transient Mood State

Arreed Barabasz, Marianne Barabasz, Rebecca Dyer, and Noël Rather

Restricted Environmental Stimulation Therapy (REST) formerly labeled sensory deprivation still suffers from misunderstanding and misconceptions. Suedfeld (1990) noted that most people learn about REST from psychology text books that report the effects of REST on the basis of early research such as the McGill studies which were confounded by such anxiety-laden procedures that it is not surprising that subjects experienced high levels of stress. The early studies produced subject reports of disorientation, tearfulness, nightmares, depression, bouts of anger, feelings of hopelessness and hallucinations (Suedfeld, 1980). In order to protect subjects, Sanders (1967) developed observational criteria for terminating REST. These include craving for stimulation, emotional lability, and impaired secondary process. With the advent of modern REST procedures, which address the experimental demand characteristics that once cued Ss to expect stressful reactions, a vastly different view of REST has emerged. Recent research and anecdotal data indicates that most subjects currently find the REST experience quite pleasant. In a review of the research,

Suedfeld (1980) noted that early termination of chamber REST is rare. Rank and Suedfeld (1978) exposed alcoholic Ss to eight hours of lying on a bed in a dark sound attenuated chamber. On a variety of measures, Ss indicated that they found the experience to be quite pleasant and in fact reported more positive experiences and fewer negative experiences than normal life.

Fine and Turner (1982) studied the effects of flotation REST and found that flotation REST induces relaxation as measured by physiological indices. Perry (1985) summarized the anecdotal data obtained in commercial REST centers which supports the impression that flotation REST is a positive experience.

Despite these widely held positive beliefs about REST, a review of the literature reveals the Rank and Suedfeld (1978) study to be the only systematic investigation of the effects of REST on the Ss' mood states which employed current REST methodology. This single study involved only alcoholics as subjects and only the chamber REST environment. The purpose of the present investigation was to test the effects of chamber REST, flotation REST and relaxation training on a measure of transient mood state.

Method

Subjects

A total of 45 subjects enrolled in upper level undergraduate and graduate level classes at a large northwestern university agreed to participate in a "relaxation and mood study." The average age for this volunteer group was 21.6 years, with a range from 19.6 to 31.4 years. There were 21 women and 24 men.

Instrument

The Profile of Mood States (POMS) (McNair, Lorr, & Droppleman, 1971) was employed as the self-report measure. The test provides descriptive data on six separate mood scales which purport to measure tension-anxiety, depression-dejection, anger-hostility, vigor-activity, fatigue-inertia, and confusion-bewilderment. The instrument uses Likert-type questions and has been shown to be reliable with internal consistency coefficients greater than .70 (Shachem, 1983). College students typically complete the test within five minutes. Several studies have used the POMS successfully to demonstrate significant mood changes in therapy (Loor, Daston, & Smith, 1967; McNair & Lorr, 1964) or in response to physical exercise (M. Barabasz, 1991; O'Neill, 1989; Wilfey & Kunce, 1986).

Apparatus

The REST tank (Floatarium Model SWS) (2.4 meters long x 1.4 meters high x 1.3 meters wide) is essentially an enclosed, sound-insulated, fiberglass tub that contains a 25 cm. deep dense solution (D = 1.30 g/cc) of tap water and epsom salts (20% solution). The solution is maintained at average skin temperature 34.5° C (±.2° C). The tank is sound attenuated and light free once the subject activated door is closed. Subjects float effortlessly in a supine position with ears submerged (subjects wore earplugs). Subject vocalizations are monitored by a built in microphone. Messages are transmitted to subjects from the monitoring room via underwater transducers. The tank is ventilated by a silent positive pressure system. Between float sessions the water is filtered and purified by an ultraviolet irradiation system. A shower is immediately adjacent to the tank for hygienic purposes immediately before and after each float experience.

The REST chamber is a sound attenuated room (2.6 meters long x 1.7 meters wide x 2.4 meters high). It has a subject or experimenter activated double door. The room is equipped with a bed upon which subjects recline in a supine position. A video camera and intercommunications system is also part of the chamber environment. Subjects use the same type earplugs employed in the tank and low level white noise is provided over padded earphones to further mask outside noises. Consistent with an earlier study (Barabasz, 1982), subjects in this experiment wore Gansfeld goggles in the lighted chamber.

Procedure

The Profile of Mood States was administered in the REST Laboratory before and after completion of treatment sessions. Subjects were randomly divided into three groups. Consistent with typical flotation REST procedure, Group A subjects (n = 15) were individually (Barabasz, 1988) exposed to two 1 hour 15 minute REST sessions in the Floatarium Brand (SWS) tank. Sessions were completed within a period of not less than two but not more than five days. Consistent with typical Chamber REST methodology (Suedfeld, 1980), Group B subjects (n = 15) were exposed to a single session of 2 1/2 hours in the chamber. Group C subjects (n = 15) were exposed to two 1 hour 15 minute progressive muscle relaxation training sessions (Kaplan & A. Barabasz, 1989) massed in the same manner as Group A sessions. Normal office levels of illumination and auditory stimulation were maintained.

Following current REST procedures (Suedfeld, 1980) all subjects were introduced to their treatment settings in a calm and reassuring manner prior to the day they were scheduled to participate in the study. All subjects were reminded at the beginning of each session that they were free to terminate the session at any time. Every subject completed their entire protocol as planned despite the need to reschedule agreed session times for two or three subjects in each group.

Results

Scores for each subscale of the POMS were calculated pre- and post-treatment. Because of the typical high degree of variability on pre-test scores among the groups, post-test scores for each subscale of the instrument were analyzed by analysis of covariance employing pre-test scores as the covariate. On the fatigue subscale analysis of covariance results indicated a significant effect ($F = 20.29$, $p < .0001$). Post hoc comparisons (Tukey HSD) revealed that the relaxation training control group reported significantly greater fatigue (M = 10.9, s.d. = 5.3) than the chamber (M = 3.5, s.d. = 3.1) or the flotation (M = 3.2, s.d. = 3.8) groups.

On the depression/dejection scale, analysis of covariance results indicated a significant effect ($F = 8.94$, $p < .001$). Post hoc comparisons revealed that the control group reported significantly higher levels of depression/dejection (M = 8.0, s.d. = 5.6) than the flotation group (M = 1.7, s.d. = 2.5). The chamber group did not differ significantly from the other two groups (M = 4.6, s.d. = 6.4).

On the anxiety subscale, analysis of covariance results indicated a significant effect ($F = 7.2$, $p < .0025$). Post hoc comparisons revealed that the control group reported significantly higher levels of anxiety (M = 7.9, s.d. = 4.7) than the flotation group (M = 2.4, s.d. = 2.2). The chamber group did not differ significantly from the other two groups (M = 4.5, s.d. = 4.6).

On the anger, confusion/bewilderment and vigor scales, analysis of covariance results revealed no significant differences (alpha = .05) among the groups. Pre- and post-treatment means and standard deviations appear in Table 13-1.

The graphic representation of the changes in the three groups from pre-test to post-test (see Figure 13-1) reveals that for both the chamber REST and flotation REST groups, the changes were in a positive direction on all but the vigor subscale. The changes were greater for the flotation REST group than the chamber REST group. Although there was high variability on pre-test scores between and within groups, it is interesting to note that inspection of the raw data revealed that Ss who showed changes in a negative direction were about the same in number (two-three) for each group. The change magnitudes were small and similar for these Ss.

Discussion

The results reported above are consistent with the anecdotal data that has been obtained in numerous REST investigations and with the

Table 13-1
POMS Means and Standard Deviations
Pre and Post All Treatments

	Chamber		Tank		Control	
	Pre	Post	Pre	Post	Pre	Post
Fatigue						
Mean	9.4	3.4	10.0	3.3	8.8	10.7
S.D.	6.1	3.0	7.7	3.8	6.8	5.2
Anxiety						
Mean	8.8	4.6	8.7	3.1	6.5	7.6
S.D.	5.6	4.6	4.9	3.0	4.6	4.7
Depression						
Mean	6.6	3.8	7.8	2.1	6.2	7.6
S.D.	8.3	6.0	6.9	2.5	5.1	5.5
Anger						
Mean	3.0	2.4	4.7	2.1	4.1	1.0
S.D.	4.7	3.7	5.9	2.9	7.2	1.4
Confusion						
Mean	7.0	5.8	6.8	3.8	6.5	3.9
S.D.	4.1	4.0	4.2	2.6	3.9	3.6
Vigor						
Mean	14.7	14.0	13.8	16.5	16.4	16.2
S.D.	6.2	8.5	7.7	6.9	5.9	6.0

reports of clients at commercial flotation Tank centers.

It is particularly interesting to find that the effects of both chamber and flotation REST on mood states were more positive than an exposure to a respected, established and widely used relaxation training procedure.

Subjects exposed to Chamber and Flotation REST reported significantly less fatigue than controls. It is important to note that the items measuring fatigue included "worn out, listless, fatigued, exhausted, weary and bushed" so this score should not be interpreted as reflecting a relaxation component. Subjects exposed to flotation REST reported

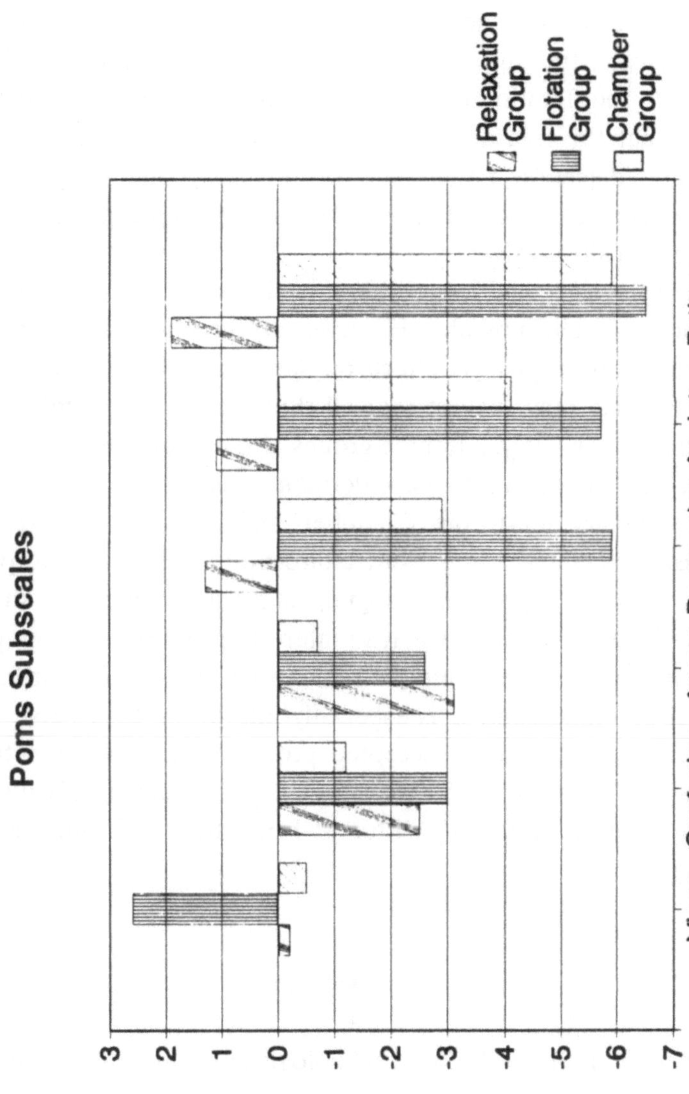

Figure 13-1. Profile of Mood States mean pre to post change score results.

significantly lower levels of anxiety and depression/dejection than subjects exposed to the relaxation training control condition. Subjects exposed to chamber REST reported consistently, but not significantly, lower levels of anxiety and depression/dejection than controls. Chamber and relaxation training control Ss demonstrated higher variability in contrast to the flotation group on these two measures. It is interesting to note that the relaxation control group demonstrated increases in depression/dejection, fatigue and anxiety suggesting a negative effect while the chamber and flotation REST groups showed decreases which indicate a positive effect.

There were no significant differences between groups on the anger, vigor or confusion subscales. However, all three groups demonstrated a tendency toward positive effects on these subscales. Decreases on the anger subscale may suggest that all three treatment conditions were experienced positively. All three groups also demonstrated a consistent decrease on the confusion/bewilderment scale.

In summary, both the Chamber and Flotation REST groups demonstrated changes in a positive direction from pre-test to post-test on the anxiety, depression, fatigue, anger and confusion subscales. These findings are particularly interesting because they provide additional evidence to refute the notion that the REST environment is stressful or unpleasant. It is especially interesting to observe that, in comparison to the widely accepted procedure of relaxation training, mood states following REST were found to be either significantly more positive or not significantly different from those following relaxation training.

Acknowledgment

The authors thank REST Technologies of Huntington, New York.

14

REST: A Key Facilitator in the Treatment of Eating Disorders

Marianne Barabasz

REST offers some unique characteristics that support it's utility in the treatment of eating disorders. REST affords the opportunity to process ones attitudes and behaviors, perhaps as never before, in a unique environment without interaction with the external environment. REST is especially suited to facilitating the reduction of conflicts between eating desires, cultural expectations, and health concerns. REST enables clients to determine their personal goals because there are no stimuli to arouse maladaptive defense mechanisms which might interfere with clients' personal goal directed processing. At the same time, adaptation to the environment includes imaginal activity which may also interfere with the evocation of cognitive defenses. REST is, perhaps, the ultimate safe non-judgmental non-directive therapeutic milieu.

Several researchers have stressed the influence of cultural factors on attitudes toward obesity and the dieting behavior of Americans (Garner & Garfinkel, 1980; Garner, Rokert, Olmstead, Johnson, & Coscina, 1985; Garner & Wooley, 1991). The category of eating disorders includes obesity and bulimia and anorexia which can be conceptualized as a fear of obesity. Cultural pressures and the norms for thinness have increased in recent decades. Garner et al. (1985) point out that the cultural pressures for a slender appearance have intensified. Models and ideals for thinness have become increasingly thinner in recent years while, during the same period, the actual mean weight of woman aged 20-29 years has increased. The cultural emphasis on thinness, and the implication that it is associated with happiness, success, and self worth have resulted in an obsession with weight control. An additional cultural stigma associated with obesity, is the attitude that it is the simple product of lack of will power or insufficient self control. These cultural attitudes and expectations leave woman in conflict between their biological desire to eat and their desire to conform to cultural pressures to obtain social approval. Many respond to this conflict with physically self damaging behaviors such as fad diets, binging, purging and laxative abuse. Anorexics literally starve themselves. The issue of control, associated with dietary restraint, becomes a major focus for obese persons who are striving to lose weight, and especially for bulimics and anorexics. For many, life is seen as a state of constant control over the desire to eat inappropriate unhealthy types and/or quantities of food. These people find themselves in conflict between two mutually exclusive desires--the desire for food and the desire to meet cultural expectations for thinness, and thus evoke feelings of attractiveness, social approval and self approval. For many eating disordered clients this produces ambivalence. Clients fluctuate between self loathing, because of lack of control, and hostility toward societal expectations expressed in bouts of overeating.

Suedfeld (1980) postulated that cognitive processing is affected in the REST environment. Subjects' ability to defend against counter-attitudinal messages is decreased. A. Barabasz (1982) showed that chamber REST subjects became involved with imaginal activity in an attempt to cope with reduced sensory input. Recently, he hypothesized that such preoccupation with fantasy involvement might serve to preclude the evocation of previously imbedded cognitive defense mechanisms. The arguments that clients historically used to justify unhealthy eating behaviors become less available and perhaps less justifiable. It has long been observed that individuals bring their own experiment to the REST experience, that is to say that participants bring their own agenda to the REST session. A person's underlying agenda might reasonably be expected to include the desire to resolve the conflicts described above. Concurrent with this agenda, REST induced preoccupations with imaginal activities may facilitate new and more appropriate resolutions to these conflicts.

Only a small minority of obese people (Garner & Wooley, 1991) have not tried to diet. For most dieters, the decreased weight is not maintained over the long-term. Brownell (1980) noted that the likelihood of maintaining ideal weight for five years is lower than the national cancer recovery rate. For many, it is an apparently endless experience of weight cycling. One diets, loses weight, and then regains the weight. This can be conceptualized as an alternation between striving to meet societal expectations and responding to one's immediate desire to overeat or eat high calorie foods. In contrast to the entire range of traditional weight loss interventions, the solitude of the REST environment facilitates a person's ability to reevaluate their conflicting behaviors and attitudes.

When people seek out professional help for eating disorders, they frequently are faced with professionals who share in the culture's pejorative view. Obesity treatment programs have frequently included social rewards for success at achieving thinness or even social shaming procedures (Garner & Wooley, 1991). Even when clients obtain professional help from an unbiased professional, they tend to assume that the therapist shares the cultural values regarding the goals of therapy--dietary control for the obese and bulimics, and renourishment for the anorexic. In the majority of therapeutic approaches, the role of the therapist is to employ interventions and strategies to achieve the stated goal. Thus, the therapist assumes the role of constantly enforcing cultural expectations, either directly or indirectly. In contrast to this obvious problem created by traditional procedures, Restricted Environmental Stimulation Therapy allows the clients to focus on and process their conflicting desires, perhaps as never before, in an atmosphere free from confrontation with cultural expectations or the expectation of such confrontation. As most therapists employing traditional treatment programs can verify, many clients respond to interventions by arguing against expectations and procedures.

It is hypothesized that REST may be a particularly effective treatment for bulimics and certain anorexics. Bulimics are uniquely high in hypnotizability (M. Barabasz, 1990; Pettinati, 1985; Pettinati, Horne, & Staats, 1985) and binging anorexics are higher in hypnotizability than abstaining anorexics (Pettinati, 1985; Pettinati, Horne, & Staats, 1985). Barabasz (1982) has shown that Chamber REST can enhance hypnotizability and that flotation REST elicits spontaneous hypnosis (Barabasz, 1990c,e) in the highly hypnotizable person. Unfortunately, clients' issues of control and expectations for infliction of the cultural values noted above, can cause resistance to hypnosis. Despite careful procedures, including information about hypnosis, debunking it's myths, viewing videotaped hypnosis sessions, and the opportunity to ask questions about hypnosis, many subjects retain their preconceived misperceptions and fears that they can be made to act against their own will or will lose self-control. These fears prevent these individuals from entering hypnosis even when the induction is attempted by a highly trained psychologist or psychiatrist. As noted above, REST and the role of the REST therapist in REST does not incite such resistance. Both chamber and flotation REST environments afford bulimics (and binging anorexics) an ideal opportunity to make use of their hypnotic ability to obtain their goals.

REST's ability to elicit hypnotic responsiveness, even without a formal induction (A. Barabasz, 1990c,e), may also be employed for obesity. M. Barabasz and Spiegel (1989) found that subjects exposed to a simple self-management technique and to a hypnotic induction with the hypnotic suggestions emphasizing specific food aversions, lost significantly more weight at a three month follow-up than subjects exposed only to the self management treatment. The specificity of hypnosis in the program was supported by a significant correlation between weight loss and a measure of hypnotizability (Stanford Hypnotic Susceptibility Scale: Form C, Weitzenhoffer & Hilgard, 1962). Since the factors that cause resistance to hypnosis in bulimics (and binging anorexics) also characterize the obese, flotation REST would be highly likely to be effective for highly hypnotizable obese persons. Of course, in cases of low or moderate hypnotizability, one could first enhance hypnotizability with six hours of chamber REST (Barabasz, 1982).

Suedfeld and Clarke (1981) did not measure hypnotizability, but found that subjects undergoing REST for smoking cessation, who were allowed to bring a few of their favorite foods into the session, consistently reported lowered preferences for those foods. In subsequent research, the authors replaced the anti-smoking message with one discussing the importance of diet and exercise in the achievement of weight loss (Suedfeld & Clarke, 1981). Subjects reported lowered preference and consumption of previously preferred foods.

In a recent true experimental design study (Dyer, A. Barabasz, & M. Barabasz, 1990; also see Chapter 15), subjects were assigned to one of four REST or one of four non-REST groups: REST with a message, REST with problem foods only, REST with a message and problems foods, REST only, or comparable non-REST groups. The investigation demonstrated that 24 hours of chamber REST, either with or without messages and consumption of problem foods, significantly lowered subjects' total caloric consumption, problem food consumption, and body fat percentage. Interview data obtained as part of the study supported the hypothesis described above. The interviews appear to suggest the conclusion that REST facilitates the resolution of conflicting attitudes and behaviors.

It appears that there are some qualities of REST that make it particularly appropriate for the treatment of eating disorders. These include the REST environments' affect on cognitive processes which may disable maladaptive defense mechanisms, the unique role of the therapist, the ability of flotation to elicit spontaneous hypnosis and the ability of the chamber to enhance hypnotizability. Furthermore, chamber REST has the ability to create specific food aversions with consequent food consumption reductions and reduced body fat percentages. Future research should investigate the specific contributions of each of these factors.

15

Twenty-Four Hours of Chamber REST Produces Specific Food Aversions in Obese Females

Rebecca Dyer, Arreed Barabasz and Marianne Barabasz

"If 'cure' from obesity is defined as reduction to ideal weight for five years, a person is more likely to recover from most forms of cancer than from obesity" (Brownell, 1980, p. 820). According to the second National Health and Nutrition Examination survey, 26% of all U.S. adults are overweight (Van Itallie, 1985). This percentage accounts for 34 million people of which 12 million are severely overweight, or obese. Successful treatments for obesity are rare (Nicholas & Dwyer, 1986; Stunkard, 1976, 1986). As with other habits such as smoking, initial improvement is most often followed by relapse (Brownell, Marlatt, Lichtenstein, & Wilson, 1986; Brownell, 1980; Collins, Rothblum, & Wilson, 1986; Colvin & Olson, 1983; Hartz, Kalkhoff, Rimm, & McCall, 1986; Stuart, 1971; Stunkard, 1976).

A hypothesized reason for the problems people face with dieting is that overweight individuals perceive themselves as having little control over their impulses with regard to food consumption (Krantz, 1979; Lowe & Fisher, 1985; Striegel-Moore & Rodin, 1986). Motivation plays a vital role in weight loss and its maintenance (Israel, Silverman, &

Solotar, 1986; Stuart, 1967; Stunkard, 1976). Many successful weight loss programs report extremely high attrition rates. Stunkard (1976) found that widely known programs such as Weight Watchers or TOPS (Take Off Pounds Sensibly) reported six month attrition rates as high as 90%. Stunkard (1976) reported that patients who completed psychotherapy for an average of two years, sometimes consisting of daily visits, eventually lost weight and kept it off, or at least were able to accept their weight. However, long term psychotherapy is not readily available to many people. Relapse prevention is the key area needing further research.

Chamber REST in combination with motivational messages has been shown to be effective with habit disorders that have varying etiologies, durations, and poor prognoses (Suedfeld, 1980). The most encouraging results have been reported in studies of smoking cessation (A. Barabasz, Baer, Sheehan, & M. Barabasz, 1986; Best & Suedfeld, 1982), weight control (Borrie & Suedfeld, 1980), and trichotillomania (M. Barabasz, 1987b). The intriguing finding, in studies that employ chamber REST as a treatment method for smoking cessation, is in the long term follow-up data (A. Barabasz, Baer, Sheehan, & M. Barabasz, 1986; Best & Suedfeld, 1982). In a one year follow up, Best and Suedfeld (1982) reported a smoking abstinence rate of 53%. At a 19 month follow up of 327 subjects exposed to seven alternative treatments at the Harvard Medical School, REST with hypnosis was the most effective treatment showing a smoking abstinence rate of 47% (A. Barabasz, Baer, Sheehan, & M. Barabasz, 1986). These data give an indication of the impressive durability of results involving chamber REST, and demonstrate that long term effects can be obtained in the treatment of habits resistant to change following a single treatment session. This finding seemed promising for the application of REST to weight control, in light of reported attrition rates from popular, well-known weight-loss programs (e.g., TOPS, Weight Watchers) (Stunkard, 1986).

An intriguing observation by Suedfeld and Clarke (1981) was that subjects undergoing REST treatment for smoking cessation who were allowed to bring a few of their favorite foods into the session consistently reported lowered preferences for those foods. In further research, the authors replaced the anti-smoking educational message with one discussing the importance of diet and exercise in the achievement of weight loss (Suedfeld & Clarke, 1981). Again, subjects reported lowered preference and consumption of previously preferred foods, a change which remained stable throughout the three month follow-up period.

M. Barabasz and D. Spiegel (1989) found that subjects exposed to a hypnosis intervention, modified to include a suggestion for specific food aversions, lost significantly more weight than subjects exposed to hypnosis with a general suggestion or to self-management techniques alone. This finding along with the Suedfeld and Clarke (1981) findings suggests that aversive reactions to problem foods produced by REST may be a valuable adjunctive treatment for the achievement and maintenance of weight loss.

Hypnosis and REST have many similarities. During REST, as with hypnosis, distracting stimuli are reduced increasing the ability of the subject to focus attention (Suedfeld, 1980). In the chamber, the only contact the subject has with the external environment is through the experimenter. Similarly, during hypnosis, the subject's contact with the external environment is maintained through the hypnotist. The increased focus of attention facilitates the subject's ability to concentrate on the motivational messages of the experimenter or therapist (Kubie & Margolin, 1944; Reyher, 1964; Suedfeld, 1980).

The purpose of the present study was to determine the effects of REST, REST with educational/motivational messages and specific problem food consumption during REST on the development of food specific aversions in obese female subjects.

Method

Subjects

Female subjects (n=48) volunteered from a large rural university community. Subjects were at least 15% above the ideal body fat percentage which is 23% for women. This was determined by standard caliper skinfold measures as defined by the YMCA criteria for physical fitness (Murray & Shephard, 1988; Golding, 1982).

Apparatus

The REST chamber is sound attenuated with 10 cm of Dow-Corning sound proofing material on wall and double door surfaces. Dimensions of the chamber are L=3 meters, W=1.7 meters, H=2.4 meters. It is equipped with a bed, portable toilet, intercommunications system, and a silent positive pressure ventilation system. Low level white noise is produced by a Lafayette 15011 white noise generator to mask background noise in the building. The white noise is broadcast through earphones placed near the bed, and is of such a low level as to be unnoticed by subjects once earplugs are in place. All subjects wore 26 decibel wax ear plugs. Subjects were monitored via an audio intercommunication system. Subjects have free access to liquid food and water through plastic tube "straws" that ran from a thermos in the adjoining psychophysiological monitoring room. The chamber is equipped with a 10 cm. diameter sound attenuated opening through which subjects' problem foods were provided.

Non-REST sessions took place in another room in the same laboratory. The room was equipped with a bed, television, video player, radio, books, magazines, study materials, and a variety of video tapes. Subjects were monitored via a video camera and an audio monitor. Consistent with the REST conditions, liquid food and water were continuously available from vacuum bottles. Problem foods were served by the experimenter to subjects in the problem food conditions.

Skinfold measurements were obtained using a Lafayette Instruments dial indicator caliper, Model 01127.

Procedure

All volunteers' body fat percentages were measured by the first investigator. Using standardized procedures, the body fat index consisted of three skinfold measures taken from the subject's triceps, abdomen, and suprailliac. The three measures were totalled and compared to a table for percentage of body fat for women (Golding, 1982) which accounts for age differences. Subjects meeting the criterion for inclusion in the study were randomly assigned to one of the eight 24-hour treatment groups: REST-message-problem food consumption (REST-MSG-PFood), REST-problem food consumption (REST-PFood), REST-message-bland liquid food consumption (REST-MSG), REST-bland liquid food consumption (REST-only), non-REST-message-problem food consumption (non-REST-MSG-PFood), non-REST-problem food consumption (non-REST-PFood), non-REST-message-bland liquid food consumption (non-REST-MSG), and non-REST-bland liquid food consumption (non-REST-only).

Consistent with Suedfeld's (1980) REST procedures, subjects in all conditions received a full orientation to the REST chamber or room, as well as all pertinent information concerning their treatment condition prior to experimental sessions.

Subjects were asked to keep a daily log of their total food consumption for a two week period, including the frequencies and the quantities of food eaten. They were informed that at the end of the two week period they would be contacted for a second interview during which time their specific problem foods would be determined. On the basis of the food log, up to three specific problem foods were identified in collaboration with the subject. Consistent with M. Barabasz and D. Spiegel (1989) the absolute quantity of food consumed was converted into absolute calories yielding two measures; total two week caloric consumption and total two week problem food consumption. To provide verification of this self-report data, subjects provided the experimenter with the name of a cohort to corroborate the information reported on the food logs (Best, Owen, & Trentadue, 1978; Best & Suedfeld, 1982).

On the day of the scheduled REST session, experimenters followed procedures similar to those outlined in Suedfeld (1980, pp. 377-380). Briefly, subjects were reoriented to the chamber or room after which the experimenter answered any questions for the subject. Each subject was reassured in a calm manner concerning any fears or apprehensions about the REST procedure and reminded that they were free to terminate the session at any time. No subjects chose early termination.

REST subjects were asked to minimize their movements during the session without going to the extreme of experiencing discomfort. After the subject was comfortably situated on the bed the following message, adapted from Barabasz (1982, p. 151), was read over the intercommunication system.

> Please feel free to tell me whatever you want about your reactions to this session. Your experiences will be helpful in understanding the results of the study. Whatever you choose to talk about will, of course, be kept confidential. Since it is contrary to the purpose of the REST session, I will not engage in conversation with you in response to your remarks over the intercommunication system. At different times, you may feel relaxed, anxious, bored, or quite comfortable and you may at times engage in problem-solving, intense fantasies, reminiscing, daydreaming, or wondering about the purpose of the REST session. You may at times feel uncomfortable, but the desire to leave is usually quite temporary. Your meals will be served periodically throughout the session. At this time the experimenter will not converse with you, but you should be sure to eat some of the foods when served and again as often as you like. (For REST-Message subjects only) During the session a message will be played for you which is designed to help you achieve your desired goal of decreased intake of your specific problem food. The message will be repeated once. After hearing the message, you should repeat the message to yourself, and then again during the session whenever you feel it necessary. You may request repetitions of the message by pressing the button next to the bed anytime after you hear the initial message. (For all subjects) Try not to sleep during the session, but if you should doze off, don't feel guilty. Do you have any questions?

After the subject's questions were answered, a taped version of the relaxation instructions from Barabasz (1977, pp. 168-169) without muscle tension contrasts was played.

Subjects in the REST-MSG-PFood (n=6), REST-PFood (n=6), REST-MSG (n=6), and REST-only (n=6) conditions were exposed to

24 hours of chamber REST. Suedfeld (1980) noted that exposure to 24 hours of REST produces the most dramatic effects in the treatment of habits. Twenty-four hours of REST is also consistent with prior REST studies on weight loss (Borrie & Suedfeld, 1980) and food aversions (Suedfeld & Clarke, 1981). The 24-hour REST period was also found to be the most effective in a study comparing 3, 6, 12, and 24 hour REST durations (M. Barabasz, A. Barabasz, & Dyer, 1990).

Subjects in the non-REST-MSG-PFood (n=6), non-REST-PFood (n=6), the non-REST-MSG (n=6), and the non-REST-only (n=6) conditions spent their 24-hour sessions in the above mentioned room in Dr. Arreed Barabasz's laboratory. These subjects were monitored throughout the session, and materials were provided to help maintain normal levels of stimulation (e.g., books, magazines, television, video cassette player). Social contact was maintained by allowing the subjects to invite friends to the session for visitation and by intermittent interruptions by the experimenter approximately every hour.

For subjects in problem food conditions, the subject's problem food was provided by the experimenter a minimum number of eight times during the session, and on demand. Time intervals were varied so that the subjects were unable to establish a relationship between the time the food was served and the time spent in the session. Subjects were encouraged to eat as much of the food as they liked, and they were allowed to request additional servings at any time. For subjects in the REST conditions, the problem foods were delivered through the opening in the chamber wall. Subjects were notified of eating times by a brief communication from the experimenter: "I'm going to serve you your foods now." Subjects in the non-REST control conditions had their problem foods served by the experimenter. In addition to the problem foods, a supply of water and the standard REST lab liquid diet was provided in order to supplement the nutritional needs of the subjects.

Subjects in the message conditions (REST-MSG-PFood, REST-MSG, non-REST-MSG-PFood, and non-REST-MSG) were alerted at the 12-hour point in the session that a tape recorded message would be played. Research has not yet determined an optimal time pattern for delivery of messages during REST (Suedfeld, 1980). At 12 hours, the subject has had a prolonged period to become comfortable with the

REST environment, to have consumed her problem food, and to have begun experiencing the REST effect of stimulus hunger (Suedfeld, 1980; Jones, 1969). The message was adapted from suggestions used during hypnotic treatments for smoking and weight loss (M. Barabasz & D. Spiegel, 1989; A. Barabasz, Baer, Sheehan, & M. Barabasz, 1986; H. Spiegel & D. Spiegel, 1978, pp. 212-213): "For my body, but not for me, (quantity and type of problem food) is a poison, I need my body to live, I owe my body this respect and protection". The message was repeated for each of the subject's specified problem foods. Following sessions, a quasi-nondirective post-experimental interview was conducted to discuss subjects' REST experiences. Subjects were then provided with a second copy of the food log for the posttreatment measure.

At 6 week, 3 month, and 6 month follow-ups, subjects were again asked to record their food consumption for two weeks. Caliper skinfold measures were obtained at these follow-up data collection periods.

Results

Data were analyzed using a Friedman two-way analysis of variance. Measures included in the analysis were subjects' two-week total caloric consumption, two-week total caloric problem food consumption, and the sum of caliper skinfold measures. Non-parametric analyses were used because the data did not meet interval assumptions and because of the subsequent inability to make predictions regarding the population distribution (A. Barabasz & M. Barabasz, 1992; Siegel & Castellan, 1988). For interest, group means (daily total caloric consumption, daily problem food caloric consumption, sum of caliper skinfold scores) computed for each of the times of measurement are shown in Figures 15-1 to 15-6.

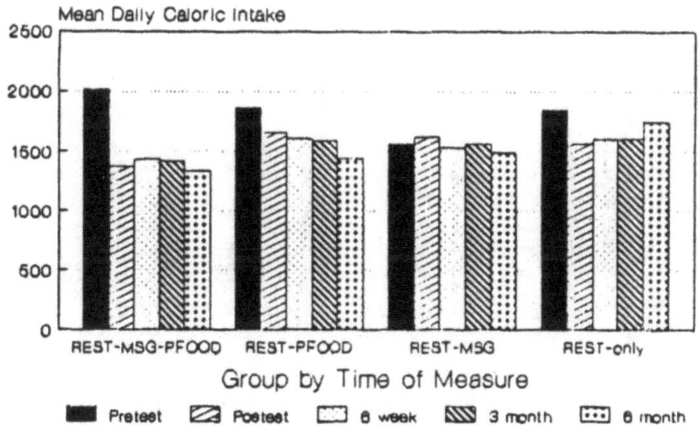

Figure 15-1. REST group total caloric results.
Mean daily total caloric intake.

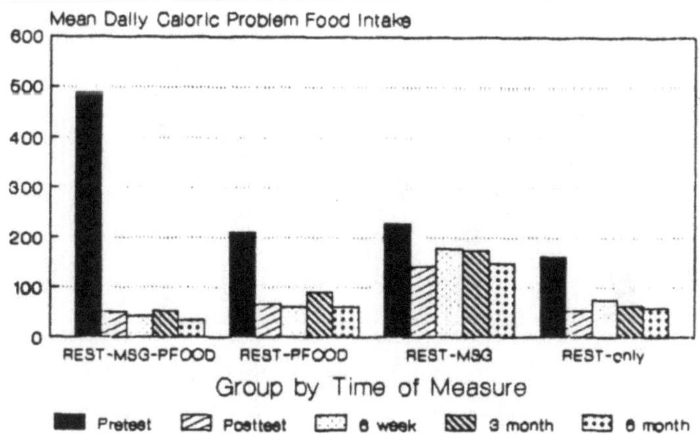

Figure 15-2. REST group problem food results.
Mean daily caloric problem food intake.

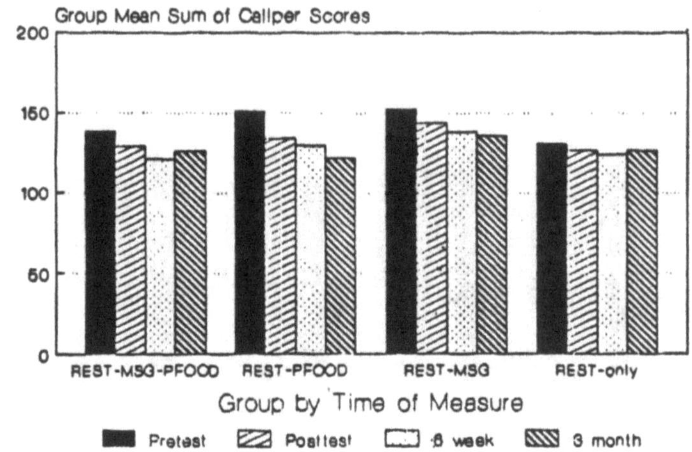

Figure 15-3. REST group bodyfat results.
Mean sum of caliper scores.

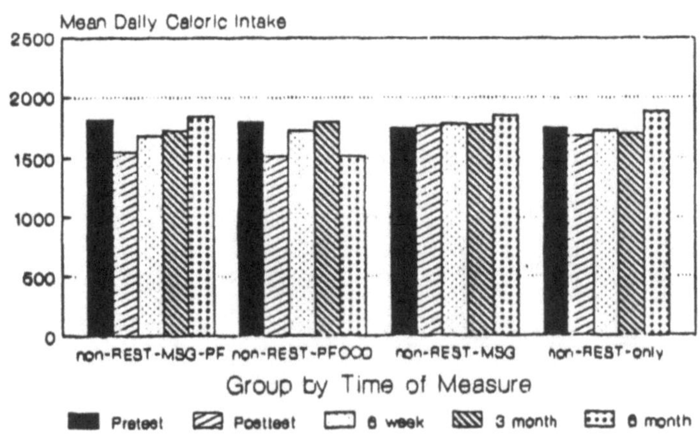

Figure 15-4. Control group total caloric results.
Mean daily total caloric intake.

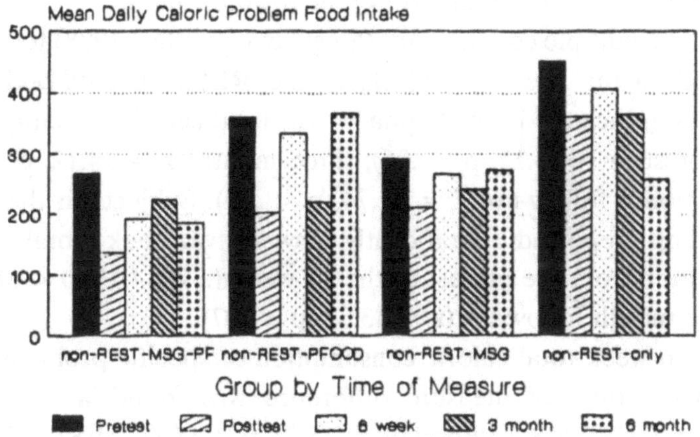

Figure 15-5. Control group problem food results.
Mean daily caloric problem food intake.

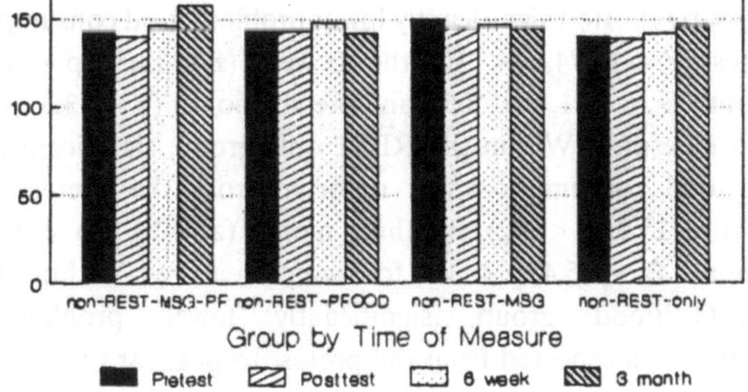

Figure 15-6. Control group bodyfat results.
Mean sum of caliper scores.

For total two-week caloric consumption, a significant time of measure difference was found within groups exposed to REST-MSG-PFood ($\chi^2 = 9.80$, $p < .043$) and REST only ($\chi^2 = 8.67$, $p < .07$). No other significant within group differences were found.

Post hoc multiple comparisons (Siegel & Castellan, 1988) found that compared to the pretest, subjects in the REST-MSG-PFood group reported significantly lower (alpha = .10) total caloric consumption at the post-test ($z = 14.12$, $p < .05$), three month ($z = 14.12$, $p < .05$), and six month follow-up ($z = 12.74$, $p < .10$). Subjects in the REST only group reported significantly lower two-week total caloric consumption from the pretest to the six week ($z = 14.11$, $p < .05$) and the three month follow-up ($z = 13.32$, $p < .07$).

For two-week total caloric consumption of specific problem foods, a significant time of measure difference was found within groups exposed to REST-MSG-PFood ($\chi^2 = 15.84$, $p < .003$), REST-PFood ($\chi^2 = 14.26$, $p < .006$), REST only ($\chi^2 = 14.8$, $p < .005$), and non-REST-MSG-PFood ($\chi^2 = 7.86$, $p < .09$). No other significant within group differences were found.

Post hoc comparisons showed that, in comparison to the pretest, subjects exposed to REST-MSG-PFood reported significantly lower problem food consumption at the posttest ($z = 15.4$, $p < .02$), six week ($z = 14.1$, $p < .05$), and six month ($z = 15.4$, $p < .02$) follow-up measures. Compared to the pretest measure, subjects in the REST-PFood group reported significantly lower problem food consumption at the posttest ($z = 12.74$, $p < .10$), the six week ($z = 15.37$, $p < .02$), the three month ($z = 14.1$, $p < .05$), and the six month ($z = 13.3$, $p < .07$) follow-up measures. Within the REST only group, significantly lower problem food consumption was reported from the pretest to the posttest ($z = 15.4$, $p < .02$), the three month ($z = 14.1$, $p < .05$), and the six month ($z = 15.4$, $p < .02$) follow-up measures. Within the non-REST-MSG-PFood group, significantly lower problem food consumption was reported from the pretest to posttest ($z = 2.57$, $p < .05$) only.

For the sum of caliper skinfold scores, significant differences were found within groups exposed to REST-MSG-PFood ($\chi^2 = 16.4$, $p < .001$), REST-PFood ($\chi^2 = 15.35$, $p < .001$), and REST only ($\chi^2 = 6.08$,

$p < .04$). No other significant within group differences were found.

For the REST-MSG-PFood group, post hoc comparisons revealed significantly lower sums of skinfold scores at the three month ($z = 11.79$, $p < .02$) and the six month ($z = 11.79$, $p < .02$) follow-up measures, in comparison to the pretest measure. For the REST-PFood group, in comparison to the pretest, significantly lower sums of skinfold scores were found at the three month ($z = 10.7$, $p < .05$) and the six month ($z = 11.8$, $p < .02$) follow-up measures. The REST only group comparison yielded a significantly lower skinfold score sum at the three month ($z = 10.02$, $p < .07$) follow-up measure, in comparison to the pretest measure.

Discussion

The present study demonstrated that 24 hours of chamber REST, either with or without educational messages and consumption of problem foods, significantly lowered subjects' total caloric consumption, problem food consumption, and body fat percentage. These dramatic effects suggest that chamber REST may be a valuable intervention for females who exceed optimal body fat limits.

Despite the exciting findings of this study, it is necessary to recognize the limitations of this investigation. The minimum criterion for inclusion in this study was that a subject had to be at least 38% body fat. Except for the exclusion of morbidly obese subjects whose weight loss program required medical intervention, there was no maximum criterion. A body fat percentage of 38% typically indicates that a subject is between approximately 10 and 20 pounds overweight, depending on the amount they exercise, bone structure and height (Metropolitan Life Insurance Company, 1984). It was apparent during the collection of follow-up data that subjects who had 25-30 pounds or less to lose were the subjects who benefitted from the REST treatments. Subjects with a greater amount of weight to lose reported initial progress (5-10 pound loss), but they reported that they were unable to maintain their diet and exercise regimens. One subject requested additional "booster" REST sessions.

Unfortunately, all of the subjects in the REST-MSG-PFood condition, all but one subject in the REST-PFood condition, and four of the subjects in the REST-only were in the 30 pounds or less group. In the REST-MSG condition, the reverse occurred in that all but one subject were more severely overweight. The control conditions had similar distributions, but this factor did not appear to account for any significant changes.

Subjects exposed to the REST-PFood condition significantly lowered their specific problem food consumption and sum of caliper scores while maintaining no significant differences in total caloric intake among the measurement periods. The interview data collected from these subjects during follow-up is revealing. Two of the subjects who were assigned to this condition reported that in addition to making post-treatment dietary changes, they also added intensive exercise programs including both aerobic exercise and body building. Although this intensive exercise regimen drastically decreased their body fat percentages, both subjects reported appetite increases. However, they reported increasing their total caloric consumption with foods that were high in nutrients and low in sugar and fat content. At the end of the follow-up measurements, these two subjects reported that they had previously experienced numerous failings to alter their eating and exercise habits before REST.

Subjects in the REST-only group lowered their total caloric consumption, their problem food consumption, and their sum of caliper scores. This finding is consistent with A. Barabasz and M. Barabasz (1992) in supporting Suedfeld's (1980) theory that subjects bring their own experiment to the REST session. However, the subjects in this condition did not maintain their lowered total caloric intake or the lowered sum of caliper scores at the six month follow-up, but did maintain their lowered problem food consumption. A closer look at the individual subject's data within this group seems to provide an explanation for this discrepancy. Although the subjects in this group typically reported lowered problem food consumption, perusal of their two week food logs showed an increase in high calorie foods, possibly indicating a substitution of alternative problem foods for the original problem foods.

The REST-MSG condition was not found to be significantly effective on any of the three measures. In fact, these subjects showed a non-significant but consistent increase in total caloric intake following the session. Furthermore, interview data showed that several subjects in this condition reported an increase in their desire for their problem foods. Suedfeld and Clarke (1981) hypothesized that depriving overweight subjects of their favorite foods may result in an increase of consumption of those foods. This study was not intended to test this hypothesis, however, the finding that subjects who were allowed to consume their desired foods during the REST session found the treatment significantly more effective suggests the need for further investigation into the effects of depriving individuals of favorite foods while involved in weight loss and/or weight maintenance programs. It is a well documented finding that popular weight loss programs which require abstinence from specific problem foods, and sometimes require that the individual purchase pre-packaged meals, have extremely high relapse rates (Nicholas & Dwyer, 1986; Stunkard, 1986). The problems with such programs occur when individuals are unable to maintain a diet regimen which is low in calories and high in nutritional value (Brownell, Marlatt, Lichtenstein, & Wilson, 1986; Brownell, 1980; Collins, Rothblum, & Wilson, 1986; Hartz, Kalkhoff, Rimm, & McCall, 1986). It would seem that helping clients lower their desire for problem foods would be a valuable adjunct to any weight loss treatment.

A major contribution of the present study to the area of REST research was the almost exclusive finding of non-significant differences within the non-REST control conditions. There was a single significant pretest-posttest decrease in the non-REST-MSG-PFood condition. Most of the control subjects reported slightly lowered food consumption between the pretest and posttest, but none of the control subjects were able to maintain a significant decrease in consumption. The post-session interview inquiry showed that subjects in the non-REST conditions were more likely to make vague statements regarding the benefit of the session to their specific weight problem than were REST subjects. However, not a single subject reported that they were aware that they were in the control condition. One control subject who was involved in a graduate program and was well aware of common research design procedures asked the experimenter "do you also have a control condition where people receive a placebo? At least I'm sure I'm not in the control group, because who would have a 24 hour control group?" The implications of the findings of non-significance within the non-REST conditions supports the specificity of REST. Placing subjects in a room with normal levels of stimulation for a 24 hour period of time is not sufficient to produce significant and enduring changes.

All subjects were asked to utilize the 24 hour sessions to focus on the importance of diet and exercise, and the role their particular problem foods had in their weight problems. Subjects in the REST-MSG-PFood condition reported that consuming the foods within the session appeared to "alter the flavor," "made the taste seem more potent", and "it was intensely sweet". They reported being surprised at how little of the food they ate during the 24 hour period compared to the amount "I would've eaten while watching TV." In particular, the subjects in this group reported far less enjoyment and desire after exposure to the message. Curiously, subjects in the REST-PFood group showed very similar patterns of problem food consumption during the treatment session. When asked to report what thoughts they had during the session regarding their problem food consumption, four of the six subjects reported that it occurred to them that eating [problem food] is poisoning my "body", "life", or "health."

In contrast to problem food consumption during REST, subjects in the non-REST-MSG-PFood condition and the non-REST-PFood condition consumed far greater quantities of their problem foods during the 24 hour session. Almost all of the subjects in these two conditions reported at the post-session inquiry that they felt sure they would be able to control their future consumption of these foods. In fact, nearly all of these subjects insisted that the experimenter keep the "leftovers." However, their food logs indicated that, although problem food consumption initially decreased for a few days, this decrease was not maintained during the two week logging period.

When questioned about their thoughts during the session about diet, exercise and problem food consumption, subjects in the non-REST conditions made vague statements regarding their knowledge of the importance of these factors. In contrast, subjects in all of the REST conditions reported that they spent time focusing on solutions to their weight problem which would be specific to their current lifestyle needs. For example, one 24-year-old subject reported that the REST session helped her develop an exercise plan which worked for her: "I've always had trouble sticking with an exercise plan because of my hectic schedule. I join an aerobics class and I'm always having to skip it for one reason or another. I came up with a plan that if I bought an exercise video tape I could hold my own class whenever it's convenient and I wouldn't have any excuse not to exercise." At the six month follow-up, this subject reported that she continued to use this plan to do aerobic exercise five times per week. Another subject, a 42-year-old mother of three, reported another solution developed during REST: "I was really fighting the notion that in order to lose weight I'd have to exercise and give up ice cream (one of her problem foods). In thinking about ice cream, and my food cupboard in general, I realized that whenever something is on sale at the grocery store I stock up. Our family can eat a lot of food! But after a while I realized that I used this logic for foods that are supposed to be treats, that's what I tell my kids, anyway. From now on, if I, or my family, want ice cream we'll go out and have one serving. The extra effort will make it taste better." In the follow-up interview, this subject reported that she and/or her husband frequently combine going out for an ice cream cone with a two to three mile walk. Not only has she lowered her overall consumption of ice cream and other problem foods, but she increased her exercise and lowered her body fat percentage.

The findings of the present study demonstrate that chamber REST in combination with specific problem food consumption and motivational messages may be a powerful treatment or treatment adjunct for moderately overweight clients who seek help for weight loss. As has been repeatedly reported in the literature, any nutritionally sound weight reduction program will work, but problems (such as weight-cycling, decreased motivation, and relapse) arise when individuals are not able to eliminate many of their established dietary habits (i.e., eating problem foods) (Brownell, Marlatt, Lichtenstein, & Wilson, 1986; Nicholas & Dwyer, 1986; Stunkard, 1976, 1986). The present study indicates that overweight individuals and treatment specialists may have an effective mechanism to combat such problems. The addition of chamber REST is inexpensive (Suedfeld, 1980) because it requires only one treatment session and produces long term results. Chamber REST is time and cost-effective (Best & Suedfeld, 1982).

16

Treatment of Trichotillomania and Smoking with Hypnosis and REST

Marianne Barabasz and Arreed Barabasz

The treatment of habit disorders has long been viewed as the domain of behavior therapy (Barabasz, 1977). In particular, both trichotillomania and smoking control have been the foci of numerous behavioral studies. Behavioral formulations view these disorders as isolated habits comparable to fingernail biting, thumb sucking and nose picking, but applied behavioral analysis (Wolf, 1978) suggests that they serve an anxiety-reducing function for thc individual and can be maintained by endogenous or exogenous antecedents with consequences of varying complexity. Conceptualizing these disorders as isolated behaviors within the behavioral paradigm, seems debatable and may account for the continuum of complexity of behavior therapy interventions.

The literature on the treatment of trichotillomania includes numerous case study reports which show a wide variety of elaborate behavioral interventions that have been attempted with varying degrees of initial success and relapse rates. Interventions have included self-monitoring with response chain interruption (Taylor, 1963); counting and recording pulls (Saper, 1971); denial of privileges (Epstein &

Peterson, 1973); aversive self-stimulation (Mastellone, 1974); covert desensitization (Levine, 1976); habit reversal (Azrin, Nunn, & Frantz, 1980); asking the client to do 15 sit ups whenever she attempted to pull her hair (MacNeil & Thomas, 1976); attention-reflection and response prevention by cutting hair close to the scalp (Massong, Edwards, Range-Sitton, & Hailey, 1980); attention-reflection combined with punishment (Altman, Grahs, & Friman, 1982); and a multicomponent treatment package combining self-monitoring, goal setting, relaxation, and stimulus control (Bornstein & Rychtarik, 1978).

These behavioral interventions are also problematic because of the high dependence on client cooperation for both trichotillomania and smoking treatments, or parental cooperation in the case of hair pulling children. Therefore, it is not surprising that treatment failures and relapses have been blamed on compliance problems. Derschewitz and Christopherson (1984) note that noncompliance heightens the effort necessary to perform the treatment.

Hypnosis has a long history of success in the treatment of habit disorders without the complexity of most of the behavioral interventions cited above. Furthermore, hypnosis does not seem to foster such problems with client compliance. In contrast to numerous studies on the treatment of smoking, minimal attention has been given to the treatment of trichotillomania with hypnosis. Nevertheless, it has, at least, shown promise with highly hypnotizable clients. Herbert Spiegel and David Spiegel (1978) used a hypnotic intervention similar to their widely used self-management-self-hypnosis smoking control procedure. Case study reports of two females in their 20s showed that the highly hypnotizable client "Responded quickly and dramatically stopping her hair pulling completely (p. 290)" while the less hypnotizable client "stopped quite gradually, and not completely (p. 288)." In another interesting case, Galski (1981) used hypnosis adjunctively during "analytically oriented" psychotherapy with a highly hypnotizable 26-year-old female. The intervention focused on "scalp sensitivity" which resulted in immediate and complete cessation of hair pulling which was maintained at a 6-month follow up. Rowen (1981) employed Cautela's (1967) covert sensitization method during hypnotic age regression with a highly hypnotizable 21-year-old male. Complete freedom from the habit was maintained 6 months after treatment. Rowen (1981) concluded that the value of the intervention "would be limited to the most highly hypnotizable (p. 197)."

A three-year study of 307 subjects treated for smoking cessation by hypnosis also showed hypnotizability to be the key predictive factor in treatment success (A. Barabasz, Baer, Sheehan, & M. Barabasz, 1986). Consistent with this data, the clinical reports discussed above suggest that success with hypnosis in the treatment of trichotillomania has been limited to highly hypnotizable clients (M. Barabasz, 1987).

Hypnotizability has been shown to be dramatically enhanced by chamber REST. Following REST, Ss initially low in hypnotizability demonstrated significantly enhanced responsiveness to suggestions for both experimental (A. Barabasz, 1982) and clinical pain control (A. Barabasz & M. Barabasz, 1989). In the clinical trials reported here, REST is combined with hypnosis in the treatment of either trichotillomania or smoking habits with clients for whom hypnosis alone was not effective.

Method

Trichotillomania clients' diagnosis-assessment of abnormal hair loss was confirmed by a physician (Price, 1978). The physician also took responsibility for the initial history taking which included information on drug intake, physical development, general appearance, duration of hair loss, history of hair disorders in other family members, and direct observations of hair pulling. In all cases, the diagnosis was considered clear, precluding the need to conduct Wood's light examination of plucked hairs (see Steck, 1979) or the trichotillo test (see Wright et al., 1979).

Smoking clients completed a medical and smoking history questionnaire prior to treatment. These individuals had made several previous attempts to quit smoking consistent with the H. Speigel and D. Speigel (1978, p. 217) "hard core smoker group". Clients reported that both of their parents were life-long smokers, a history common to those most resistant to treatment.

Procedure

All clients were seen in out-patient clinics. Initial 1.25 hour to 1.75 hour sessions for hypnosis included the following: 1) Onset, duration, present condition, and history of duration were reviewed from the written reports; 2) As in a previous clinical study (A. Barabasz et al., 1986), hypnosis was discussed. Details are reported elsewhere (see Barabasz et al., 1986); 3) Clients were introduced to hypnotic experience via two to four brief inductions featuring motoric responses. The aim of this procedural step was to help maximize or plateau client hypnotic responsiveness; 4) The Stanford Hypnotic Clinical Scale (SHCS) of Morgan and Hilgard (1975) was administered and discussed with an emphasis on items successfully passed; 5) Hypnosis was induced using the eyeball set technique (eyes rolled up while remaining closed) followed by relaxation induction instructions from the SHCS. For trichotillomania clients, posthypnotic suggestions targeting hair-pulling behavior were then given as follows:

> You will be acutely aware whenever you put your hand to your head, then it is entirely up to you, you have the power, the control, no one else, no habit controls you. You can pull your hair if you want to or you can choose to control the habit.

Smoking clients were given post hypnotic suggestions as prescribed by H. Spiegel and D. Spiegel (1978, pp. 212-213) and found to be successful with clients of adequate hypnotizability (A. Barabasz, et al., 1986). The hypnotic suggestions emphasized that a client was "for" his or her body rather than merely against smoking.

Since hypnosis alone was not effective, clients were then exposed to a REST session (See individual cases) and followed by a hypnotic induction and the suggestions cited above.

Apparatus

The REST chamber is a small room equipped with 2.5 cm. of Dow-Corning coated fiberglass sound attenuating material on the walls, ceiling, and both sides of the door. The sound of the ceiling vent air flow also serves to help mask any sounds external to the chamber. The sound attenuating characteristics are adequate to prevent the transmission of voices, music, or secretarial activity sounds. During REST sessions, efforts are made to minimize the possibility of clinic door slamming. This occasional sound of the clinic door slamming is not completely attenuated by the chamber sound proofing measures. The room is kept light free while clients recline on a lazy-boy type chair. Reassuring explanations of the procedure (Suedfeld, 1980) precede all sessions. Clients are aware of the presence of an open intercom which the psychologist uses as a monitor. Clients are reminded that they are free to terminate the session at any time. In this study no one chose early termination.

The REST tank (Floatarium Model SWS) (2.4 meters long x 1.4 meters high x 1.3 meters wide) is essentially an enclosed, sound-insulated, fiberglass tub that contains a 215 cm. deep dense solution (D=1.30 g/cc) of tap water and epsom salts (20% solution). The solution is maintained at average skin temperature 34.5° C (±.2° C). The tank is sound attenuated and light free once the subject activated door is closed. Subjects float effortlessly in a supine position with ears submerged (subjects wore earplugs). Subject vocalizations are monitored by a built-in microphone. Messages are transmitted to clients from the monitoring room via underwater transducers. The tank is ventilated by a silent positive pressure system. Between float sessions the water is filtered and purified by an ultraviolet irradiation system. A shower is immediately adjacent to the tank for hygienic purposes before and after each float experience.

Cases

Trichotillomania

Case T1

Ms. K., age 21, was referred by her family physician. She reported a history of mild hair plucking which started before she entered high school. Her condition at the time of the initial session was described as "no better--no worse." Hair length was about four inches, with no prominent bald areas.

Her SHCS score was 2. Hair pulling continued at pre-treatment levels immediately after the initial hypnosis session. A second session was conducted four days later. The one-hour session emphasized additional experience with hypnosis in an attempt to further maximize responsivity and included supportive counseling with a focus on hope for a successful outcome. Despite these efforts, and an apparently well-motivated client, hair pulling continued at the usual level until the next session eight days later.

On the basis of previous experimental research demonstrating enhancement of hypnotizability (A. Barabasz, 1982) and clinical research showing enhanced treatment outcomes in smoking cessation (A. Barabasz et al., 1986), the next session employed chamber REST. After reassuring explanations of the procedure (Suedfeld, 1980), the client reclined on a lazy-boy type chair in a sound attenuated chamber for a period of two hours. Before leaving the chamber, the SHCS was administered with the addition of the posthypnotic suggestion package targeting hair-pulling behavior. At this administration her SHCS score was 4, showing an increase of two points. The client telephoned nine times over the next several weeks noting that she had caught herself touching her hair but found it easy to resist the urge to pull her hair. She was seen 4 months and 12 months after the REST/hypnosis session to confirm the telephone follow ups. At 12 months she proudly showed her long-length hair style.

Case T2

Ms. L., a 34-year-old woman with three children and a "very successful husband," wore a wig to cover her nearly bald head. Regular hair plucking began two years earlier. Before attempting to deal with the client's hair-plucking behavior, 12 weekly one-hour counseling sessions were devoted to teaching this client responsible assertion skills, hypnosis for relaxation, stress management, and consistency in the behavioral management of her children. The client's husband, reportedly, cooperated fully in instituting the new child management policies but refused to attend therapy. Despite many improvements in the client's perceived level of stress and general evidence of improved coping, she still continued hair plucking at the precounseling rate. Session 13 was the first devoted to hypnosis for hair plucking using the standardized procedure outlined above. The client's SHCS score was 3. Since she had experienced a total of 31 hypnotic inductions prior to testing, her hypnotic responsiveness was considered fully plateaued at testing. Following administration of the standard post hypnotic suggestions for hair pulling and termination of hypnosis, the client expressed worry as to whether or not the procedure would be successful. Therefore, the following day the chamber REST intervention was conducted as outlined in the previous case. During the intervening period between the hypnosis only and the REST sessions, the client reported abstinence from hair plucking "but it took all the control I had--I am a nervous wreck now--I doubt this (REST) will make any difference." Although she was strongly motivated to attempt REST and further hypnosis she thought she might have to leave the REST chamber in 10 or 15 minutes. After 2.5 hours of REST, the SHCS induction and hair-plucking suggestions were administered. Her new SHCS score was a clear 4 points. She emerged from the chamber claiming she felt more relaxed and more refreshed than she could recall. Despite no problems with hair-plucking control, at the client's request the REST-hypnosis procedure was repeated about one week later. Counseling sessions continued bi-weekly for the next three months, but no further interventions aimed directly at hair-pulling behavior were conducted. The client was seen briefly at 6 and 12 months after the first REST session to confirm telephone reports of complete abstinence from hair pulling.

Case T3

Ms. M., age 19, was referred by her psychiatrist specifically for hypnotic treatment of trichotillomania. The client had been seeing her psychiatrist for psychoanalytically oriented therapy once a week for the past 30 months. The client reported hair plucking continued to increase in severity during this period. It was agreed that psychotherapy would continue as usual, and the intervention for hair pulling would be strictly limited to an immediate focus on the habit. Ms. M. had been engaging in hair plucking repeatedly since puberty. Hair length at our initial session was about 2.5 cm. with two 25 square cm. areas with less than 6 mm. of hair growth. The client did not wear a wig. She refused to provide the usual details during a review of her history because of fears it might interfere with her progress in psychotherapy.

Despite some success on the pretesting hypnotic experiences, the client's SHCS score was 0, Because of the client's SHCS score, the usual induction for hair pulling was postponed until a chamber REST session could be scheduled. Six days later a 2.5 hour REST session was conducted as outlined for Case T2, and the SHCS and posthypnotic suggestions for hair pulling were administered. After REST, Ms. M. reported she felt "surprised to feel so relaxed." Her post-REST SHCS score was 2. At 10:00 p.m. that evening an "emergency" telephone call was received from the client. She complained that she "couldn't pull her hair" and that the "tension was unbearable." The client was reminded of the wording of the posthypnotic suggestions emphasizing awareness of the habit and the choice as to whether or not hair is then plucked. Brief progressive muscle relaxation instructions (Barabasz, 1977) were then administered. Ms. M. reported feeling "more relaxed, in control" and having "no particular concerns about touching my hair."

After discussing the advisability of continued hypnotic/REST treatment with Ms. M.'s psychiatrist, Ms. M. was seen for four more sessions during the following three weeks. At the second session the client reported having reduced hair pulling "by at least 50%." The REST/hypnosis procedure was readministered at this session; one week later Ms. M. reported she had not pulled a single hair since the previous session and that she could not believe how easy it was after so many years. Hypnosis was repeated without REST. Evidence of increased hair length and density was clear. Ms. M. canceled her next scheduled session less than one hour before the appointed time leaving the message that she had started plucking her hair again but "not as badly as before." In the client's final session she reported how she had learned in psychotherapy just how important hair pulling was to her and that she was not "ready to quit." Hair-pulling behavior at the time of the last session was apparently at the baseline prehypnotic pre-REST intervention level. Telephone follow ups at six and nine months also suggested that hair pulling continued at the baseline level.

Smoking

Case S1

Mr. C, age 45, had been seen by the second author eight years earlier for hypnosis for smoking (2 1/2 to 3 packs per day) using standardized procedure (A. Barabasz et al., 1986). The client reported smoking abstinence for the seven years immediately following hypnosis. He then began smoking again,increasing rapidly to two packs per day. The client noted, "I was doing just fine, didn't miss it at all. Then I had some financial reversals, thought I'd have just one (cigarette); now I'm two packs a day... I tried the self-hypnosis you taught me years ago but it didn't work." The client, who resided over 2,000 miles from this psychologist (A.B.), was urged in a telephone discussion to see a local psychologist trained in hypnosis using a similar procedure. Prognosis was considered good since hypnotizability is normally a highly stable talent and the client's SHCS score, measured eight years earlier, was 4 out of the maximum of 5 points. Mr. C. saw the local psychologist one week later noting, "He was really good at it (hypnosis); he used the same instructions you did, it just didn't work this time. Please let me fly up and see you."

The client was seen for a single session of 3 1/2 hours duration. SHCS retesting revealed the identical score (4) as from eight years earlier with passes on the identical items. The standard procedure was used but the client smoked immediately after hypnosis. After a 10 minute break, the client was exposed to a one-hour session of flotation REST. The H. Spiegel and D. Spiegel (1978, p. 212-213) hypnotic suggestions for smoking cessation were again administered, after 45 minutes of flotation REST. Telephone follow ups at two days, two weeks, three months, and six months provided client reports that smoking abstinence had been "easily" maintained "but I still didn't feel hypnotized." Cotinine levels obtained independently at about six months confirmed abstinence from smoking.

Discussion

Consistent with the major goals of a clinical report (Fromm, 1981), the present paper details interventions to facilitate further clinical and experimental research. Hypnosis combined with REST was effective in all but one case. Efforts were made to obtain direct physiological confirmation of client reports. In the successful cases, treatment results were maintained in long-term follow up. As in a previous clinical study (A. F. Barabasz et al., 1986) and experimental research (A. F. Barabasz, 1982), chamber REST appeared to enhance hypnotic responsiveness both in terms of SHCS scores and treatment outcomes. Earlier clinical reports of the use of hypnosis suggested successful outcomes might be limited only to highly hypnotizable clients. The addition of REST may serve to extend the intervention to a much wider range of clients. This new intervention for the treatment of trichotillomania needs further testing in controlled experiments using subjects fully plateaued for hypnotic responsiveness. The successful outcome in the treatment of smoking is consistent with previous data (A. Barabasz et al., 1986) which used chamber REST. However, the findings are intriguing because a simple hypnotic/REST intervention achieved long-term results with clients exhibiting extended habit histories. The findings appear to contrast sharply with a number of complex behavioral interventions requiring client self-management, compliance, and considerably more therapy time.

Experience in the failure Case T3 suggests that hypnosis combined with REST may be a powerful intervention, even with less motivated or ambivalent clients. It also suggests some of the potential difficulties of accepting a referral in the midst of another form of on-going therapy. Among other considerations, a careful preparation of the client for the referral would seem advisable as well as a sensitive exploration of his/her expectations and of the meaningfulness of the symptoms.

Recent experimental studies (A. Barabasz, 1988, 1990c,e) suggest that flotation REST elicits spontaneous hypnosis in subjects known to have hypnotic talent. The smoking case reported above suggests that flotation REST may have potential clinical usefulness as an adjunctive procedure for high hypnotizables who have experienced relapse.

Acknowledgment

The authors would like to thank REST Technologies Corp. of Huntington, New York, and Prof. Dennis Warner.

17

Motivational Factors in Alcohol Consumption: Extending Hull's Model

David DiRito

The Self-awareness Model of Alcohol Consumption

Hull (1981) proposed that alcohol functions to reduce self-awareness following failure. A failure experience is likely to produce a state of negative self-evaluation. Such a state is aversive and escape from it will be sought. That alcohol is capable of interfering with this state and thereby providing a means of escape is sufficient to induce and sustain alcohol consumption.

Hull (1981) drew upon two lines of research on cognitive processes. One is that alcohol has been shown to interfere with higher-order encoding of information (e.g., Hartley, Brinbaum, & Parker, 1978). The other is research on cognitive prototypes which has shown that the self acts as a schema for encoding information (e.g., Markus, 1977). Since processing information in a self-relevant manner involves higher-order encoding and since alcohol interferes with higher-order encoding, alcohol would interfere with self-relevant information processing (Hull, 1981).

Hull and his associates conducted a series of empirical studies to test his model (Hull & Young, 1983). The findings were strongly supportive. For example, subjects who received failure feedback on an intelligence task drank significantly more wine than subjects given success feedback.

Thus, a particular cognitive state of self-awareness following failure is the determinant of alcohol consumption. Arousal is simply a product of self-awareness, but it does not act upon self-awareness. Alcohol is consumed specifically to interrupt negative self-relevant information processing. The reduction of arousal that is subsequently experienced is the result of interruption of these cognitive processes rather than from any direct effect alcohol may have on arousal.

Arousability and Alcohol Consumption

In contrast, Adams (1988) proposed that alcohol is consumed specifically to reduce arousal. More precisely, persons who have chronic excessively elevated arousal are prone to alcohol consumption as a means of reducing arousal to more tolerable levels (M. Barabasz et al., 1990). Support for this proposition was provided by empirical studies of three widely used measures which have been successful in distinguishing alcoholics from non-alcoholics. These are the MacAndrews Alcoholism Scale (MAC) of the MMPI (MacAndrew, 1981), the Zuckerman Sensation Seeking Scale (SSS) (Zuckerman, 1979), and computerized measures of EEG fast brain-wave activity (Gabrielli, Mednick, Volavka, Pollock, Schulsinger, & Itil, 1982).

High scorers on the MAC have been described as being "characterized by the presence of strong emotions which are easily aroused" (MacAndrews, 1981, p. 622). The same persons are either at risk for alcoholism or already are alcoholic. A similar coincidence was observed in high scorers on the SSS. These individuals are described as having the tendency to become overly aroused to levels beyond the optimal range. They are also prone to alcohol abuse and other addictive behaviors (Zuckerman, 1979).

Fast EEG activity is known to be a distinctive characteristic of alcoholics (Jones & Holmes, 1976). This pattern has been shown to be genetically transmitted (Propping, 1977) and was found in the sons (11- to 13-years-old) of alcoholics (Gabrielli et al., 1982). Such an EEG pattern is associated with tension and anxiety (Kiloh & Osselton, 1961) and administration of alcohol has been shown to slow brain activity (Propping, 1977). Alcohol may be consumed to escape the unpleasant state associated with fast EEG activity (Gabrielli et al., 1982).

A pilot study by Cooper, Adams, and Scott (1988) seemed to show that Restricted Environmental Stimulation Therapy (REST) was effective in reducing alcohol intake of heavy social drinkers. Subjects were exposed to one 2 1/2 hour chamber REST session. Follow-ups revealed dramatic decreases in alcohol consumption from baseline levels. Consumption in a control group slightly increased during the follow-up periods.

The authors (Cooper et al., 1988) concluded that these effects were caused by a reduction of arousal and a slowing of excessively fast brain wave activity. This conclusion was based upon previous research showing that REST produced slowed EEG and decreased arousal (c.f., Suedfeld, 1980; Zubek, 1969a; Zuckerman, 1979). Other research has shown that training to slow brain wave activity of alcoholics produced similar dramatic reductions of alcohol consumption at follow-up (Peniston & Kulkosky, 1989).

M. Barabasz et al., (1990) completed a very carefully controlled study of the effects of chamber REST on alcohol consumption, testing session lengths of 3, 6, 12, and 24 hours of REST. Pre- and post-REST alcohol consumption data was corroborated and confirmed. Twenty-four hours of REST was found to be effective in producing marked alcohol consumption reductions.

An Integrative Model

Perhaps arousal and self-awareness interact with one another to produce a state conducive to alcohol consumption. Schachter (1964) demonstrated that cognitive and physiological processes interact to produce emotion. Zillman (1983) demonstrated that residual arousal from one activity can combine with and intensify subsequent emotional states. Gollwitzer, Earle, and Stephan (1982) demonstrated that residual arousal from an exercise task served to increase egotistical performance attributions following success and failure feedback.

In the Gollwitzer et al. study (1982), subjects were randomly given either success or failure feedback from a previous social skills test. The feedback was given either 1, 5, or 9 minutes after the exercise. It was found that subjects in the 5 minute condition made greater egotistical attributions for their performance than subjects in the other two conditions. That is, those who received failure feedback attributed their failure to external factors such as task difficulty or luck. Those given success feedback attributed their success to internal factors like ability or effort. These effects were more pronounced in the 5 minute condition, demonstrating that arousal from the exercise had influenced the attribution process.

Gollwitzer and his associates (1982) measured reactions to success and failure by measuring performance attributions. Hull measured reactions to success and failure by measuring alcohol consumption. Both studies indicate that individuals attempt to escape the aversive state produced by failure or enhance the pleasant state produced by success by whatever means are available to them. Gollwitzer and associates (1982) additionally found that egotistical attributions were enhanced under conditions permitting the transfer of arousal from a previous task to the arousal produced by the performance feedback. This, then, is an empirical demonstration of the interaction of self-awareness and arousal to influence subsequent behavior.

Failure feedback created the cognitions of negative self-evaluation and the amount of arousal not attributable to other causes determined the intensity of the negative experience. Apparently, the degree of arousal provides information about the degree of importance to be attributed to the failure. The greater the arousal, the more serious the failure. The more serious the failure, the greater the motivation to escape, alcohol consumption being one such means of escape. Furthermore, the amount consumed may be proportional to the seriousness of the failure such that, the more serious the failure, the more consumed.

Since pre-existing arousal from irrelevant sources can influence the self-evaluation process (Gollwitzer et al., 1982), failure experiences would be especially adverse for those individuals who suffer from chronically elevated arousal (Adams, 1988). Interpretation of the elevated pre-existing arousal in terms of the failure may lead to the conclusion that even minor failures implied serious self-deficits for these individuals. It is not surprising that many of these individuals are prone to use alcohol for relief.

If some individuals are prone to excessively elevated arousal perhaps they are also prone to chronic negative self-evaluation. Indeed, this is the case. Certain individuals have been found to engage in more intense self-focus on their mistakes and failings than others. They are described as possessing a trait known as Negative Affectivity or Neuroticism (Watson & Clark, 1984). Recent research has found that the presence of both negative affectivity and arousability in individuals is strongly predictive of the development of substance abuse problems (Adler, 1990; McKirnan & Peterson, 1988). Apparently, these individuals are engaged in a vicious cycle of dwelling on their shortcomings, escaping through drink, and returning to self-condemnation for drinking.

Conclusions

The major premise of this model is that cognitive and physiological processes interact to produce a particular emotional state conducive to drinking. That state is produced by the process of negative self-evaluation which is experienced as aversive. The intensity of the aversion is determined by the amount of arousal attributed to the self-evaluation. The motivation to drink is to escape the aversive experience.

Individuals with drinking problems are prone to excessive arousability and chronic negative self-evaluation (Adler, 1990). They are also known to be quite resistant to enter and engage in treatment. In terms of this model, that one needs treatment is, in itself, an indication of deficiency and failure. It is also well known that treatment involves intense focus upon one's deficiencies. This is precisely the thing that these individuals cannot tolerate and so desperately avoid.

REST has recently been postulated as an effective alternative treatment for the treatment of alcohol problems (Adams, 1988) and has recently been demonstrated as dramatically effective (M. Barabasz et al., 1990). It is said to be effective by lowering arousal to more tolerable levels. That it does so is not questioned here, but perhaps more is involved (M. Barabasz et al., 1990). The effect of REST upon cognitive processes has not yet been empirically examined in great detail. It may influence cognitive processes in a number of ways to ameliorate drinking problems.

REST may permit the consideration of negative self-relevant information during lowered arousal. If so, the quality of the experience may be quite different when arousal is decreased than elevated. Rather than being aversive, it may be tolerable, even interesting. There may be an inclination to remain in the experience and become involved with it. This may allow information processing to occur on deeper and more extensive levels than before. Higher-order cognitive structures such as self-concept, self-esteem, and self-confidence may be beneficially and lastingly altered as a result. Changes in these important structures may be just as crucial in overcoming drinking problems.

The ability to confront problems without seeking to escape them has been shown to be beneficial in itself. Self-esteem improves and symptoms disappear when one confronts, rather than escapes, their problems (Bednar, Wells, & Peterson, 1989). REST may facilitate this process. Self-evaluation during REST may increase positive self-regard simply because the self-evaluation occurred without an attempt to escape it. These and other possibilities seem worthy of investigation, especially since they may lead to improved techniques for treating alcoholism and other substance abuse problems.

18

Chamber REST Reduces Alcohol Consumption: 3, 6, 12, and 24 Hour Sessions

Marianne Barabasz, Arreed Barabasz, and Rebecca Dyer

Helzer (1987) emphasized the urgent need for studies that focus on the prevention of alcoholism. Selzer (1987) noted that alcoholism is the third most serious health problem in the United States after cardiovascular disease and cancer. In a study of middle aged men (Halldin, 1985) concluded that 28% of all hospital inpatient days were associated with alcohol related or influenced conditions, and 31% of all deaths were estimated to be alcohol related. The significance and importance of an emphasis on the prevention of alcoholism seems further magnified by the findings of the recent Epidemiological Catchment Area Survey (Helzer, 1987) demonstrating the high prevalence of alcoholism relative to other mental disorders.

Stimulus reduction is a powerful means of eliciting changes in a variety of psychological and behavioral processes. Restricted Environmental Stimulation Therapy (REST) has outlived its misconstrued association with "sensory deprivation". Researchers are beginning to apply the technique to solving problems of individual human beings (Suedfeld, 1980). Several recent investigations have shown chamber REST in combination with educational messages to be dramatically efficacious in the treatment of a variety of severe habit disorders with varied etiologies, extended histories and poor prognoses. Some major breakthroughs have recently been achieved using single chamber REST sessions ranging from 6 - 24 hours duration.

REST has generated smoking abstinence rates of 53% in a one year follow up at the University of British Columbia (Best & Suedfeld, 1982), 47% abstinence at 19 months follow up at Harvard Medical School (A. Barabasz, Baer, Sheehan & M. Barabasz, 1985, 1986), and 87% abstinence at one year follow up in a clinical setting (Tikalsky, 1984). Suedfeld (1987) recently reported the scientific literature now shows 11 replications of the smoking abstinence data using chamber REST interventions. The best abstinence rates are associated with the 24 hour long REST sessions. In addition to these systematic attempts to use REST in the alteration of habits of non-institutionalized adults, there have been several additional studies. In general, these later studies represent a single foray into an area which was not followed up by further research. The results, in virtually all cases, were positive enough that further investigation seems warranted (Suedfeld, 1980).

The research on smoking has clear implications for the treatment of alcohol abuse (Suedfeld, 1980). While sensorially isolated rats chose to drink alcohol solution rather than pure water (Cole & Goldstein, 1971), isolated human subjects have demonstrated a suppression of alcohol use (A. Barabasz & M. Barabasz, 1971; Griffiths, Bigelow & Liebson, 1973; Lobb & Schaefer, 1971). In contrast to these findings, both social and environmental stimulation have been shown to increase human alcohol consumption (A. Barabasz & M. Barabasz, 1971; Bigelow, Cowen, Liebson & Faillace, 1972; Cowen, Liebson & Faillace, 1972; Griffiths, Bigelow & Liebson, 1973).

Two studies have established alcoholics' tolerance for REST. Jacobson (1971) demonstrated alcoholics to have no difficulty in tolerating one hour of monotonous stimulation. Dissatisfied with this short duration, Rank and Suedfeld (1978) used 8 hours of lying on a bed in a dark, sound attenuated chamber with 10 self-declared alcoholic volunteers. No data on Ss' alcohol consumption was collected, however, subjects indicated, on a variety of measures, that they found the experience to be quite pleasant. Interestingly, they indicated more frequent positive experiences and less frequent negative experiences than normal life. This finding suggests that REST may be as acceptable a treatment for alcohol abusers as it has been for other populations.

Adams, Cooper, and Scott (1987) employed chamber REST with early prodromal alcoholics (heavy social drinkers) and demonstrated promising results. The first study exposed male and female college students, meeting prodromal alcoholic criteria, to 2 1/2 hours of chamber REST. During the REST session, they were exposed to prerecorded anti-alcohol educational messages aimed at reducing alcohol consumption. After two weeks, their alcohol intake levels dropped significantly (more than 55%) from baseline levels. Control subjects showed no significant changes. In a replication of this study, experimental REST subjects heard a revised version of the most effective anti-alcohol message used in the initial study. Two weeks later, their alcohol intake dropped significantly (56%) from initial baseline levels. These reductions in alcohol intake were fully sustained at follow up 3 months and 6 months later. Untreated control subjects showed increased alcohol intake, increasing progressively and significantly, across the three data collection periods. The results of these pilot studies were fully supportive of earlier preliminary exploratory work using REST and alcohol intake reports among those who rated themselves as heavy social drinkers (Cooper, McGraw, Pasternak, Paznak & Adams, 1977).

Cognitive theory provides an explanation as to why chamber REST may be an effective means of initiating behavior change. The restriction of external stimulation forces the organism to increase his/her focus on internally generated material, including memories, awareness of problems, and ways of solving those problems (A. Barabasz, 1982; Robertson, 1961a,b; Schultz, 1965). As Suedfeld (1980) points out, material is normally kept from consciousness by the availability, urgency, and impact of environmental inputs. As the individual becomes more and more preoccupied with his/her own consciousness, the thoughts, emotions and residual stimuli become increasingly separated in context and other structural anchors. In REST one becomes less critical of any remaining input. If this input consists of educational messages, being less critical means being less defensive (Suedfeld, 1980; A. Barabasz, 1982). REST temporarily eliminates the bombardment of irrelevant stimuli, thus making relevant ones such as educational messages, more salient and more likely to be processed.

As noted above, the REST environment should also be relatively pleasant for alcoholics or prodromal alcoholics, since the stimulus overload that characterizes their experience in "normal conditions" is alleviated. Since REST has been shown to be a general disrupter of complex cognitive functioning (Suedfeld, 1972; Koslin, Pargament & Suedfeld, 1971), one may extrapolate that under such conditions it would have destabilizing effects on resistance to information such as that which occurs in the typical alcoholic defense mechanism of denial. REST brings about the "unfreezing" stage of the attitude change process (Suedfeld, 1980, 1969a; Tetlock & Suedfeld, 1976). Once an attitude structure is unfrozen to some extent, the individual is able to reevaluate without the distortions resulting from that structure and is more likely to change their behavior. Cognitive disorganization theory suggests that clients would be more likely to change or abandon attitudes supporting their unhealthy activities and, consequently, to abandon the self defeating activities themselves, when appropriate educational messages are presented in the REST situation (Suedfeld 1980).

The exciting and promising findings of the preliminary REST alcohol studies certainly seemed to warrant further research which considered the use of more typical chamber REST periods ranging from 6 to 24 hours as used in the fully replicated habit control studies (A. Barabasz, Baer, Sheehan & M. Barabasz, 1986; M. Barabasz, 1987b; Suedfeld, 1980, 1985, 1987; Tikalsky, 1984). Consistent with the level of sophistication evident in other current areas of REST investigation, alcohol studies should employ control conditions which include plausible procedures rather than simple no treatment conditions. Pre-post experimental dependency measures needed to be improved to provide data beyond simple self reports of alcohol intake. Emrick and Hanson (1983) argued for the use of multiple outcome data as measured by the Student Alcohol Questionnaire, Alcohol Attitude Questionnaire or the Alcohol Use Inventory. The present study was designed to address these methodological considerations.

Method

Subjects

At the present, 40 male and female volunteer subjects from a large northwestern university have provided complete data. Additional subjects were volunteering and others were due to provide follow-up data for the study at the time this report was prepared. Persons interested in volunteering for the study were asked to keep a log of the type, quantity and frequency of alcohol consumption over a 14-day period. Indices of quantity and frequency of alcohol consumption were calculated. Consistent with prodromal alcoholic criteria applied in the previous studies (Adams et al., 1987), students with moderate-heavy (three-four drinks at least once a week, or five or more drinks at least once a month) or heavy (five or more drinks more than once a week) (Engs, 1977; Werch & Gorman, 1988) levels of alcohol consumption were employed as subjects.

All subjects were asked to complete the Alcohol Use Inventory (AUI) (Wanberg & Horn, 1987). The AUI consists of 24 scales designed to measure patterns of behavior, attitudes, and symptoms pertaining to the use of alcohol. The Alcohol Use Inventory (AUI) is based on an empirically supported theory that distinct conditions are found among persons broadly considered alcoholic. The AUI provides a basis for describing different ways in which individuals use alcohol, major benefits derived from such use, the negative consequences associated with its use, and the degree of concern individuals express about the use and consequences of using alcohol. It is considered useful in identifying and understanding different types of individuals with alcohol problems. Since it provides reliably independent measures of distinct features of alcohol use it may help identify Ss' characteristics associated with differential benefits from exposure to REST.

Apparatus

The REST chamber is sound attenuated with 10 cm. of Dow-Corning sound proofing material on wall and double door surfaces. Dimensions of the chamber are L=3 meters, W=1.7 meters, H=2.4 meters. It is equipped with a bed, intercommunications system, lighting, video camera, and a silent positive pressure ventilation system. Consistent with previous investigations (A. Barabasz, 1982; A. Barabasz & M. Barabasz, 1990; A. Barabasz & Kaplan, 1989), REST Ss wore Ganzfeld goggles. Low level white noise provided by a Lafayette 15011 white noise generator served as a masking sound. All Ss wore 26 decibel wax ear plugs.

The chamber is equipped with a portable toilet which is situated so as to provide complete privacy for the subject. Subjects' nutritional needs were met by providing liquid food and water in thermos bottles (Suedfeld, 1980). This avoided the auditory, tactile, and kinesthetic input from unwrapping, handling, and chewing the food. Free access to the food and water was available through plastic tube "straws" that ran from each thermos and were attached to the bed sheet near the pillow.

Procedure

Consistent with current REST methodology (Suedfeld, 1980, p. 377), Ss were given a "full orientation to the chamber coupled with detailed reassuring instructions administered by calm and supportive personnel prior to the day each subject is scheduled for REST."

Group 1 Ss (n=8) were exposed to three hours of chamber REST. Group 2 Ss (n=8) were exposed to six hours of chamber REST. Group 3 Ss (n=9) were exposed to 12 hours of chamber REST. Group 4 Ss (n=6) were exposed to 24 hours of chamber REST. Preliminary studies demonstrated significant decreases in alcohol consumption following exposure to one 2 1/2 hour chamber REST session (Adams, Cooper & Scott, 1987), however, Suedfeld (1980) notes exposure to 24 hours of REST has been demonstrated to be the most effective in application to other habit disorders. This study was intended to compare alternative lengths of exposure to Chamber REST.

Group 5 Ss (Controls) (n=9) spent three hours in the REST Chamber but normal levels of stimulation were maintained. The Ganzfeld goggles and earplugs were not used. Only one of the double doors was closed. Normal outside noise levels were maintained in the chamber via an open intercom hidden in the ventilator (Barabasz & Barabasz, 1989). The bed was removed. A radio and variety of reading/ study materials were provided. Social contact was maintained by Es' entry to the chamber every 45 minutes "to see how things are going."

On the day of their exposure to the treatment or control condition, Ss were reoriented to the chamber according to the procedure outlined by Suedfeld (1980, pp. 377-380).

Consistent with human subject guidelines, each S was reminded that he or she was free to terminate the session at any time. Once comfortable on the REST chamber bed, experimental Ss were asked to restrict movement to the minimum required to maintain comfort. Control Ss were not asked to restrict movement.

The following instructions were read over the intercommunications system to all subjects (adapted from Barabasz, 1982, p. 151).

> Please feel free to tell me whatever you want about your reactions to this session. Your experiences will be helpful in understanding the results of the study. Whatever you choose to talk about will, of course, be kept confidential. Since it is contrary to thc purpose of the REST session, I will not engage in conversation with you, in response to your remarks over the intercommunication system. During the session an educational message will be read to you which is designed to help you achieve your desired goal of decreased alcohol intake. You may request repetitions of this message by pressing the button. Try not to sleep during the session, but it you should doze off, don't feel guilty about it. Do you have any questions?

After answering any questions, the monitor read a standard set of relaxation instructions (Suedfeld, 1980) consistent with standardized chamber REST procedures.

Ss were monitored continuously. Research assistant monitors were trained in the criteria developed by Sanders and Reyher (1969) which indicate when REST should be terminated. These criteria have been successfully employed by these investigators (Barabasz, 1982; Barabasz & Barabasz, 1989). There was no need to terminate a REST session in this study on the basis of Sander's & Reyher's (1969) criteria. One subject requested termination of his 24 hour session at 22 hours.

At the midpoint of each session the following message was read to Ss over the intercommunication system:

> Alcohol use in the U.S. is a major public health problem. Ten million hard core alcoholics and thirty million problem drinkers far outnumber all other dangerous drug abusers combined. The association of alcoholism with crimes of violence is far greater than that of hard narcotics users. Alcoholics represent 20% to 30% of first admissions to psychiatric hospitals and are responsible for 50% of traffic fatalities. Alcoholics drain more than fifteen billion dollars a year from the economy.
>
> Although alcoholism is often described as a lower class vice, two-thirds of our alcoholics and problem drinkers come from conventional middle class backgrounds. Most began with casual social drinking; many had good jobs and were respected by families and co-workers alike. In spite of their many strengths and assets, alcohol abuse unmasks in the users many unattractive character traits. The typical alcoholic is an expert in self-deception, denying the extent of alcohol dependency and revealing qualities of maudlin sentimentality, selfish dependency, and thoughtless hostility. As these traits become more pronounced, friends and family are coerced into becoming unwilling accomplices in covering up the alcoholic's deterioration and postponing the day he or she must admit to this weakness and self-indulgence.
>
> In later stages, sympathy turns to disgust and rejection. The alcoholic continues to kid himself (for males), herself (for females), blaming his/her drinking on the nagging and misunderstanding of family and former friends, rather than seeing the loss of friendships and support as the consequence of self-destructive alcohol abuse. By the time alcoholics bottom out and are willing to admit that drinking and its consequences are their own self-created problems, loss of job, breakup of family, and damage to kidneys, liver, pancreas, and brain leave very little to rehabilitate.
>
> The typical alcoholic begins to drink in his/her late teens or early twenties. The alcoholic drinks socially for ten years and

> abuses alcohol as a problem drinker for another ten years. Finally, in his late forties or early fifties, he or she begins to lose control every time a drink is taken, ushering in the full alcoholic syndrome. From this time deterioration is rapid and, without treatment, death will occur eight years earlier than his or her normal life span. For any friends and family who are still around to watch, the death of the personality seems to precede by years the final collapse of the body. Alcohol abuse accomplishes its work slowly it fully deserves its reputation as our most dangerous drug. (Adams, Cooper & Scott, 1987).

Following termination of the treatment or control session, Ss met with one of the primary investigators to discuss their experience.

Subjects were asked to log their alcohol consumption (type, quantity and frequency) during the subsequent 14 days. At 3 months, 6 months and 12 months following treatment, Ss were asked again to log their alcohol consumption (type, quantity and frequency) for a period of 14 days. At the 6 month follow-up Ss were asked to complete the AUI.

Results

Alcohol log data (14 days each), converted to absolute total ounces of alcohol per data collection period, have been analyzed using the complete data for pre-treatment, immediate post treatment, 3 month and 6 month follow-ups for control (n=9), 3 hour REST (n=8), 6 hour REST (n=8), 12 hour REST (n=9) and 24 hour REST (n=6) groups. A between-within groups split plot ANOVA was not significant for the control group, 3 hour REST group or 6 hour REST group for any of the data collection periods. The results for the 12 and 24 hour REST sessions contrast dramatically with those of the other treatment conditions. Univariate ANOVA's for Ss exposed to 12 hours of REST showed a significant reduction in alcohol intake following REST (pre M = 30 oz. S.D. = 22.3, vs post M = 16.3 oz., S.D. = 14.99, F = 6.4, $p < .03$) and at the 3 month follow-up (pre M = 30 oz., S.D. = 22.3 vs 3 mo. M = 15.9, S.D. = 15.1, F = 7.5, $p < .02$). At the 6 month follow-up, the mean alcohol consumption was still lower but an increase in variance (some Ss dropped alcohol consumption to zero while others returned to baseline) precluded significance (pre M = 30, S.D. = 22.3, vs 6 mo. M = 14.6, S.D. = 19.5, F = 4.0, p < .07).

Despite an N of only 6, the 24 hour REST session generated even more dramatic results, both statistically and clinically, at immediate post-treatment (pre M = 40.7 oz., S.D. = 17.8, vs post M = 23.3, S.D. = 25.6, F = 9.87, p < .025) at the 3 month follow-up (pre M = 40.7 oz., S.D. = 17.8 vs 3 mo. M = 16 oz., S.D. = 22.6, F = 18.0, p < .008) and at the 6 month follow-up (pre M = 40.7, S.D. = 17.8, vs 6 mo. M = 12.7, S.D. = 19.9, F = 29.0, P < .003). The clinical significance of these alcohol consumption reductions over time is demonstrated in Figure 18-1.

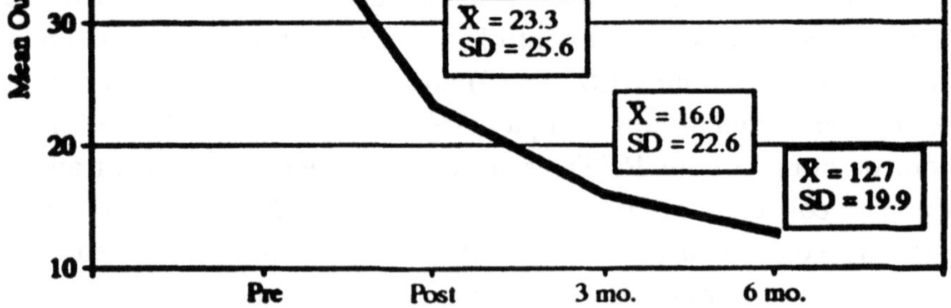

Figure 18-1. Alcohol intake reductions after 24 hours of REST.

The reduction in alcohol consumption at the three follow-up periods is consistent with 24 hour REST interventions for obesity. Borrie and Suedfeld (1980) found support for the durability of REST with educational messages in behavior change. At the three month follow-up, REST with educational messages was found to be twice as effective as REST without educational messages or control conditions with, or without educational messages while at the six month follow-up it was three times as effective.

The findings of this preliminary investigation seem to support Suedfeld's (1980) formulation of cognitive disorganization theory as a foundation as to why REST with educational messages is a profoundly effective means of producing behavior change. Independent post experimental inquiry data, to date, also support the plausibility of the non-REST and shorter duration REST interventions as active treatments. The exciting and remarkably strong findings would certainly seem to warrant further investigation.

Acknowledgment

This investigation was supported in part, by funds provided for Alcohol and Drug Abuse Research by the State of Washington Initiative Measure #171.

19

Psychophysiological Comparisons of REST and Hypnosis: Implications for Future Research

Helen Crawford

Although one would not equate Restricted Environmental Stimulation Technique (REST) and hypnosis, a consideration of the similarities between the two and the resulting experiential phenomena may permit us better to understand individual differences in cognitive and physiological functioning in the two conditions. Such an evaluation may sensitize us to experimental and theoretical issues that can be addressed in future research. In both REST and hypnosis there is typically a decrease in external stimuli with a redirection towards internal stimuli or more narrowly focused external stimuli (A. Barabasz, 1982; J. Hilgard, 1979). The hypnotic experience usually occurs in a quiet room with another individual (the hypnotist) if it is heterohypnosis, or alone if it is self hypnosis. By contrast, the REST experience occurs in controlled environments that strive for a dramatic reduction of external stimuli by attenuating light and sound in a temperature-controlled flotation tank or chamber. In addition, the REST experience all but eliminates interpersonal contact for various lengths of time. The REST experience may be much longer in duration, from 1 to 24 hours, than the typical hypnotic experience which is usually one hour or less.

A review of the common experiential reports in the two conditions reveals several similar phenomena (A. Barabasz, 1990). There are major shifts in focusing of attention from external to internal stimuli, with possible accompanying shifts in attentional processes (e.g., changes in focused and sustained attention). Individuals often report substantial increases in internally generated stimuli (fantasies, thoughts, etc.) that internally are more vivid and involving. These may be accompanied by a decrease in generalized reality testing. For certain individuals there is a shift in cognitive processing strategies away from analytic, sequential and verbal thought processes and towards more nonanalytical, holistic and imaginal thought processes. Suggestibility is temporarily enhanced following hypnotic inductions (for review, see E. R. Hilgard, 1965) and sensory isolation (Zubek, 1973). For instance, enhanced suggestibility has been reported after wintering-over isolation in the Antarctica (A. Barabasz, 1980), laboratory (A. Barabasz, 1982), and clinical REST conditions (A. Barabasz & M. Barabasz, 1989). Flotation REST appears to potentiate suggestibility in hypnotically responsive individuals (A. Barabasz, 1990c,e), whereas the longer lasting Chamber REST may enhance suggestibility regardless of prior hypnotic susceptibility level (A. Barabasz, 1982; A. Barabasz & Kaplan, 1989). Enhanced responsiveness to suggestions has been demonstrated after several months of wintering-over, in the dark isolation of Antarctica (A. Barabasz, 1980a), but did not occur after a brief summer Antarctic isolation experience with 24 hours of daylight per day (M. Barabasz, A. Barabasz, & Mullin, 1983). Such isolation experiences may reactivate or potentiate already existing mental processes that are associated with imaginative involvement, and thereby lead to greater suggestibility (A. Barabasz, 1984).

In general, REST researchers have not evaluated the importance of moderating factors such as specific personality and cognitive traits or styles on the types of REST experiences reported, however, there are a few exceptions (A. Barabasz, 1990b,c; A. Barabasz & M. Barbasz, 1992). By contrast, most hypnosis researchers emphasize the importance of the trait of hypnotic susceptibility and correlated cognitive abilities, such as absorption, sustained attention, and imagery vividness, as major moderators of experiential shifts and shifts in attentional and cognitive processing following a hypnotic induction (e.g., for reviews, see Crawford, 1982, 1989; Hilgard, 1965; Sheehan, 1979). While hypnotic susceptibility may be considered an isolated personality/cognitive trait, our research argues that it is representative of a more pervasive and important underlying individual difference that moderates performance and experiences in numerous situations.

REST and hypnosis researchers should be attentive to the moderating effects of individual differences in cognitive flexibility. Cognitive flexibility is "the degree to which an individual has and uses one or several available types of information processing strategies or styles during different tasks (Battig, 1979), as well as different states of awareness" (Crawford, 1989, p. 155). Our research (e.g., Crawford, 1982, 1989; Crawford & Allen, 1983) supports the hypothesis that highly hypnotizable individuals have greater cognitive flexibility than do low hypnotizable individuals, as assessed on standardized scales of hypnotic susceptibility. Highs can shift with greater ease from one cognitive strategy to another, and from one state of awareness to another. They shift more easily from reality to nonreality, and from analytic, detail-oriented processing to nonanalytic, holistic, and imaginal processing strategies. They shift more easily not only from waking to hypnosis, but also from waking to sleep (e.g., Evans, 1979). Similarly, highly hypnotizable individuals also shift more easily into altered states of awareness during REST (A. Barabasz, 1983, 1984a, 1990c; A. Barabasz & M. Barabasz, 1992; M. Barabasz, A. Barabasz, & Mullin, 1983).

During hypnosis highly hypnotizable subjects demonstrate substantially greater cognitive and perceptual changes than do low hypnotizables. For instance, enhanced imaginal processing of information, particularly when the information to be remembered is literal or untransformed representations, has been shown to occur during hypnosis among hypnotically susceptible individuals in visual memory studies (e.g., Crawford & Allen, 1983; Crawford, Nomura, & Slater, 1983; Crawford, Wallace, Nomura, & Slater, 1986; Wallace, 1978). There are shifts toward more holistic and imaginal processing strategies during hypnosis in hypnotically susceptibile individuals (e.g., Crawford, 1989; Crawford & Allen, 1983). While individuals who are responsive to hypnosis demonstrate greater skills in sustained and focused attention (e.g., Crawford, Brown, & Moon, 1991; Tellegen & Atkinson, 1974), increases in vigilant or focused performance during hypnosis have been reported inconsistently (e.g., Atkinson, 1991; Fehr & Stern, 1967; Kissen, Reifler, & Thaler, 1964). Thus, based upon this research and other studies not reviewed herein, it is proposed that hypnotic susceptibility level could moderate changes in cognitive and perceptual performance observed in REST contexts, and is worthy of further investigation.

Given the evidenced enhanced imagery and holistic processing that occurs during hypnosis, a commonly espoused hypothesis since the 1970s is that hypnosis involves greater right-hemisphere involvement. Attempts to identify possible electrocortical correlates of hypnosis as moderated by hypnotic susceptibility have produced quite mixed findings (Barabasz & Lonsdale, 1983; Crawford, 1991; Sabourin, 1982; Sabourin, Cutcomb, Crawford, & Pribram, 1990; Sarbin & Sable, 1979). Recently, with more sophisticated methodology and instrumentation, there is growing evidence that there are 1) psychophysiological differences between low and highly hypnotizable individuals, and 2) psychophysiological differences between waking and hypnosis conditions that are moderated by hypnotic susceptibility level. Some of the findings directly relevant to REST researchers are discussed below.

A surprisingly robust finding is the occurrence of differences in characteristic patterns of electrocortical (EEG) hemispheric arousal associated with hypnotic susceptibility. In the waking condition highly hypnotizable individuals sometimes show greater EEG hemispheric specificity in the alpha band or overall total power at several bipolar recording sites: their EEGs are more activated in the left hemisphere when doing analytical tasks such as math, while more activated in the right hemisphere when doing holistic, visuospatial tasks (DePascalis & Palumbo, 1986; DePascalis, Silveri, & Palumbo, 1988; Karlin, Goldstein, Cohen, & Morgan, 1980; MacLeod-Morgan & Lack, 1982; Meszaros, Banyai, & Greguss, 1985). Differential bipolar fronto-central and parieto-occipital asymmetries in low and high alpha bands during waking and hypnosis have been reported for low and high hypnotizables during rest, math, and imaginal tasks (Crawford, 1989; Meszaros,

Crawford, Szabo, Nagy-Kovacs, & Revesz, 1989). Sabourin et al., (1990) found during waking rest conditions, hypnosis rest, and suggestion conditions highly hypnotizable subjects generated substantially more beta power in the left hemisphere than in the right hemisphere at frontal, central and occipital monopolar recording sites. Low hypnotizable subjects showed no significant beta asymmetry in the left and right hemisphere recording locations. In a study of induced happy and sad emotional memories during waking and hypnosis, Crawford, Clarke, Kitner-Triolo, and Olesko (1989) found that highly hypnotizable subjects had substantially more right hemispheric power, while low hypnotizable subjects showed no significant asymmetry, in high theta, low and high alpha, and low and medium beta Hz bands. Thus, we have evidence that the trait of hypnotic susceptibility can moderate the degree of EEG asymmetries in varying EEG Hz bands during cognitive processing. Such research suggests that highly hypnotizable individuals may show greater EEG hemispheric asymmetries, with a greater capacity to shift hemispheric dominance across tasks, due to their greater attentional absorption in the tasks at hand. Much more research must be carried out in order to understand fully the generalizability of these findings and their theoretical implications.

During hypnosis, shifts towards greater right hemisphere relative to left hemisphere involvement have been suggested in studies of bipolar derivations of occipito-parietal alpha (MacLeod-Morgan, 1982), occipito-temporal total power (Karlin, Cohen, & Goldstein, 1982; LaBriola, Karlin, & Goldstein, 1987), and fronto-occipital alpha and beta (Banyai, Meszaros, & Csokay, 1985; Meszaros et al., 1985). However, the use of laterality ratios in these studies can be criticized since the relative contribution of left and right hemisphere activity cannot be determined (e.g., Beaumont, Young, & McManus, 1984). Thus, more recent studies include hemisphere as a factor in their analyses. Chen, Dworkin, and Bloomquist (1981) reported total energy output of both left and right hemispheres at fronto-parietal locations to decrease, with a greater decrease in the left hemisphere in theta and alpha bands, in a patient who was undergoing dental surgery with hypnosis as the sole anesthetic. Crawford, Meszaros, and their associates (Crawford, 1989; Meszaros et al., 1989) found alpha and beta power increases in the right parieto-occipital location during hypnosis in rest, math and imaginal tasks in high, but not low, hypnotizable individuals. By contrast, monopolar recordings during rest and hypnotic suggestions (Barabasz & Lonsdale, 1983; Sabourin et al., 1990) and during induced sad and happy emotional states (Crawford et al., 1989) found no hemispheric shifts in power at anterior, central, and posterior (parietal or occipital) locations.

Research from electrodermal (skin conductance), haptic, electrocortical and divided visual field studies demonstrates that both the left and right hemispheres are involved in shifts from waking to hypnosis in hypnotically responsive individuals (e.g., Gruzelier, 1987, 1990; Gruzelier, Brow, Perry, Rhonder, & Thomas, 1984; Gruzelier, Thomas, Brow, Conway, Golds, Jutai, Liddiard, McCormack, Perry & Rhonder, 1987). Such research suggests that at the very first the focal attentional processes of the left hemisphere are engaged and then there is selective inhibition of the left hemisphere as planning functions and reality testing decrease when an individual enters hypnosis. Subsequently there is an increased engagement of the right hemisphere which "coincides with the emergence of primary process thinking, visual imagery, sensory memory and hyperamnesia" (Gruzelier et al., 1987, pp. 15-16). A final stage is entered if there are specific cognitive demands during hypnosis. Gruzelier (1990) reported neuropsychological test evidence for the hypothesis that during hypnosis in hypnotically responsive individuals, the left anterior region of the brain is inhibited while activation of the right posterior region is increased. This is supportive of earlier research (e.g., Crawford, 1989; Meszaros et al., 1989) suggesting a greater involvement of the right parietal region which has been associated with imaginal processing (e.g., Farah, 1988). Such research findings provide quite testable hypotheses about the localization of brain activation patterns which future research can investigate. Such research will clarify our understanding of underlying neurophysiological correlates of hypnosis as moderated by hypnotic susceptibility level and other cognitive abilities.

Hypnosis may involve enhanced cognitive effort even though an individual shows greater muscle relaxation. Crawford, Skolnick, Gur, Benson, and Gur (1986; see also Crawford, 1989) studied the effects of rest, ischemic pain without suggested analgesia, and ischemic pain with suggested analgesia in conditions of waking and hypnosis upon regional cerebral blood flow as measured by the xenon inhalation method. Low and high hypnotizables had similar regional cerebral blood flow metabolism patterns during waking conditions, regardless of pain or not. While low hypnotizables had essentially the same pattern across frontal, temporal, parietal and parieto-temporal regions in waking and hypnosis, highs showed dramatic shifts. High hypnotizables showed increases from 13% to 28%. The highest shifts in regional cerebral blood flow were in the temporal regions of both hemispheres, during hypnotic rest, and pain with and without suggested analgesia conditions during hypnosis. We believe that the enhanced cerebral metabolism is reflective of the enhanced cognitive effort and absorption that accompanies hypnosis in highly responsive individuals.

Increments in theta (approximately 3 to 7 Hz) EEG activity are associated with many problem-solving, perceptual processing and cognitive tasks, as well as with the production of imagery (Schacter, 1977). This is interpreted as representing what Vogel, Broverman, and Klaiber (1968, p. 172) refer to as "Class II inhibition", which is associated with attentive performance and represents "a selective inactivation of particular responses so that a continuing excitatory state becomes directed or patterned". This state is in contrast with "Class I inhibition", associated with general inactivity or drowsiness. Interestingly, highly hypnotizable individuals generate more mean theta power than low hypnotizable individuals, often in both waking and hypnosis (e.g., Galbraith, London, Leibovitz, Cooper, & Hart, 1970; Tebecis, Provins, Farbach, & Pentony, 1975; Sabourin et al., 1990; Ulett, Akpinar, & Itil, 1972) which may be reflective of their greater absorptive and sustained attentional abilities. In a study of waking rest, hypnotic rest, and hypnotic suggestions, Sabourin et al. (1990) found that stringently screened, highly hypnotizable individuals generated substantially more mean theta power than lows at occipital, central, and frontal locations (See Figure 19-1). Both low and high hypnotizable subjects showed a substantial increase in mean theta power during hypnosis, although highs continued to generate more power than lows. Similar enhancements in theta power have been reported during

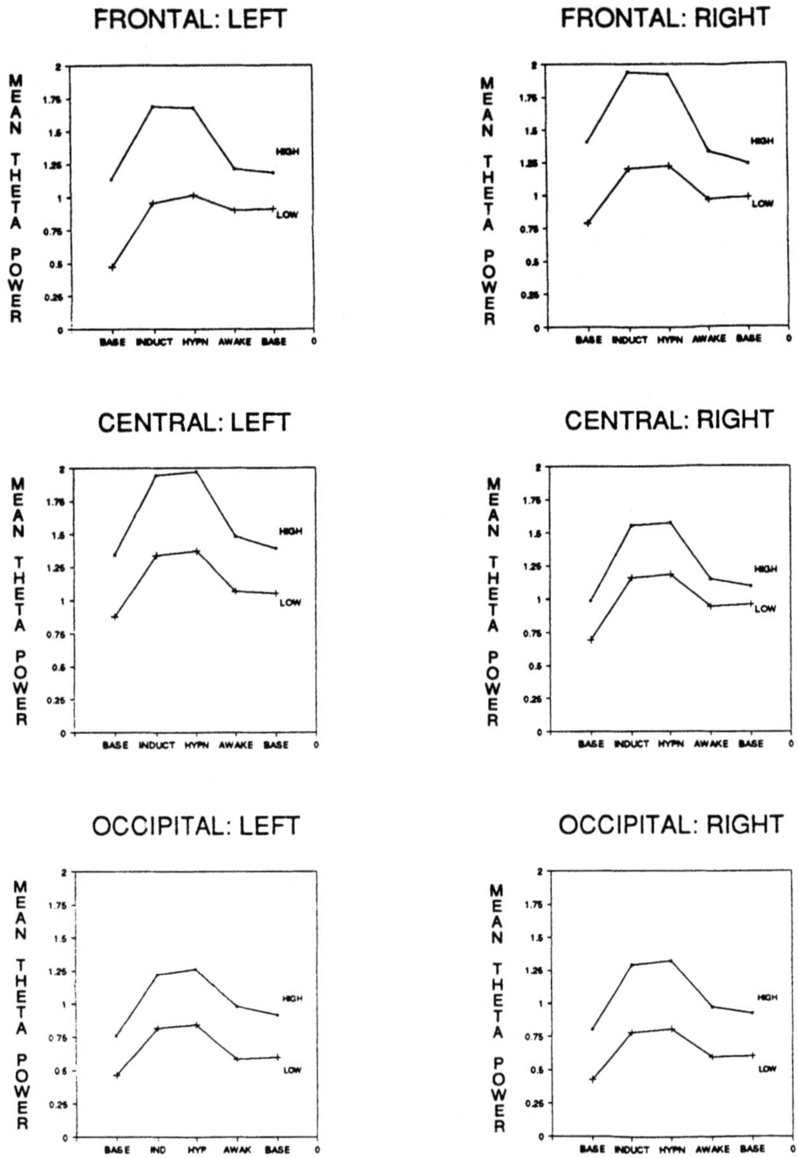

Figure 19-1. Mean power for theta band: Comparison of low and high hypnotizables during waking rest, hypnosis rest, and hypnotic suggestions (adapted from Sabourin et al., 1990).

sustained, quiescent meditative states in experienced meditators (e.g., Banquet, 1973; Corby, Roth, Zarcone, & Kopell, 1978; Hebert & Lehmann, 1979; Saletu, 1987; Taneli & Krahne, 1987). A. Barabasz (1990b) reported significant enhancements of theta power after exposure to one hour of flotation REST. Most interesting, and consistent with our own work, the theta power increase occurred only in highly hypnotizable individuals.

Hypnotically responsive individuals who can eliminate the perception of pain through suggestion generate substantially more theta power than those who cannot control pain (Larbig et al., 1982; Crawford, 1990a,b). Larbig et al. (1982) reported that an Indian fakir generated substantially more theta at a parietal location (Pz), but not at a vertex location (Cz) on the scalp, in comparison to controls during pain control conditions. Crawford (1990a,b, 1991) studied low and high hypnotizable subjects who were stringently screened for hypnotizability level. They were trained in a two-hour session to reduce pain when placing their left arm into ice cold water for 60 second dips. To participate in the final pilot study high hypnotizables had to be able to eliminate completely all perception of pain during this preliminary session. Monopolar recordings at frontal, temporal, parietal and occipital regions with references to balanced earlobes were obtained in counterbalanced conditions of waking and hypnosis with the following experimental manipulations: prerest baseline, pain dip with no analgesia, suggested analgesia without pain, suggested analgesia with pain dip, and postrest baseline. Only the hypnosis findings are reported here. As anticipated, the four highly hypnotizable subjects exhibited significantly greater power than the lows within the high theta range (5.5 - 7.5 Hz). The most clear and fascinating results are found in a comparison of hypnotic pain dips with and without suggested analgesia, as is shown in Figure 19-2. During pain and suggested analgesia dips, the seven low hypnotizable subjects showed no significant theta power asymmetries between the left and right hemispheres at frontal, temporal, parietal, and occipital locations, whereas the highs did in certain locations. Particularly in the temporal locations, but also in the parietal locations, the highs were significantly more left hemisphere dominant in the pain dip when they were experiencing pain, and then

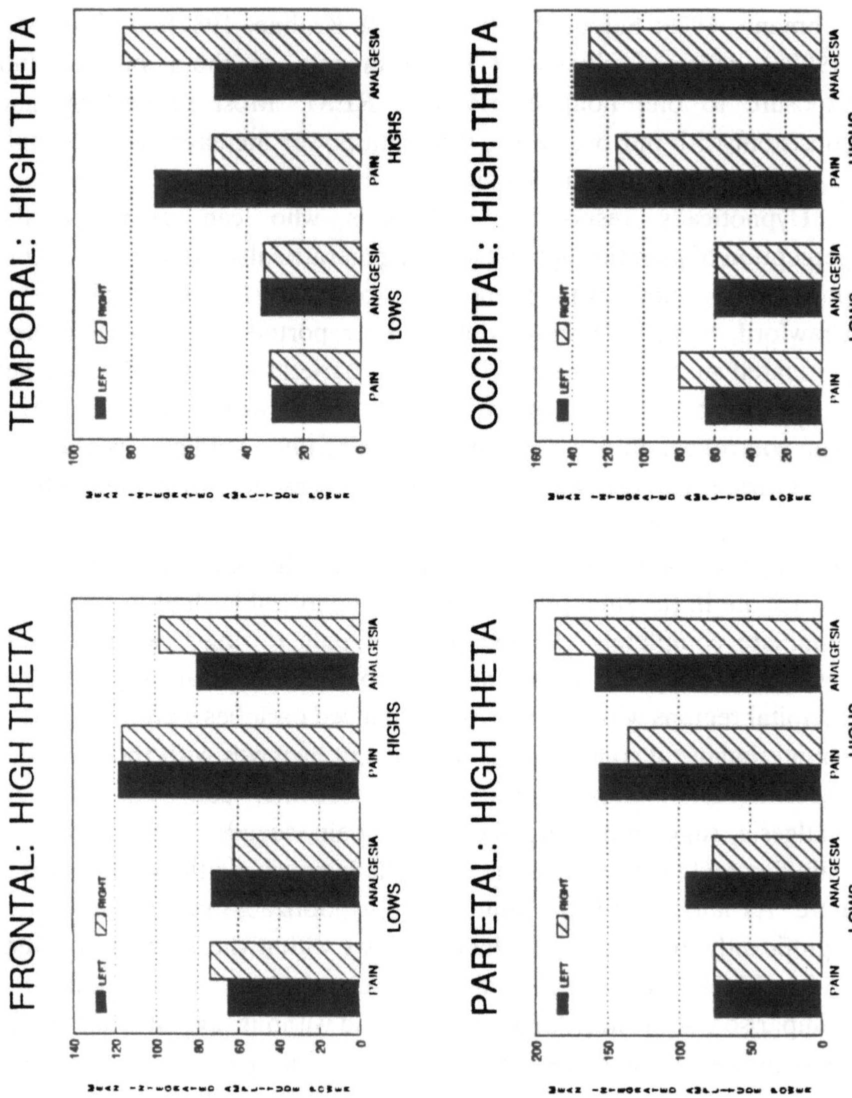

Figure 19-2. Mean power for high theta (5.5 - 7.5 Hz) band: Comparison of low and high hypnotizables during cold pressor pain and hypnotic analgesia.

showed a significant decrease in left-hemisphere theta power and a significant increase in right-hemisphere theta power during hypnotic analgesia. These dramatic shifts in hemispheric dominance appear to be correlative of different attentional states: attend to versus disattend to noxious stimuli. Thus, they may represent underlying neurophysiological shifts in the fronto-septo-hippocampal system which may be involved in selective attention and disattention mechanisms accompanying sustained attentional activities.

Only further research will delineate the relationships between theta (and other EEG Hz bands) and cognitive and attentional performance. Such work is important to REST, hypnosis, and meditation researchers--as well as to those involved in attention research in both applied and experimental situations. At both applied and theoretical levels, it is extremely important that we determine under what conditions theta power is associated with enhanced attentional and cognitive effort, as well as enhanced performance. The importance of hemispheric shifts in theta power accompanying task performance has only recently been noted (Crawford, 1990a,b, 1991) and must be clarified. Finally, we need to investigate how individual differences in sustained and divided attentional skills, as well as hypnotic susceptibility and possibly other cognitive abilities, moderate overall theta power, as well as hemispheric specificity and shifts in hemispheric dominance.

Until now, studies of the EEG responses to the REST experience have been quite limited in scope, often have been handscored rather than spectral analyzed with computerized techniques, and have not considered the moderating factors of hypnotic susceptibility level, attentional, or other cognitive abilities. Zubek (1969b) suggested that there was a progressive slowing of alpha, but more recent REST studies (Barabasz, 1979, 1980a, 1982; A. Barabasz & M. Barabasz, 1985) emphasizing a reduction in anxiety producing experimental cues (Suedfeld, 1980), have demonstrated a consistently significant increase in EEG alpha density from pre- to post-REST that was not progressive. Rather, mid-REST EEG alpha densities (8.5 to 12.5 Hz) were significantly lower than pre- and post-REST levels. More recent work by Barabasz (1990b) reported increases of theta power after one hour of flotation REST. Whether the chamber and flotation restricted environmental stimulation techniques produce different attentional states in a subject has yet to be investigated thoroughly.

In conclusion, it can be said that we are only now beginning to reap the fruits from combining cognitive and physiological research in the fields of REST and hypnosis. It is clear that individual differences in cognitive flexibility, attentional processing and hypnotic susceptibility play important moderating roles in cognitive performance and experiential phenomena in both flotation and chamber REST as well as hypnosis contexts.

Acknowledgment

Portions of the research reported herein were supported by grants from The Spencer Foundation and a NIH Biomedical Grant to Helen Crawford.

20

REST in the Treatment of Persistent Psychophysiological Insomnia

Elizabeth Ballard

Every year between 33% and 42% of adults experience insomnia (Bixler, Kales, Soldatos, Kales, & Healy, 1979; Mellinger, Balter, & Uhlenhuth, 1985). The inability to get adequate sleep is a symptom that can be either primary or secondary in nature. Seven of nine subclasses are considered secondary. Only two are thought of as primary insomnias; that is, insomnias with no obvious underlying cause, such as a medical or psychiatric condition (Association of Sleep Disorder Centers [ASDC], 1979). The second most common insomnia to be treated is "persistent, psychophysiological insomnia" (Coleman, Roffwarg, & Kennedy et al., 1982).

Patients who suffer persistent, psychophysiological insomnia are characterized as having chronic, somatized tension-anxiety as well as negative conditioning in their normal sleep environment. The tension and anxiety are generally experienced as "restlessness, motor tension, . . . automatic hyperactivity, apprehensive expectation, ruminative thoughts, hypervigilance, and excessive visual scanning" (ASDC, 1979, p. 24).

These characteristics make persistent, psychophysiological insomnia amenable to treatments that incorporate relaxation therapies. Behavioural treatments such as progressive muscle relaxation or autogenic training disrupt the cognitive ruminations, and focus attention on sleep-inducing stimuli. Research shows that these treatments have been successful in easing the somatized tension-anxiety and in reducing the conditioned arousal associated with persistent, psychophysiological insomnia (Borkovec, 1982; Borkovec & Hennings, 1978; Nicassio & Bootzin, 1974; Van Oot, Lane, & Borkovec, 1983; Woolfolk, Carr-Kaffashan, McNulty, & Lehrer, 1976). It appears that the common element in the relaxation therapies is their ability to distract attention from the racing thoughts. Patients learn to focus on pleasant, soothing sensations and calm mental representations (Borkovec, 1982).

REST researchers are familiar with the relaxation properties associated with flotation REST. For example, floaters in research facilities experienced a significant decrease in plasma cortisol (Turner & Fine, 1983), and achieved significant decreases in blood pressure, plasma levels of aldosterone, renin, and urinary cortisol (Turner, Fine, McGrady, & Higgins, 1987). Hypertensives showed that flotation REST led to clinically significant decreases in both systolic and diastolic blood pressure.

Self-report data support the same conclusion. Floaters at a commercial facility significantly decreased their subjective feelings of stress and reported feeling calm, still, at rest, alert, and acquiescent after flotation REST (Suedfeld, Ballard, & Murphy, 1983). Normotensives, who floated multiple times and heard a guided relaxation exercise showed both subjective and objective signs of improved relaxation. They felt deeply relaxed. Their systolic and diastolic blood pressure decreased significantly more than subjects who only heard the guided relaxation tape multiple times (Jacobs, Heilbronner, & Stanley, 1984).

These REST studies demonstrate that flotation REST is effective in assisting individuals to experience deep relaxation, psychological calmness, and decreases in blood pressure and adrenal hormones. These features suggest that flotation REST might be an effective treatment for persistent, psychophysiological insomnia.

This study attempted to address the methodological shortcomings of earlier research. First, both subjective and objective sleep data were collected. Second, this study focused on long-term (rather than immediate) therapeutic efficacy. Third, to increase generalizability, participants were recruited from the community at large. And finally, to avoid confounding primary and secondary symptomatology only one subclass of insomnia was treated.

The purpose of this study was to test the long-term efficacy of flotation REST as a treatment for persistent, psychophysiological insomnia. The major questions addressed by the research were: 1) Is flotation REST effective in decreasing sleep latency over the long term? 2) Is flotation REST as effective as autogenic relaxation in reducing sleep latency?

Method

Subjects - Volunteers who: a) were between the ages of 19 and 45 years; b) were receiving neither medication nor therapy for either a medical or psychiatric disorder; c) estimated regularly taking an hour or more to fall asleep; and d) did not work shifts, were recruited from the community via newspaper, television, and radio advertisements to participate in a free insomnia treatment study. Two screenings (over the phone and by a clinician at the Sleep Disorders Clinic) took place to assure that the volunteers met the Association of Sleep Centers' (1979) criteria for persistent, psychophysiological insomnia.

The final sample of 20 women and 16 men ranged in age from 24 to 44 years, with a mean of 33 years. The group's mean duration of insomnia was 15 years. Prior to treatment, sleep onset latency means and standard deviations for the sample were self-reported as 67 (32) minutes but objectively measured as 50 (28) minutes.

The Relaxation Environments and Autogenic Relaxation Exercise

Tank - The Float-to-Relax Brand flotation tank resembled a large, enclosed, fiberglass bathtub. A sliding door in the top half allowed easy opening from both inside and outside the tank. The inner dimensions were approximately 2.4 m. long by 1.2 m. wide by 1.2 m. high. The tank was filled to a depth of about 30 cm. with a solution of water and $MgSO_4$ with a specific gravity of approximately 1.26 and a temperature of 34° C. An intercom outside the tank allowed auditory monitoring of the floater and voice communication with the experimenter. Speakers for playing tape-recorded material were housed in the tank's shell.

The REST chamber was a quiet, dimly lit room manufactured by the Industrial Acoustics Corporation. The walls and ceiling were sound absorbent. To add to the restful ambience, the floor was carpeted and a large landscape poster hung. A speaker and intercom were attached to the wall just behind the head of the bed. During the autogenic relaxation treatment sessions the door was closed and the participant was instructed to remove shoes, eyeglasses, large pieces of jewelry, and to loosen tight clothing before reclining on the bed which was made up with a pillow, fresh linens, blankets, and a comforter.

Budzynski's (1974) script (30 minutes) for the autogenic relaxation exercise was used. Key phrases focused on the arms and legs feeling heavy and warm. One, audio taped, version was for use in the REST chamber and the other, amended slightly for use in the REST tank.

Sleep Monitoring Instruments

Subjective - Pollak's (1979) sleep log was used to estimate sleep latency and sleep duration reports.

The SOMTRAK (Farrell Instruments Co.), or sleep assessment device (SAD) consisted of a timing device and an adjustable tone generator attached to a cassette tape recorder. Just before going to bed on each night of use, the participant recorded the time and date, then pushed the "start timing" button. The controls were set so that the first one-second tone would go off 10 minutes after starting time and then every 10 minutes throughout the night. Immediately prior to the tone, the tape recorder would begin recording for a 10-second period. If the person was awake and heard the tone, a response of "Hello" or "I'm awake" was given during the 10-second recording time. The tape was transcribed and coded for sleep latency and for total sleep duration.

Baseline Phase

During an initial interview participants completed questionnaires, viewed the REST chamber and flotation tank, and scheduled the dates for the baseline sleep-monitoring phase. They were also shown how to use the SAD machine and fill in the sleep log. Participants went home and monitored their sleep behaviour for 14 nights using the sleep log. On the last four of these nights they also used the SAD machine. Upon completing the baseline, the participants were randomly assigned to one of four conditions. The participants who were assigned to the delayed treatment control condition were told that their treatment would begin 13 weeks later and that because of the long time between their baseline and their treatment it would be necessary to reevaluate their sleep one week before treatment began.

Treatment Phase

Four treatment sessions were given over a 14-day period, with at least one day between any two sessions. Each occurred in the morning to avoid thinking of the treatment as a bedtime ritual. All treatments took place in the REST Laboratory at the University of British Columbia, where the flotation tank and the REST chamber are located.

All participants were told that the two goals of the treatment sessions were: a) to help them develop a personal standard of relaxation; and b) to help them concentrate so that they could focus on their relaxation standard. The idea was to experience a deeply relaxing sensation that could be recreated at bedtime. Brief homework assignments in cognitive focusing were given between each treatment.

On the first day of treatment subjects were told about normal sleep, about the cognitive and the physiological hyperarousal hypotheses concerning the mechanisms underlying insomnia. They also learned how relaxation therapies try to reduce cognitive and physiological arousal by a) distracting attention from any mental activity that is incompatible with sleep, and by b) focusing attention on the experiencing of sleep-conducive sensations.

Before questionnaires were administered in sessions 2, 3, and 4, therapeutic progress was discussed. Any problems related to the homework and any questions about the treatment procedure were dealt with during this period. After treatments and post-treatment measures had been administered, an inquiry was made into the degree of relaxation experienced and thoughts about the sensations. This subjective response to the experience was elicited to help develop the images and sensations of relaxation that would make up subjects' personal standard of relaxation. Finally, the homework assignment was reviewed.

On the last day of treatment participants were given two handouts. One was a list of sleep hygiene suggestions, with stimulus conditioning instructions embedded in it (Bootzin, 1972). The other was chapter 12 from *The Complete Book of Sleep* (Hales, 1981). These handouts provided information on good sleep habits and their relation to sleep.

Homework

Participants were instructed to practice cognitive focusing four times daily for two minutes each time. They were to start with a concrete object, such as a pencil, and concentrate on it as if seeing it for the first time. Whenever they noticed their attention drifting, they were to acknowledge the drift and bring their mind back to the object. Over the course of treatment, practice shifted from focusing on the physical object to focusing on a mental image of the object.

The participants were asked to try to recall the sensations they experienced during their treatment sessions and to rehearse their relaxation exercise. People receiving autogenic relaxation, whether in the chamber or in the tank, focused on key phrases from the exercise. People in the REST-only condition focused on the physical sensations of relaxation that they recalled passively experiencing during their floats. The idea was to practice paying attention to pleasant, monotonous, relaxing experiences and sensations which, because they were physiologically soothing, were conducive to sleep. The focused attention also served as a distraction from sleep-incompatible thoughts and images.

Treatment Conditions

Upon entering the tank or chamber all participants were instructed to do four cycles of a deep breathing exercise. They breathed in deeply to a slow count of four, held it for four counts, released their breath, held it, then repeated the cycle three more times.

REST only (R) ($n=9$). People in this group received four 45-minute floats in the REST flotation tank. Before each float, the floater was reminded to focus on feelings of relaxation, and to look for evidence that muscle tension had begun to be released.

REST and autogenic relaxation (RA) ($n=9$). Before each of the four 45-minute floats, participants in this group were reminded to focus on the key phrases in the prerecorded autogenic relaxation exercise. The autogenic relaxation tape began two minutes after entering the tank. It lasted for 30 minutes. Each floater was told to rehearse the key phrases from the exercise at least once after the tape had ended.

Autogenic relaxation (A) ($n=9$). People in this group received four 45-minute treatments while reclining comfortably on a bed in the dimly lit REST chamber. The autogenic relaxation instructions were the same as in the RA condition. The exercise tape was played over the speaker at the head of the bed.

Delayed treatment control (C) ($n=9$). People assigned to this group did two baseline sleep monitoring phases. The first was identical to that of the three treatment groups. The second baseline occurred 12 weeks later. A seven night sleep log was kept and on the last three of those nights SAD recordings were made.

After the second monitoring period, the people in this group received two autogenic relaxation and two REST-only treatments plus three post-treatment assessments. Only the two baseline data sets were analyzed for this study.

Post-treatment Assessments Phase

To assess the long-term effectiveness of the treatments, evaluations of subjective and objective sleep latency were made 12 weeks after the last treatment session. This assessment is referred to as the follow-up. For the control group the follow-up occurred 12 weeks after the baseline evaluation. Because the pattern of change for the three treatment groups was also of interest, two other assessments of sleep latency were also made. They occurred one week and four weeks after the last treatment session and are referred to as the 1-Week and 4-Weeks Post-test, respectively. They represent an immediate and a short-term evaluation of improvements in sleep latency. To avoid confounding elapsed time with the effects of sleep monitoring, the control condition did not receive these additional assessments. Each assessment involved seven nights of sleep log monitoring, with SAD recordings occurring on the last three of those nights.

Subjects' debriefing interview included a description of the other treatments in the study. All participants were offered the opportunity to take four treatments of their choice.

Results

Question 1

Does flotation REST significantly decrease sleep latency in persistent psychophysiological insomniacs as long as 12 weeks after treatment? A two-way factorial design, with flotation REST (present, absent) crossed with autogenic relaxation (present, absent), was used to answer this question. When referred to individually, the conditions are labelled: REST only (R), REST and autogenic relaxation (RA), autogenic relaxation only (A), and control (C). When used to describe analytic effects, REST (R and RA) refers to both the REST only condition and the REST and autogenic relaxation condition, while AUTO (A and RA) refers to both the autogenic relaxation condition and the REST and autogenic relaxation condition.

A two-way, multivariate analysis of covariance (MANCOVA) was computed on the follow-up (12 weeks) means for all four sleep variables: a) subjective sleep latency, and b) objective sleep latency, and

c) subjective sleep duration, and d) objective sleep duration. All four baseline sleep variable means were covaried. The test of significance used was Wilks' Lambda (L).

The MANCOVA yielded a significant AUTO main effect [FJJ(4,25)J = J5.20, pJ < J.01, L = .546] and a significant REST by AUTO interaction [FJJ(4,25) = 2.80, pJJ < J.05, L = .691]. The REST main effect was nonsignificant [FJJ(4,25) = 1.34, pJ > J.25, L = .823].

To probe the significant effects of the MANCOVA, two-way univariate ANCOVAs were performed in turn on the follow-up means of each of the four sleep variables using the single corresponding baseline measure as the covariate. The results from the univariate ANCOVAs are shown in Table 20-1.

There was a significant main effect for autogenic relaxation on subjective sleep duration as well as a significant REST by AUTO interaction. The results of the analyses with respect to objective sleep duration were all nonsignificant.

In summary the main effect of REST on both subjective and objective sleep latency is difficult to interpret in light of the significant REST by AUTO interactions. The planned comparisons discussed below will help to clarify these results.

Likewise, the significant interaction makes the main effect of autogenic relaxation in subjective sleep duration hard to interpret. The planned comparisons below will also help to explain these findings.

Question 2

Does flotation REST and flotation REST combined with autogenic relaxation training differ from autogenic relaxation training in decreasing sleep latency in persistent psychophysiological insomniacs as long as 12 weeks after treatment? For the two sleep latency variables, planned comparisons were conducted on the follow-up adjusted group means, with alpha set to .05. All comparisons were mutually orthogonal. The comparisons were: a) flotation REST (R and RA) versus autogenic relaxation (A); b) treatment (R, RA, and A) versus no treatment (C);

Table 20-1

Results of Univariate Analyses of Covariance of Four Sleep Measures Taken 12 Weeks After Treatment

Group[a,b]		Sleep Latency Subjective	Sleep Latency Objective	Sleep Duration Subjective	Sleep Duration Objective
R[c]		27.6	21.3	371.8	382.7
RA		45.9	32.1	394.8	383.3
A		44.4	31.2	414.5	390.5
C		67.4	57.0	335.4	351.9
MS (df = 31)		441.13	533.77	1063.41	2612.37
F-ratio for Effects					
REST[d]	F	5.63	5.01	.58	.48
	P	< .05	< .05	> .05	> .05
AUTO	F	.52	.89	22.26	1.59
	P	> .05	> .05	< .001	> .05
Interaction	F	4.65	5.71	6.46	1.42
	P	< .05	< .05	< .05	> .05

Note: For each dependent variable analyzed the baseline score on the same variable was used as covariate.

[a] The group means are adjusted (for the effect of the covariate) means.

[b] n = 9 per group.

[c] R = REST only; RA = REST and autogenic relaxation; A = autogenic relaxation only; CJ = control.

[d] REST = R and RA; AUTO = A and RA; Interaction = REST by AUTO.

and c) REST only (R) versus REST and autogenic relaxation (RA). The tJ-values for the subjective sleep latency comparisons were: a) R and RA versus A, t J(31) = ^^.71, pJJJ > J.10; b) JR, RA, and A versus C, tJJ(31)J = J2.92, p J < J.01; and c) R versus RA, tJJ(31)J = J^^1.81, p > .05. The t^^ values for the objective sleep latency comparisons were: a) R and RR versus AR, t (31) = J-.47, p > .10; b) R, RA, and A versus C, tJJ(31)J = J3.16, p < .01; and c) R versus RA, tJJ(31)J = J^_.96, p J > .10. The results of the first and third planned comparisons were nonsignificant for both latency variables. The results of the second set of comparisons were significant for both latency variables.

Summary

These results indicate that flotation REST and autogenic relaxation are equally effective in reducing sleep latency in persistent, psychophysiological insomniacs and that they are more effective than just letting time pass. They further suggest that the main effect for REST found in the univariate ANCOVAs on the sleep latency variables may be interpreted as supporting the assertion that flotation REST significantly reduces sleep latency over the long term.

Three planned comparisons were carried out on the follow-up (12 weeks) adjusted group means for the subjective sleep duration variable only. Alpha was set at .05. All comparisons were orthogonal. The comparisons were the same as the three conducted on the two latency variables. The t^^ values for the subjective sleep duration comparisons were: a) R and RA versus A, t J(31) = J^^2.31, p J < J.05; b) R, RA, and A versus C, t J(31) = J^^4.58, pJ < J.01; and c) R versus RA, t J(31) = J^^1.47, pJJ > J.10. These comparisons demonstrated that receiving any of the treatments in this study led to significantly longer self-reported sleep duration than receiving no treatment. However, the autogenic relaxation appeared to be more effective in increasing self-reported sleep duration in persistent, psychophysiological insomniacs than was flotation REST. There was no difference between the two flotation REST groups in ability to increase sleep duration. None of the main effects tested earlier with the objective sleep duration variable were significant.

A set of one-way, univariate analyses of covariance (ANCOVA) was conducted on the subjective sleep latencies at the 1-week post-test [F (2,23) = 0.023] and the 4-week post-test [F (2,23) = 0.152] and objective sleep latencies at the 1-week post-test [F (2,23) = .616] and the 4-week post-test [F (2,23) = 1.036] to look at the immediate and short-term effects of treatment. Only the three treatment groups were included in these analyses. All comparisons were nonsignificant. Although there were clinical decreases in subjective and objective sleep latency none of the decreases were statistically significant.

Discussion

Over the long term flotation REST significantly reduced both self reported and objectively recorded sleep latency in people with persistent, psychophysiological insomnia. Although sleep latency decreased over time, the reduction did not reach significance until 12 weeks after the end of treatment.

Over the long term the flotation REST treatments did not differ significantly from the autogenic relaxation treatment in ability to reduce sleep latency. The findings indicate that any one of the three treatments given in this study led to a greater reduction in sleep latency than when no treatment was given.

The observation that flotation REST is as effective as autogenic relaxation in decreasing sleep latency raises an interesting question as to why they did not differ. It might be because autogenic relaxation is actually a minimal form of self-induced REST. Consequently, all three treatment effects might really be REST effects. As Suedfeld (1980) pointed out, there are some strong similarities between REST and autogenic relaxation. For example, they share a common goal of reducing afferent and efferent impulses. The difference between the two techniques is in the method of achieving the reduction. REST is more stimulus-bound, achieving the reduction with the help of environmental control. On the other hand, autogenic training requires a quiet, non-stimulating environment in which to practice gaining cognitive control over the same impulses. For the autogenic relaxation condition in this study the training was limited to a prerecorded set of procedures played over a speaker into a dimly lit REST chamber. The participant heard these instructions while reclining comfortably on a bed. In other words, the environment used for autogenic relaxation training was very similar to a standard chamber REST environment.

Why there were no significant differences between the two flotation REST treatments in their ability to reduce sleep latency is another question. Perhaps "messages" (i.e., any verbal material presented to the participant during the REST session) do not always enhance the therapeutic effect of the REST environment. Evidence to support this view comes from chamber REST research. Suedfeld and Baker-Brown (1987) found that reductions in the number of cigarettes smoked after treatment did not differ between a group receiving therapeutic messages during their 24 hours in chamber REST and a group that received no messages. On the other hand, there are examples of messages enhancing the therapeutic outcome. Borrie and Suedfeld (1980) found that chamber REST plus messages led to a significantly greater weight loss in obese women six months after treatment than did REST without messages.

What is the Effect of Treatment on Sleep Duration?

Self-reported sleep duration was longer at follow-up for the treatment groups than for the control group. Also, sleep duration was longer at follow-up in the autogenic relaxation condition than in either of the flotation REST conditions. Thus, not only did sleep latency decrease in all three treatment groups, but subjective sleep duration also increased in each. Because there were no significant effects for objective sleep duration, it is difficult to argue that treatment actually did lead to increased sleep duration. The role of extraneous factors, such as expectancy and demand characteristics, in contributing to this pattern of effects should not be overlooked.

The Sleeper Effect

The observation that no statistically significant improvements were noted in sleep latency prior to the 12-week follow-up could be dubbed a "sleeper effect". The differential effect of treatment on the components of persistent, psychophysiological insomnia might account for this interesting phenomenon. Persistent, psychophysiological insomnia consists of chronic, somatized tension-anxiety and negative conditioning to internal or external factors which lead to disturbed sleep. If this accurately describes the disorder experienced by the participants in this study, then the relaxation treatment they received may have helped reduce the degree and chronicity of the somatized tension-anxiety that they experienced. Consequently, a reduction in sleep latency--due to their more relaxed state--would be expected after treatment. However, the magnitude of reduction may be a function of such factors as practice and conditioning.

As the participants practiced and became more skilled at eliciting their own personal standard of relaxation, they may have become more proficient at reducing the somatized tension-anxiety which was assumed to be associated with their prolonged sleep latency. Then if treatment reduced the chronic, tension-anxiety component, the insomniac may have gradually developed a new association. An association containing more relaxed, sleep-conducive features. This new, relaxing association could then have replaced the negative and arousing association that previously helped maintain the sleep problem.

Although reductions in sleep latency were found at one week and four weeks after treatment they were not statistically significant. But by 12 weeks the reduction had reached significance. The complete two-step process of first reducing the somatized tension-anxiety and next changing the negative conditioning may take longer than four but less than 12 weeks. If this is true, the "sleeper effect" could account for the observed delay in achieving significant therapeutic outcome.

Alternative Theoretical Explanations for the Observed Reductions in Sleep Latency

All treatments led to improvement in sleep latency by 12 weeks after treatment. Although the two-step process may explain the findings, there are alternatives.

One theoretically-based explanation for the positive psychotherapeutic changes is based on the effort justification paradigm (Cooper, 1980). The paradigm explains change in terms of the reduction of cognitive dissonance. If someone voluntarily takes part in a therapy procedure that requires considerable effort, then the goal of the therapeutic intervention (in the present case, latency reduction) becomes more attractive. The effortful therapy is assumed to arouse cognitive, emotional, or physical tension which can be reduced by achieving the desired goal. According to the effort justification hypothesis, any psychotherapy that involves significant participant effort and that is undertaken voluntarily would be likely to induce clinical improvement via the arousal and subsequent reduction of cognitive dissonance.

To the extent that participation in the present insomnia study was both effortful and voluntary, it is indeed possible that effort justification accounts for the therapeutic outcome. Unfortunately, there was no way of predicting when the arousal (which is predicted to lead to cognitive dissonance) would likely occur. Thus the probability of capturing changes which would have demonstrated a reduction in cognitive dissonance was small. As a result, no evidence was collected that would allow rejection of the effort justification account of the outcome.

Another explanation for the outcome may be the effect of the instructions to try to remain awake during the treatment sessions. These instructions parallel those for the paradoxical intention paradigm. In that paradigm, insomniacs are asked to try to stay awake instead of trying to fall asleep. This switch in performance requirements is intended to relieve the anxiety created when the insomniac tries but fails to fall asleep. With a reduction in anxiety, the person should find it easier to fall asleep.

Seven of the nine people in the autogenic relaxation condition reported falling asleep at least once during their four treatment sessions. This may have helped them reduce their anxiety about their ability to fall asleep in their own bed. However, only four of the 18 people who received either form of flotation REST treatment reported that they may have fallen asleep during the float. Therefore, the REST people were not learning to reduce their performance anxiety by falling asleep in a sleep-conducive environment. The fact that the treatment groups did not differ from each other in their ability to reduce sleep latency over the long term further suggests that the paradoxical intention paradigm is not an acceptable alternative explanation.

Incidental Beneficial Effects

Eleven of the 18 people who received flotation REST spontaneously reported unanticipated benefits after their treatment. These benefits included: acquiring the ability to recognize the onset of tension during the day and the ability to reduce the tension by recalling the sensations experienced in the tank; taking up piano lessons after imagining playing the piano during a float (this person had wanted to learn to play throughout her adult life); perceiving a reduction of sinus pressure; deciding to seek professional advice and counseling concerning an intimate personal relationship; deciding to confront a family member over childhood abuse; changing a heavy-drinking lifestyle to one of moderation, even in the face of ridicule from drinking buddies; initiation of an active search for a new job; significant attitude changes in one individual which led to a decrease in angry outbursts, a perceived increase in patience, and the development of an entrepreneurial idea.

Only two of the nine people in the autogenic relaxation condition spontaneously reported positive side effects of their treatment. One person felt motivated to make significant lifestyle changes, such as expanding cultural exposure, and thinking about starting a handyman business. The other person considered of a major career change to accommodate a desire to work in a service position. These anecdotal reports suggest that flotation REST, like chamber REST, provides additional benefits beyond improvements in the target behaviour.

Future Directions

A new line of thinking, concerning the possibility that flotation REST is an analogue of rapid eye movement (REM) sleep, was stimulated by the observation of a simple physical similarity between the two states. Both in REM sleep and while floating, the mind is very active, but the body is functionally immobile. Beside this physical similarity some of the cognitive effects of flotation REST (based on anecdotal reports from the floaters) appear to parallel the type of imagery found in nighttime cycles of REM sleep (see Roffwarg, Herman, Bowe-Anders, & Tauber, 1978). Furthermore, an unpublished study at the University of British Columbia REST Laboratory found motor evidence suggesting that an hour of floating led to decreased differences in interhemispheric activity, which in turn implies increased interhemispheric synchrony. This is an exciting finding because increased interhemispheric EEG synchrony is a characteristic of REM sleep (e.g., Armitage, Hoffmann, Loewy, & Moffitt, 1988). This particular REST finding should be substantiated by electroencephalographic recordings. Should flotation REST turn out to be an analogue of REM sleep, we may begin to ask some new questions about the nature of REM sleep and we may be able to develop a more complete theoretical explanation for the effects of flotation REST.

21

Differential Effects of Wet and Dry Flotation REST on EEG Frequency and Amplitude

Thomas Fine, Donna Mills and John Turner, Jr.

During the last decade there have been numerous studies examining physiological processes altered during human exposure to brief flotation REST. These studies have examined heart rate (Turner & Fine, 1985a; Belinson & Forgays, 1985), muscle tension (Jacobs, Heilbronner, & Stanley, 1985; Fine & Turner, 1987), blood pressure (Fine & Turner, 1982; Jacobs, Heilbronner, & Stanley, 1985; McGrady et al., 1987; Turner et al., 1989) and various plasma and urinary endocrine measures (Turner & Fine, 1983, 1985, 1991; Turner et al., 1987; McGrady et al., 1987). Except for a study of EEG theta (Barabasz, 1990b), electrocortical activity in flotation REST has not been studied. Since it has been repeatedly demonstrated that brief flotation REST affects subjective experience and physiological processes it seems reasonable to postulate that it also may have somewhat specific effects on the electrical activity of the brain. Barabasz (1990b) found significantly increased theta after flotation REST.

Previous studies carried out during the first wave of sensory deprivation research indicated that short duration periods of sensory reduction did lead to significant changes in EEG activity. Studies carried out by Dutch researchers (van Wulfften Plathe, 1958, 1959, 1962) demonstrated the predominance of low, slow dysrhythmic activity in the theta and delta frequency. Cohen, Silverman, and Shmavonian (1962a,b) examined the effect that the subjects' body field orientation had on EEG activity during short duration sensory reduction. Their studies demonstrated an interaction between subjects' performance on Witkins rod and frame test (a measure of an individual's relative dependence on external visual and proprioceptive cues in perceiving spatial relations) and the type of EEG activity present during sensory restriction. Field oriented subjects showed increased beta and decreased alpha activity, while body oriented and middle group subjects showed decreased beta and increased alpha activity.

There are no published reports of EEG changes during flotation REST. Barabasz (1990b) presented the findings of his controlled experimental study at the International Congress of Psychophysiology in Budapest. There is also an unpublished report of EEG changes that took place within a session (Stern, 1980). In this study an increase of alpha and theta activity was reported after a one hour flotation REST session. Although this was an uncontrolled pilot report, it was suggestive of the types of changes reported above, and evidence that further exploration of the changes in EEG during flotation REST would be worthwhile.

This pilot study examines the changes in central frontal monopolar EEG and frontal EMG during flotation REST (F-WET) as compared to a "Dry" flotation condition (F-DRY), and a non-REST control (MAT).

Materials and Methods

Nine subjects, five female and four male, were run in each of three 60 minute sessions. Each session was in a different condition. Subjects were all medical students on summer break.

The conditions were: F-WET, F-DRY, and MAT. F-WET was an ovoid fiberglass chamber (Enrichment Enterprises, Inc., Huntington,

New York) 2.5 m. long, 1.8 m. wide and 1.1 m. high. Subjects floated in a saturated epsom salt solution (specific gravity 1.28). The tank temperature was maintained at 34.5° ± 0.3° C. The chamber was completely enclosed, eliminating light. Subjects floated nude in a supine position. In this position the ears were submerged, resulting in a marked reduction of sound perception.

F-DRY was a rectangular chamber (Relaxation Dynamics, Inc., Boulder, Colorado) similar in dimensions and conditions to REST-Wet with several exceptions. First, a pliable, 15 mm. plastic polymer membrane separated the floater from the fluid, a $MgSO_4$ solution at 1.20 sp. gr. This condition was associated with tactile stimulation and low humidity. Second, subjects wore under-clothing in the chamber. Third, thermoneutrality (comfort, with no perspiring) was approximately 29.5° C in this environment. Fourthly, although the sound level in the air was <20 db, the ears were exposed to the air, i.e., hearing was not attenuated by submersion. The MAT condition consisted of lying on a mat in a dimly lit room. Subjects were randomized across conditions with respect to order of condition.

Physiological Measurements

EEG: A frontal monopolar electrode placement was used; this involves attaching one active electrode mid-forehead approximately 2.5 cm. above the eyebrow line, one active electrode to nasal cartilage, and the reference electrode to nasal cartilage. This placement was used for its superior performance in F-WET. EEG measurements were made on an Autogen 120, with filter settings of 8-13Hz and 4-8Hz. The Autogen has meter readings for average frequency, average amplitude, and percent time in filter range. Readings were taken every five minutes by the technician.

EMG: A frontal placement was used; the EMG electrodes were placed just slightly lower than the EEG frontal placement. EMG measurements were made on an Autogen 1700. The machine has a meter reading for average Uv amplitude of the EMG signal. Readings were taken every five minutes by the technician.

Results

EMG: First trial EMG amplitudes were much higher in MAT than the other two conditions. Average EMG amplitude decreased across time periods in MAT, rose slightly in F-DRY and decreased slightly in F-WET. All of the EMG amplitude levels fell within the resting to relaxed range with the lowest amplitude in the F-WET. EMG results are presented in Figure 21-1.

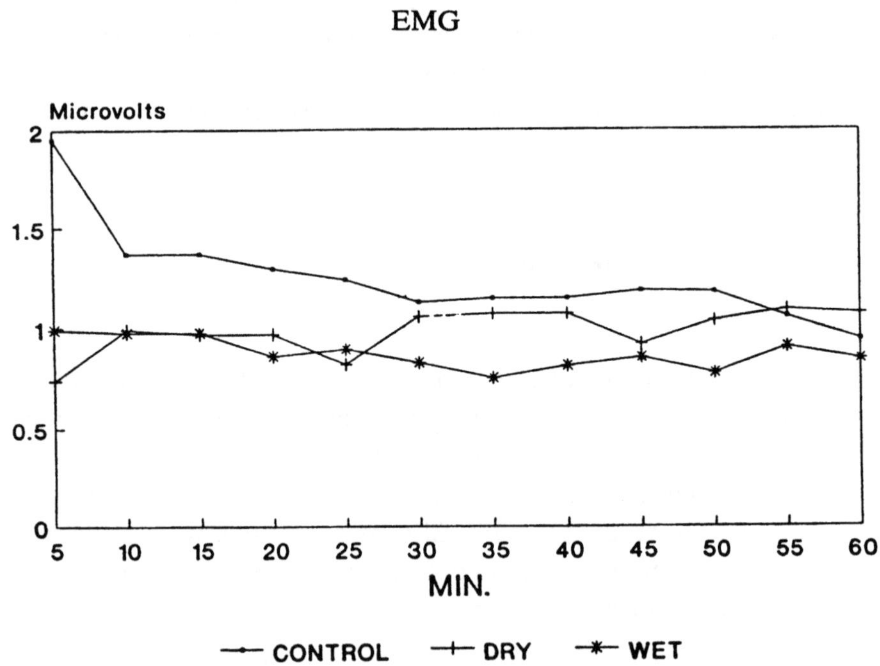

Figure 21-1. Frontal EMG levels across sessions for all conditions.

EEG: Average Frequency: Data are presented in Figure 21-2. Average frequency declined across time periods in all three conditions. MAT produced a fairly uniform linear decline beginning at 12.8Hz and ending at 11.3Hz. F-DRY followed a similar course until 30 minutes into the session when there was a drop in frequency followed by a slow rebound to 11.2Hz. F-WET began slightly higher than the other two conditions, but fell rapidly with frequency dropping to 11Hz by 15 minutes. Frequency rebounded to 12Hz by 25 minutes, once again dropping to around 11Hz by 40 minutes and remaining at that level to the end of the session.

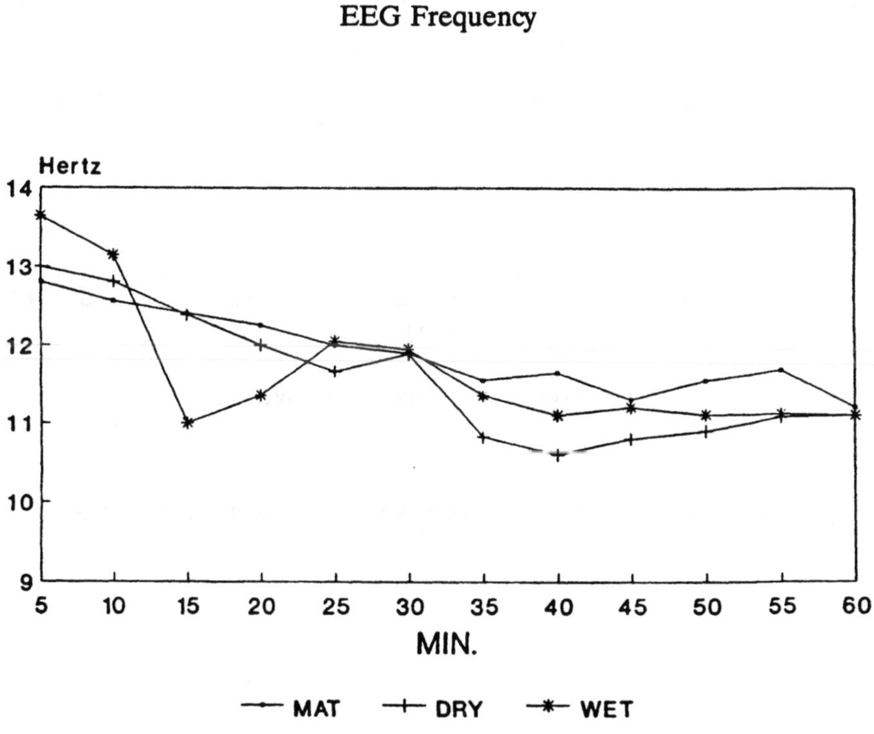

Figure 21-2. Average frequency across sessions for all conditions.

Average Amplitude: Amplitude increased in all three conditions. However, amplitude increases were more rapid and much larger in F-WET. Average amplitude results are presented in Figure 21-3.

EEG Amplitude

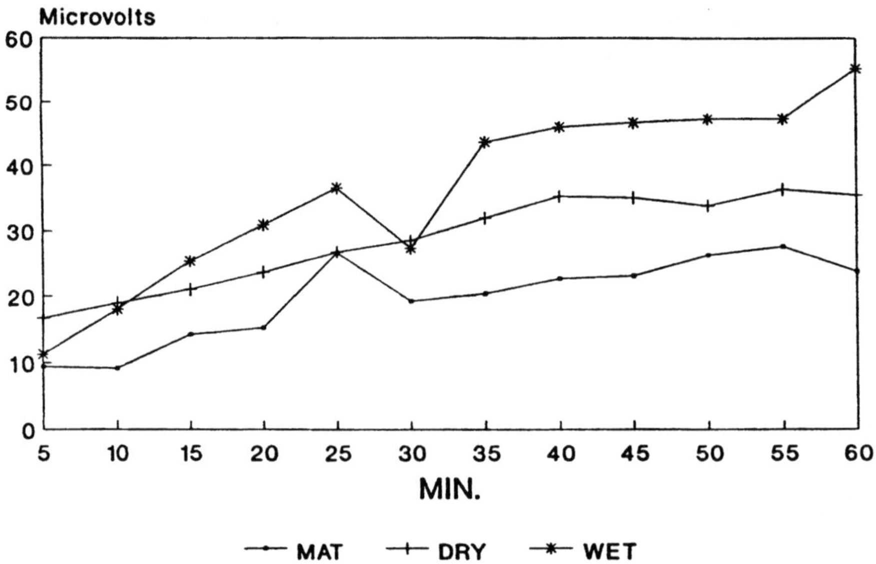

Figure 21-3. Average amplitude across sessions for all conditions.

EEG percent alpha: The percent time the EEG was in alpha or theta during a particular time period was measured. The percent time in alpha was similar for MAT and F-DRY for the first 20 minutes of the session. At 20 minutes, the percentage of Alpha began to increase in F-DRY, while it remained level for MAT. At 40 minutes, percent Alpha began decreasing slightly in both of these conditions. F-WET had a much lower percent alpha than the other two conditions. F-WET percent alpha remained relatively flat until 35 minutes into the session at which time it began rising slightly. EEG percent alpha results are presented in Figure 21-4.

EEG Percent Alpha

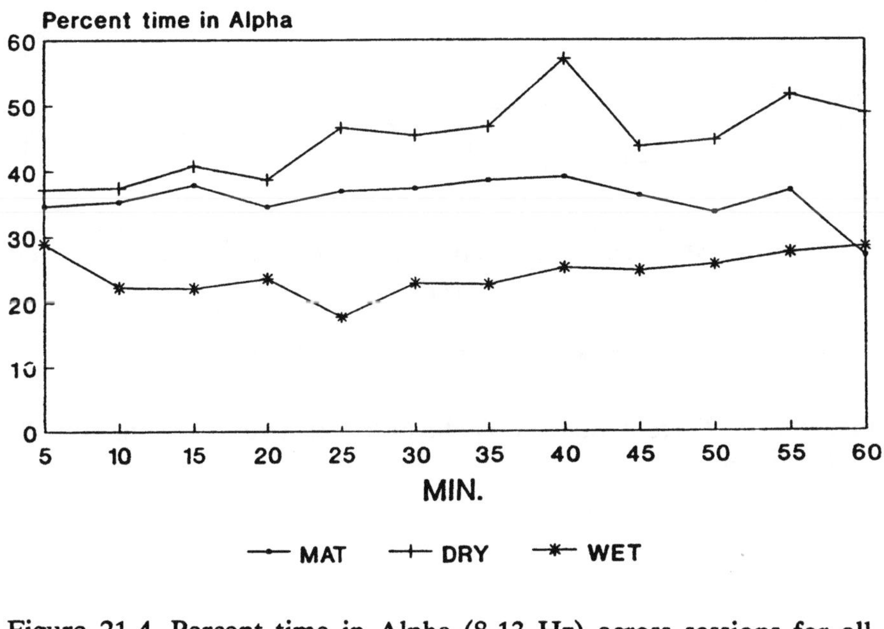

Figure 21-4. Percent time in Alpha (8-13 Hz) across sessions for all conditions.

EEG percent Theta: The percent time in theta rose slightly in both MAT and F-DRY, with MAT being larger than F-DRY; while percent time in theta rose sharply in F-WET and remained much higher than the other two conditions throughout the time period. EEG percent Theta results are presented in Figure 21-5.

EEG Percent Theta

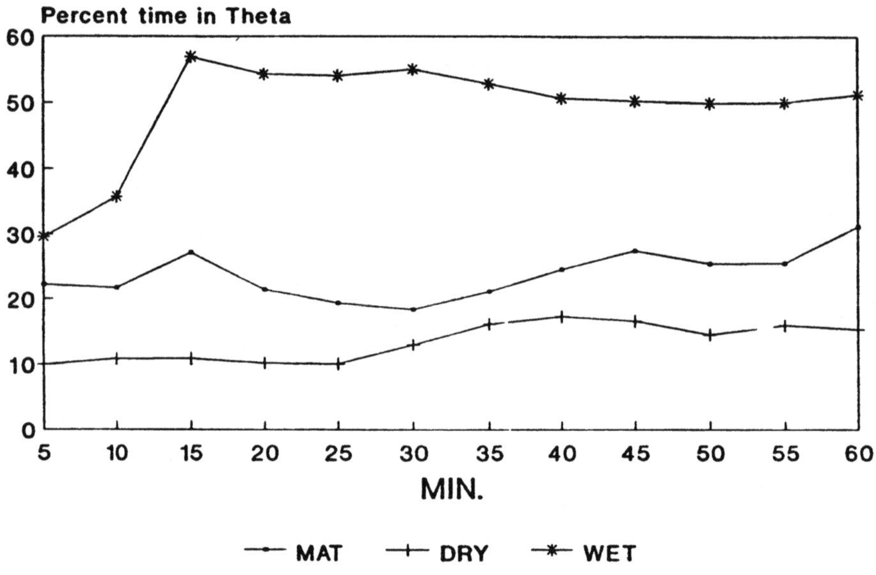

Figure 21-5. Percent time in Theta (4-8 Hz) across sessions for all conditions.

Discussion

Although average frequency was similar in all three conditions; average amplitude, percent time in alpha and theta were quite different. F-WET was dominated by higher amplitude, theta frequency components; while the MAT and the F-DRY were dominated by lower amplitude, alpha frequency components.

These preliminary data suggest F-WET is qualitatively different than either the F-DRY or lying on a mat in terms of the CNS electrical activity. F-WET produced the lowest state of arousal, F-DRY the next lowest, and the highest state of arousal was on the MAT. The activity observed in the wet tank condition is similar to the "twilight learning state" (Budzynski, 1976), a state induced through hypnotic trance, and Stage 1 sleep.

Most interesting was the difference between F-WET and F-DRY, since the environments both dramatically reduce environmental stimulation. Another study has demonstrated differential effects of these two environments on plasma cortisol, with F-WET affecting a decrease in mean values while F-DRY did not. The differences between the two conditions are humidity, temperature, and the amount of tactile stimulation available to the subject. It is unknown which factors or combination of factors might have contributed to the EEG differences.

The results of this study suggest that further investigation of EEG activity during flotation REST is worthwhile. The progressive increase in alpha in the F-WET condition is consistent with an earlier chamber study (A. Barabasz & M. Barabasz, 1985). The similar increases in theta are consistent with Barabasz (1990b). One intriguing aspect of the changes reported in this study was the small amount of time required for subjects to reach the very high percent time in theta, only 20 minutes. This lends support for the use of brief sessions (20 to 25 minutes) for relaxation training. Future studies using more sophisticated EEG placements and analysis, and more complex subject selection, will provide important basic data for our understanding of the flotation REST experience.

22

The Physiological Effects of Flotation REST

John Turner, Jr. and Thomas Fine

There is an emerging research and clinical tool which may facilitate the exploration of interrelationships between mind and physiology. This tool is Restricted Environmental Stimulation Technique or (REST). This chapter will introduce you to the psychophysiological framework of REST by presenting some basic human research studies which we have performed over the past 10 years. There are several REST formats which have been investigated, with the two most common being chamber (room) REST and flotation REST. In the former, an individual is in solitude in a room with greatly limited external contact for an extended period (24 hours). In flotation REST, the individual lies supinely for 30-60 minutes in thermoneutral, buoyant fluid with minimal photic, auditory and tactile stimulation.

Early studies of sensory isolation, performed in the 1950s and 1960s by researchers such as Donald Hebb (1955a) and John Zubek (1969b), demonstrated that this condition could be highly stressful. However, even in these endurance studies lasting from eight hours to days, monitored parameters such as blood pressure (BP), heart rate (HR), respiration rate, electromyogram (EMG), and measures of adrenal activity indicated that the first 60-90 minutes of these isolation experiences were relaxing. John Lilly, one of these early investigators, recognized this and designed the first flotation REST environment for the purpose of deep relaxation. Subjective reports by many users of Lilly's environment, then called "the tank," described the experience as deeply relaxing (Lilly, 1977). In the context of this background, we set out to examine the psychophysiology of flotation REST (henceforth, REST).

The REST environment used in all of these studies was a plastic or fiberglass chamber, approximately 1.1 m. x 1.3 m. x 2.5 m., filled to a 25 cm. depth with saturated epsom salts ($Mg\ SO_4$) solution having a specific gravity of 1.28 and temperature maintained at 34.5° C. The chamber was light-free and the sound level was <10 decibels, with further attenuation due to submersion of the ears in the solution. The general protocol consisted of 30-40 minute sessions repeated approximately every third day with a total number ranging from 4 to 20 sessions per study.

Both within-session and across-session assessments were made. With a few exceptions subjects were normal, healthy students ranging in age from 20-35 years and REST was compared to a relaxing control condition in which subjects reclined on a bed or reclining chair in a quiet (<30 db) dimly lit (<20 lumens) room.

The first parameter we addressed was the subjective report of the REST experience. Indices of subjective reports included the Spielberger state anxiety scale, Zuckerman multiple affect adjective checklist (Turner & Fine, 1990a), profile of mood states (POMs) (Turner et al., 1989) and subjective rating scales of relaxation. Marked pre-post and across-session changes indicating relaxation were found in all studies. In addition, an analysis of well over 1,000 descriptions of the REST experience, indicated more than 90% of subjects found REST deeply relaxing.

In choosing physiological parameters of the REST effect on relaxation, we simply worked from the basic physiological and biochemical hormonal changes associated with stress responding. Physiological parameters measured included BP, EMG, and HR.

Hormonal parameters included adrenal axis hormones such as ACTH, epinephrine, norepinephrine, cortisol and aldosterone and hormones not mediating stress responding (luteinizing hormone and testosterone). Both within and across-session decreases have been observed in various hormones. Hormones directly associated with stress responding (cortisol, ACTH and epinephrine) showed decreases during REST, whereas luteinizing hormone, which was not associated with stress responding showed no change (Turner & Fine 1983). Likewise, across-session decreases were observed in adrenal-associated hormones (cortisol, aldosterone, renin activity) while a hormone unrelated to stress responding (testosterone) did not shown across-session changes (Turner & Fine, 1990a). Furthermore, cortisol, which has received more attention than the other hormones, and BP, have been shown to maintain the REST effect after cessation of repeated REST sessions (Turner & Fine, 1983). This phenomenon suggests that the REST effect may be more than a simple, immediately reversible response.

Interestingly, in comparing hormonal and BP changes in REST with these changes in another relaxation condition (biofeedback), REST consistently showed greater hormonal effects but similar BP effects to biofeedback-assisted relaxation (McGrady et al., 1987). This led us to consider that REST was either mechanistically different from the biofeedback (since it affected cortisol levels when other methods did not) or was simply more powerful (i.e., REST reached the threshold for cortisol change but biofeedback did not).

Can we determine which of these possibilities is true or are both true? Direct proof is very difficult in the face of the many variables. However, several considerations seem worth examining. Some data would support the "power difference" hypothesis. Decreased plasma or urinary cortisol has been reported in association with transcendental meditation or biofeedback in some studies (Jevning et al., 1978; Michaels et al., 1976; McGrady et al., 1979, 1981), suggesting that these methods are, under some conditions, capable of reducing cortisol and several other hormones. In addition, the responses were usually greater in subjects who had prior training in the method. In contrast, REST subjects showed these hormone reductions whether the subjects were experienced or naive. In addition, significant Pearson correlations have been shown for BP and cortisol decreases in REST, although no cause-effect relationship has been established (McGrady et al., 1987). In support of the consideration that REST may be mechanistically different from biofeedback is the difference in the process between the two methods, with biofeedback effectiveness requiring the learning of a task and REST effectiveness being the consequence of reduced environmental demands.

Another consideration of possible mechanistic differences between REST and biofeedback comes from a preliminary electroencephalographic (EEG) study. Single channel monitoring of EEG frequency and amplitude using a frontal (forehead) monopolar active electrode and two bipolar reference electrodes on the nose demonstrated in 10 subjects a marked domination of theta activity. This was reflective of decreased arousal (stage-1 sleep) as compared to two other relaxation conditions (non-REST) showing more alpha (greater arousal than theta) activity. One condition was lying on a mattress while the other consisted of lying in a modified REST environment in which a pliable 15 mm. polymer membrane separated the floater from the fluid (henceforth, REST-Dry). This condition was associated with considerable tactile stimulation and low humidity, and subjects wore underclothing. Thermoneutrality (i.e., comfort, no sweating) was approximately 29.5° C. Sound levels were <20 decibels in the air, and the ears were not submerged.

The marked EEG differences between standard REST (henceforth, REST-Wet) and REST-Dry prompted us to investigate exactly what aspect or aspects of sensory reduction were essential for the REST-Wet effect. Because it was the simplest manipulation, our first effort in this direction examined the effect of the presence or absence of light, using BP and plasma cortisol as endpoints. One group experienced repeated REST-Wet with a 15 watt incandescent light illuminating the chamber, while the other group experienced REST-Wet without light. Both BP and plasma cortisol decreased significantly across sessions in both groups, suggesting no effect of *dim* light or illumination on the REST experience. It is possible, however, that light of higher intensity could have an effect.

Are there other aspects of the reduced stimuli which can be pinpointed as essential for the REST effect? For example, how important are tactile stimulation, quiet, buoyancy and thermoneutrality? To begin addressing these questions, we compared blood pressure and plasma cortisol responses in REST-Wet (n = 10) and REST-Dry (n = 9). Across eight sessions BP decreased in both groups but plasma cortisol decreased only in REST-Wet (Turner et al., 1991a).

Clearly, REST-Wet is associated with greater overall sensory reduction than REST-Dry. Of the variables mentioned above, tactile stimulation is probably the one which is most different between REST-Wet and REST-Dry. Further studies in this direction are needed before conclusions can be made regarding the minimum degree and type of sensory reduction necessary to permit the deep relaxation response.

The need for examining another aspect of the REST response has emerged from our analysis of subjective reports which indicated that up to 80% of floaters experience feelings ranging from an enhanced sense of well-being to mild euphoria immediately after a REST session. This led us to consider a possible REST effect on the endogenous opioid system. In a preliminary double-blind study, four experienced floaters each experienced four REST sessions. At the outset they received a Naloxone (opioid receptor blocker) injection or a saline placebo injection. Treatment was random, but each person received two injections of each type across the four sessions. After each session they guessed which type they had received, and pre and post session they filled out a Zuckerman mood checklist. All subjects guessed correctly in all cases and all showed mood improvement only in the placebo sessions (Turner & Fine, 1990a). These results suggested that the REST experience either increased CNS availability of opioids or the ability of the floater to distinguish between the two injections.

We, therefore, performed an experiment to measure within and across-session changes in plasma beta-endorphin in REST (n = 15) and a relaxing control (n = 12) condition. Although no pre-post session changes were observed, endorphin decreased across-sessions in REST but not in the control condition (unpublished results).

While within-session changes may have been masked by large inter-sample variability, the across-session effect clearly demonstrated a REST effect on endogenous opioid activity.

The decrease was not unexpected since adrenal activity is decreased with REST, and adrenocorticotropin (ACTH) and pituitary beta-endorphin which are part of the same parent pituitary hormone, are released concomitantly (Guilleman et al., 1977). Furthermore, the decrease peripherally may not be contradictory to the hypothesis that REST increases central beta-endorphin activity since there are data from several laboratories which indicate that central and peripheral beta-endorphin pools can be separate and inversely related in activity (Muller & Genazzani, 1984; Rossier et al., 1977). The implication of the REST effects on endogenous opioids in terms of potential applications to pain therapy and immunoenhancement therapy is significant, and further examination of this phenomenon is warranted.

To date, most REST studies have focused on pre-post and across-session changes in the parameters measured. We felt that it could greatly enhance the potential for understanding REST if we could monitor biochemical changes *during* the REST experience. We, therefore, set about developing a method for continuous blood sampling during REST.

Plasma cortisol was monitored in each of four normal subjects experiencing a baseline (non-REST, waterbed) session followed by four REST sessions (Turner et al., 1991b). All sessions were 60 minutes with continuous blood sampling occurring for 40-60 minutes in the baseline and in the fourth REST session. An intravenous (i.v.) line was placed in the dorsal forearm vein. The line was heparinized (outside of the body) by infusion of heparin at 51 units/min. and blood was removed continuously at a rate of 1.4 ml/min. via peristaltic pump. The i.v. site was kept out of the $MgSO_4$ solution by resting the hand on a small buoyant pad. Subjective relaxation rating scales indicated no differences between sessions with and without sampling. Although no within-session changes in cortisol were observed, all cortisol values were in the normal range. In addition, cortisol values in the fourth REST session were lower than in baseline, a response consistent with other studies.

We are hopeful that the continuous sampling methodology will provide us with a new window for observing REST, including the opportunity to monitor acute subject responses to challenges and tasks presented during REST.

This brings us to a point of some synthesis on the nature of the REST experience. Based on our data, we have developed a simple psychophysiological model for the actions of REST within the context of cybernetic theory. At a given moment an individual exists physiologically in a state ranging from Physiology UP to Physiology DOWN and from Attention EXTERNAL to Attention INTERNAL (to self). In REST, by virtue of reduced external input, the situation is Physiology DOWN and Attention INTERNAL. The extreme degree of input reduction permits extreme down regulation of physiological function and associated opportunity for unhindered self-attention. The combined relaxation and self-attention processes enhance the opportunity for integration and improved self-regulation. Included in this process is a cognitive feedback loop for appraisal of the experience. If appraisal moves toward ACCEPTANCE, the REST experience will achieve maximum potential. If appraisal moves toward REJECTION, the REST experience will be hindered. We hypothesize that repeating the exposure to REST helps to move appraisal toward acceptance.

Is there evidence to support this hypothesis or parts of it? Certainly the Physiology DOWN part of the model has been documented. One experiment which we have performed may contribute to evaluating the attention portion of this hypothesis. We have demonstrated in a controlled study that the ability of subjects to increase or decrease heart rate is greater in REST than in a control relaxation condition. In 21 subjects maximum change in HR was greater and latency to maximum change was shorter in REST than in the control condition. Furthermore, when correlations of HR and psychological data were made, interesting information on self focus emerged. Subjects were divided into repressors and non-repressors based on their coping style, with repressors defined as individuals who reported experiencing little distress in everyday situations and are inaccurate in their perceptions (i.e., are deceiving themselves, using a repressive copying style) (Schwartz, 1990). Based on this concept, repressive subjects would not only be less aware of self processes, but also would be less able to attend to controlling them due to the detraction of active repression. In the present study repressors relative to non-repressors showed poorer control of HR in control relaxation, as expected, but performed like non-repressors in the REST condition (Turner & Fine, 1985a). This suggests that REST may have interfered with the normal repressive coping style, i.e., repressors become less repressive in REST.

Assuming that self-attention occurs in REST, is there any evidence of enhanced self-regulation in REST? We have completed one study which addresses the possible contribution of REST to self-regulation. In cybernetic theory, the amount of variability around a mean value of a parameter can be considered a reliable measure of the regularity or "well being" of the loop. In general, decreasing variability means better regulation. In a study of REST effects on plasma cortisol, we observed a decrease in both mean cortisol levels and their variability across REST sessions, but not across control relaxation sessions.

Determination of coefficient of covariance demonstrated that this effect was not due to lower cortisol levels per se (Turner & Fine, 1991). These data, combined with the data showing maintenance of effect beyond treatment suggest that REST can influence the dynamic regulation of physiological systems and their organization. Regarding appraisal, we have no data as of yet. Evaluation of this critical component of our model will receive high priority as we continue to explore the REST phenomenon.

Despite years of research in several laboratories, REST remains poorly understood. It is our opinion that the psychophysiological changes which have been observed in association with REST are substantive and representative of the powerful potential of REST. We hope that this chapter will help to manipulate your attention to a focus on REST.

Acknowledgment

Partial funding of the study was provided by Needmor, Inc., Boulder, Colorado.

23

Effects of Flotation REST on the Immune Response: T-Cells, B-Cells, Helper and Suppressor Cells

Patricia Ruzyla-Smith and Arreed Barabasz

Psychoneuroimmunology researchers are attempting to clarify how stress influences the immunologic process. It appears that assisted relaxation may be one psychological approach which may alter immune system responses. Peavy (cited in Achterberg, 1985) demonstrated the effects of biofeedback-assisted relaxation on immune function. When individuals, naive to immune function and the purpose of the study, learned to relax there was an enhancement effect on immunity. Achterberg (1985) observed that:

> Through many examples and varied processes, then, the filters that prevent direct mental access to the physical body can be lifted. Most of the ways have in common a means of either removing, or significantly altering, or even competing with the demands the external environment makes on the brain (p. 137).

Restricted Environmental Stimulation Therapy (REST) exposes the participant to an environment of reduced external stimuli for specified periods of time. Both chamber and flotation REST methodologies have been shown to produce relaxation responses (A. Barabasz, M. Barabasz,

Dyer, & Rather, 1992), while reducing distractibility (Zubek, 1969b). Participants become more open to new information (Suedfeld, 1980), and may enter the hypnotic state (Barabasz, 1990c,e).

Turner and Fine (1985b) investigated the effects of flotation REST assisted relaxation on the plasma levels of several hormones including cortisol, ACTH, luteinizing hormone (LH), and urinary cortisol. Subjects (n=12) were randomly assigned to either REST assisted relaxation or a similar procedure without REST. The experiment consisted of three phases: 1) the baseline phase of two 35 minute sessions, each one day apart; 2) the REST and nonREST relaxation phase of a 35 minute session for four consecutive days; and 3) the follow-up phase, four or five days after treatment, identical to the two session baseline procedure. Blood samples were obtained before and after sessions 1, 2, 5, and 8. There were significant changes in plasma cortisol and ACTH but not LH. Decreases in both cortisol and ACTH were demonstrated only in the REST assisted relaxation group. Cortisol showed a significant, progressive decrease across sessions in the REST group only while ACTH showed trends of decrease across sessions in both groups. REST assisted relaxation was associated with a specific decrease in activity of the pituitary-adrenal axis.

Later, Fine and Turner (1987) used a cross-over control design in which subjects used REST assisted relaxation with EMG biofeedback during one condition and control relaxation with EMG biofeedback in the other condition. Plasma cortisol was measured to compare the effects of treatment. Cortisol levels during the REST condition and the control condition were found to be significantly lower than baseline levels. However, there was no difference between conditions. It was concluded that perhaps both control relaxation and REST conditions were equally effective in producing physiological relaxation.

Recent research on voluntary immunomodulation emphasizes strategies such as hypnosis, relaxation, imagery, and biofeedback (Hall, 1989, p. 85). Often, the suggestion to relax is combined with vivid imagery. Janoski and Kugler (1987) compared the effects of relaxation alone and relaxation with imagery on selective indices of the immune function. The study attempted to determine whether either or both major neuroendocrine (pituitary-adrenocorticoid and sympathetic adrenomedullary) pathways were associated with immune function. Subjects (n = 28) were prescreened and identified as high in the capacity for imaginative involvement which is related to hypnotic capacity (Barabasz, 1984). Subjects were randomly assigned to one of three conditions: 1) progressive muscle relaxation, 2) progressive muscle relaxation and imagery for enhanced immune function, and 3) a vigilance task control. Salivary immunoglobulin A (SIgA), an index of immune function, was significantly enhanced by relaxation alone.

The relationship between REST and hypnosis has recently become a focus of study (Barabasz, 1988, 1990c,e, 1992). Hypnotizability, typically a very stable trait (Barabasz, 1982) provides a new way of explaining subjects' responses to REST. Hypnotizability can be enhanced by chamber REST (A. Barabasz, 1982; A. Barabasz & M. Barabasz, 1989) but not flotation REST (Barabasz & Kaplan, 1989). However, flotation REST elicits spontaneous hypnosis in subjects who already possess hypnotic talent (Barabasz, 1990c,e).

Experimentally-induced cold pressor pain has been used to test for the possible occurrence of spontaneous hypnosis in flotation REST (Barabasz, 1990c,e). High hypnotizables (n = 10) and low hypnotizables (n = 10) were exposed to three conditions in random order. Condition A consisted of a flotation REST session where subjects remained in the tank without a hypnotic induction. After 45 minutes of REST, cold pressor pain data were obtained. In Condition B, subjects were seated comfortably and exposed to a hypnotic induction during administration of cold pressor pain. In Condition C (controls), subjects were treated as in Condition B but no hypnotic induction was used. Results showed significant pain reduction effects for both REST (A) and hypnosis (B) conditions compared with the control condition for both high and low hypnotizables. However, pain reduction was significantly greater for subjects capable of high levels of hypnosis compared to the lows. Consistent with A. Barabasz, M. Barabasz, Dyer, and Rather (1990), all subjects reported the flotation REST sessions to be relaxing. However, only the high hypnotizables added hypnosis-like descriptions of the experience. It was hypothesized that while pain reduction for lows may be due to relaxation, the greatly enhanced pain reduction for highs may be due to both relaxation and hypnosis. Consistent with Hilgard's

(1977) neodissociation conceptualization of hypnosis and J. R. Hilgard's (1974) imaginative involvement findings, Barabasz (1990c) hypothesized that flotation REST produces spontaneous hypnosis in subjects known to have hypnotic talent.

The purpose of this investigation was to determine the effects of flotation REST on the immune response. It was considered important to control for subjects' hypnotizability level.

Method

Subjects

Ss (n = 44) consisted of student volunteers (18-56 years of age) enrolled at large rural university located in the Pacific Northwest United States. Subsequent to a prescreening medical questionnaire, subjects were oriented to hypnosis, maximized in hypnotizability, and divided into high or low hypnotizability groups on the basis of Stanford Hypnotic Susceptibility Scale: Form C (Weitzenhoffer & Hilgard, 1962) scores (highs >7, lows <5). No subjects reported blood disorders, malignancy, auto immune disorder, active virus, allergy, immuno-suppressant medication, or life styles that would prohibit blood donation.

Instrumentation

A self-administered computerized version of the Symptom Checklist-90-R (SCL-90-R) (Derogatis, 1977) was employed. Ninety items are rated on a 5-point scale of distress from "not at all" to "extremely." Scores are obtained for 10 primary symptom dimensions (somatization, obsessive-compulsive, interpersonal sensitivity, depression, anxiety, hostility, phobic anxiety, paranoid ideation, and psychoticism). Three global indices of distress are also calculated: Global Severity Index (GSI); Positive Symptom Distress Index (PSI); and Positive Symptom Total (PST). Raw scores were transformed into T-scores using non-psychiatric norms and a "cut off" GSI score of 70 was established in order to exclude subjects who reported life stresses which might be likely to confound immune function data.

Assay Process

Peripheral blood was obtained by venipuncture. Each of three samples per subject consisted of 16cc of blood. Assays were performed at the Microbiology Laboratory at Washington State University. The Ficoll-Paque method for in-vitro isolation of lymphocytes was used on fresh blood samples. White blood cell counts were performed by standard hematologic techniques (Jackson & Warner, 1986). Due to the complex nature of T- and B-cell function, a pilot study was conducted to determine which subsets of lymphocytes were likely to manifest proliferation. The use of monoclonal antibodies (Becton-Dickinson, 1986) permitted targeting and marking of T-, B-, and T-cell subsets of helper and suppressor cells. The cell staining procedure followed the protocol for Simultaneous Two Color Enumeration of T-Helper/ Inducer and T-Cytotoxic/Suppressor cells, and Human T- and B-cells in peripheral blood (Becton-Dickinson, 1986). The standardized modification technique for multiple plate samples was used. Flow cytometry was employed to facilitate analysis.

Apparatus

A Becton-Dickinson FACS 440 flow cytometry system was used to detect electronic and optical signals from cells which were illuminated by laser light. Simultaneous multiparameter analyses of surface characteristics, cell volume, and cell size were obtained (Jackson & Warner, 1986). Surface antigens present on retrieved peripheral blood lymphocytes were bound and labelled by specific mouse monoclonal antibodies, developed to detect T-cells, B-cells, helper T-cells, and suppressor T-cells. Fluorescent dyes, conjugated to the antibodies, were distinguished by flow cytometry to facilitate identification and enumeration of specified cells. Color dot plot graphs were generated which yielded percentages of T-, B-, and T-cell subsets of helper and suppressor cells.

Skin conductance response (SCR) was determined for each subject immediately prior to each venipuncture blood sampling using standardized procedure (Barabasz, 1977, p. 131-132). SCR was monitored by using a Lafayette Instruments 76100-30 Barabasz Desensitization Quantifier. A "cutoff" SCR was established during the pilot study to determine the arousal SCR stress level associated with venipuncture which would likely confound immune function. Two subjects with measurements beyond cutoff were excluded from the study.

The REST tank, Floatarium Brand SWS, is an enclosed, sound-insulated, fiberglass tub containing a 24 cm. deep solution of tap water and epsom salts ($MgSO_4$, 20% solution). The solution was maintained at 34.5° ± .2° C. Ventilation was provided by a silent positive pressure system. Subjects wore 28 decibel attenuating wax earplugs and floated supine with ears submerged. Subjects were monitored throughout the session via a built-in microphone. Subjects showered immediately before and after sessions.

Procedure

Subjects were randomly assigned, within high and low hypnotizability groups, to either flotation REST or control conditions. All subjects received written pre-treatment instructions which included refraining from excessive exercise, caffeine, dieting, and being abstinent from alcohol and nicotine. Subjects were asked to get adequate sleep within 24 hours prior to scheduled sessions. A pre-treatment blood sample was obtained from all subjects immediately prior to the first session or at the first scheduled meeting with control subjects. Each 16 cc. blood sample included two heparinized tubes, one EDTA tube, and one serum tube. Each subject was given a code number identifying their blood sampling series so blood analyses could be conducted blind with respect to treatment group. SCR was measured during each blood drawing to account for the impact of venipuncture-related anxiety (Olness, 1988). All subjects were first given an orientation to the immune response via a short videotaped presentation which gave an overview of the major components and functions of the human immune system.

Subjects in the REST group received an orientation to the flotation tank (Suedfeld, 1980) and were told that they would be monitored throughout each session. Prior to preparation for the one-hour flotation tank experience, subjects took the SCL-90-R, self-administered computerized version. The one-hour flotation REST experience was uninterrupted with the exception that subject inquiries were responded to by the experimenter at the start of each session. Blood samples were taken at the end of the session. The second session followed in one week. Prior to REST Treatment 2 the SCL-90-R was again administered. A third blood sampling and SCR measure followed the REST session.

Control subjects were scheduled and run at the same times used for REST treatment subjects. At the first session, control subjects took the SCL-90-R and pretreatment blood samples were obtained. Blood samples were again obtained one hour later. These subjects were then scheduled for a second session one week later, during which the SCL-90-R was readministered and third blood sample taken.

After the second REST treatment and second control session, an independent post-experimental inquiry was conducted. This semi-structured interview was intended to evaluate subjects' experiences and identify extraneous factors that may have impacted immune function (i.e., development of life stressors or infectious conditions during the course of the study). In addition, comments from subjects in the REST group were evaluated to provide data on the possible occurrence of spontaneous hypnosis (Barabasz, 1990c,e).

A two-week post-experimental follow-up telephone contact also was made with all subjects to determine whether an active infection was developing during participation in the study. This procedure was intended to eliminate data from subjects whose immune systems may have been impacted by responses to infections.

Results

The data were analyzed by a 2 (Treatment = REST, Control) X 2 (Hypnotizability = Hi, Lo) X 3 (Time = Pre-treatment, Post-treatment 1, Post-treatment 2) ANOVA with repeated measures. Due to wide variations in pre-treatment measures of immune response ANCOVAs were also used to analyze between subjects data. An alpha level of .10 was selected as suggested by Orne and Scheibe (1964) for data of the kind generated in this study. Significant between subjects results emerged from this analysis for the following: 1) T-cells: Treatment X Hypnotizability $F(1,30) = 4.39$, $p = 0.45$; and 2) Absolute T-4 cells X Hypnotizability $F(1,27) = 3.45$, $p = .074$. Post hoc follow-up revealed a significantly lower percentage of T-cells for REST subjects high in hypnotizability compared to REST subjects low in hypnotizability and Control subjects low in hypnotizability. Post hoc tests for Absolute T-4 cells revealed that, regardless of treatment, subjects low in hypnotizability demonstrated significantly greater T-4 cell counts than subjects high in hypnotizability. Significant within subjects results were found for the following indicants: 1) B-cells: Hypnotizability X Time $F(2,62) = 2.96$, $p = .059$; 2) H-cells: Treatment X time $F(2,62) = 2.82$, $p = 0.67$; 3) Absolute T-4 cells: Time $F(2,56) = 2.61$, $p = .082$; Treatment X time $F(2,56) = 3.54$, $p = .036$; Treatment X Hypnotizability X Time $F(2,56 = 2.50$, $p = 0.91$; 4) H/S ratio: Treatment X hypnotizability X Time $F(2,62) = 3.17$, $p = .049$. Post hoc comparisons showed that, regardless of treatment, there was a significantly greater percentage of B-cells in subjects high in hypnotizability from Pre-treatment to Post-treatment 2. Subjects low in hypnotizability demonstrated a significant decrease in percentage of B-cells from Pre-treatment to Post-treatment 2. Follow-up analysis for the two-way interaction of Treatment and Time for percentage of H-cells showed a significant increase for REST subjects from Pre-treatment to Post-treatment 2. Control subjects decreased in percentage of H-cells from Pre-treatment to Post-treatment, although not significantly. Overall, subjects showed a decrease in Absolute T-4 cells from Pre-treatment to Post-treatment 2. Follow-up analyses revealed that REST subjects decreased in Absolute T-4 cells from Pre-treatment to Post-treatment 1 and Post-treatment 2. REST subjects high in hypnotizability had the greatest decrease from Pre-treatment to Post-treatment 2. The three way interaction follow-up analysis for H/S ratio revealed that REST subjects high in hypnotizability showed a significant increase from Post-treatment 1 to Post-treatment 2. See Tables 23-1, 23-2, and 23-3.

Discussion

This was the first study to use monoclonal antibodies to mark and enumerate lymphocytes as a measure of immune function in Ss exposed to REST. Our findings suggest that flotation REST may enhance immune function. However, the data must be regarded as very preliminary. There was considerable variability in immune function data, despite prescreening of subjects to meet the criteria of a healthy, normal, non-stressed population. Apparent changes in a direction of enhancement or suppression must be interpreted with caution. This reflects both the homeostatic nature of the human body and the more subtle effects of flotation REST in altering the physiology of the immune response. It is noteworthy that in Peavy's (cit. Archterberg, 1985) study of biofeedback assisted relaxation and immune function, subjects selected were those under high levels of stress manifesting low levels of immunity as measured by white blood cell counts and neutrophil function. When these highly stressed subjects learned to relax, there was a direct but selective effect on immunity. Neutrophil function increased following treatment, suggesting relaxation may enhance immune function toward homeostasis in an immune suppressed sample. Turner and Fine (1987) suggested that since REST produced a decrease in pituitary-adrenal axis activity its effects seem to be more than a simple response to relaxation. They also observed that REST is associated with the release of endogenous opioids. These findings are consistent with the current psychoneuroimmunology research which implicates endorphins, interferon, interlukins, and

Table 23-1

B-Cell and T-Cell Results for High and Low Hypnotizables

Indicancy	Tx/Hyn	+/-	N	Mean Rank	Z	P (2 tailed)
B-Cell	REST HI	INC	8	(6.4)	-1.60	0.10
		DEC	3	(5.0)		
			11			
	REST LO	INC	3	(5.0)	-0.88	0.37
		DEC	6	(5.0)		
			9			
	Control HI	INC	4	(5.5)	-0.05	0.95
		DEC	5	(4.6)		
			9			
	Control LO	INC	5	(3.6)	-0.00	1.00
		DEC	3	(6.0)		
			8			
T-Cell	REST HI	INC	7	(6.1)	-0.88	0.37
		DEC	4	(5.7)		
			11			
	REST LO	INC	5	(4.8)	-0.17	0.85
		DEC	5	(5.2)		
			10			
	Control HI	INC	7	(5.0)	-1.48	0.13
		DEC	2	(5.0)		
			9			
	Control LO	INC	2	(3.0)	-1.68	0.09
		DEC	6	(5.0)		
			8			

Table 23-2

H-Cell and S-Cell Results for High and Low Hypnotizables

Indicants	Tx/Hyn	+/-	N	Mean Rank	Z	P (2 tailed)
H-Cell	REST HI	INC	7	(5.4)	-0.44	0.65
		DEC	4	(7.0)		
			11			
	REST LO	INC	5	(5.0)	-0.29	0.76
		DEC	4	(5.0)		
			9			
	Control HI	INC	5	(4.8)	-0.17	0.85
		DEC	4	(5.2)		
			9			
	Control LO	INC	1	(1.0)	-2.38	0.02
		DEC	7	(5.0)		
			8			
S-Cell	REST HI	INC	3	(6.6)	-1.15	0.24
		DEC	8	(5.7)		
			11			
	REST LO	INC	5	(4.3)	-1.12	0.26
		DEC	6	(5.3)		
			11			
	Control HI	INC	2	(6.5)	-1.12	0.26
		DEC	7	(4.5)		
			9			
	Control LO	INC	6	(5.5)	-2.10	0.03
		DEC	2	(1.5)		
			8			

Table 23-3

Absolute T-4 Cells and H/S Ratio Results for High and Low Hypnotizables

Indicates	Tx/Hyn	+/-	N	Mean Rank	Z	P (2 tailed)
Absolute T4	REST HI	INC	0	(0.0)	-2.52	0.01
		DEC	8	(4.5)		
			8			
	REST LO	INC	2	(6.5)	-1.12	0.26
		DEC	7	(4.5)		
			9			
	Control HI	INC	5	(5.6)	-0.65	0.51
		DEC	4	(4.2)		
			9			
	Control LO	INC	2	(5.5)	-0.98	0.32
		DEC	6	(4.1)		
			8			
H/S Ratio	REST HI	INC	7	(5.5)	-0.53	0.59
		DEC	4	(6.7)		
			11			
	REST LO	INC	6	(5.1)	-1.00	0.31
		DEC	3	(4.6)		
			9			
	Control HI	INC	6	(4.3)	-1.12	0.26
		DEC	2	(5.0)		
			8			
	Control LO	INC	0	(0.0)	-2.20	0.02
		DEC	6	(3.5)		
			6			

peptides as chemical messengers in the two-way communication feedback loop of the body-mind.

The findings reported here used hypnotizability as a blocking variable in an attempt to better understand REST effects. Another aspect of the research, which exposed additional subjects to hypnotic inductions and self-hypnosis, demonstrated that hypnosis enhanced immune function results well beyond those produced by REST. This data (Ruzyla-Smith, A. Barabasz, M. Barabasz, & Warner, in preparation) will be reported elsewhere.

The production of a significantly higher percentage of T-cells by the low hypnotizability REST subjects compared to high hypnotizability REST subjects is difficult to explain. In an attempt to explain the findings of significantly enhanced hypnotizability following six hours of chamber REST, it was hypothesized that "REST forces the organism to focus, perhaps as seldom before, on internally generated imaginal activity" (Barabasz, 1982; p. 162). Barabasz (1982) conceptualized this response as a dissociative reaction which serves to maintain neuronal integration in the organization of brain functions. Sean Mee (see Chapter 2) elaborated on Barabasz's conceptualization of the phenomena within Hilgard's (1977a,b) neo-dissociation theory. During the postexperimental inquiry for the present study, all flotation REST subjects reported subjective feelings of deep relaxation. However, only the high hypnotizables described enhanced perceptual experiences. The highs noted, "I was more aware of what was going on in my body", "Images were coming, going, and changing a lot", "Pictures came to me in vivid colors", "I went on an exciting (imaginary) adventure... the time in the tank seemed like only a few minutes".

The second author has been attempting to determine whether the lack of specific suggestions in flotation REST with high hypnotizables may cause paradoxical hyper arousal as suggested by the arousing perceptual experiences described above, the occurrence of reduced EEG alpha, and increased electrodermal activity during mid-REST (A. Barabasz & M. Barabasz, 1985). Perhaps the absence of a positive descriptive suggestion to enhance the immune response, produced a hyperarousal state in the high hypnotizables thus mitigating REST relaxation effects and, thereby, precluding immune response enhancement. As recently demonstrated (Barabasz, 1990e) (also see Chapter 5), flotation REST elicits spontaneous hypnosis in high hypnotizables. The highs in the present study may not have shown immunoenhancement because the relaxation effects of flotation REST, experienced by the normal population, were not manifested by the highs because of their active engagement in satisfying and stimulating imaginative involvements (Barabasz, 1984). The findings of a significantly lower percentage of T-cells in the high hypnotizable REST subjects seems to support this speculation and suggests further investigation. Assigning subjects high in hypnotic susceptibility to a REST group with a positive suggestion to enhance the immune response and then comparing results to a REST only group would be an initial step towards understanding the interactive effect of REST and hypnotizability. Perhaps the low hypnotizables, who were incapable of entering hypnosis, responded to the relaxation effects of the tank showing cell counts consistent with immunoenhancement.

It would seem that researchers of voluntary immunomodulation should be sure to consider hypnotizability and study the effects of relaxation combined with imagery on immune function enhancement. This research should employ imagery that "is consistent, at least metaphorically, with actual immunological functioning" (Hall, 1989, p. 87). The selection of immune function indices should be related to the accuracy of imagery used as well as the choice of a component that shows reactivity to psychological interventions. Several questions regarding immunological measures remain including: 1) When should post-treatment samples be taken? 2) What individual differences may be linked to enhancement or suppression of the immune response? and 3) What effect does invasiveness of obtaining samples have on the results?

Explorations of mind/body interactions are multifaceted and often complex. In seeking the truth, nonsignificant findings also add to this growing field of knowledge. The significant findings, observed trends, and nonsignificant findings suggest the following areas for future research.

1. Comparing Ss, grouped by hypnotizability, in flotation REST with hypnosis to enhance immunological function with other flotation REST

Ss without hypnosis.

2. Comparing stressed and/or immune suppressed Ss, with Ss meeting criteria for nonstressed and/or immune suppressed using the above treatments.

Undertaking this type of study may have far reaching multidisciplinary implications in light of advances being made in the fields of health psychology, psychoneurology, neuroendocrinology, immunology, and REST.

Acknowledgments

Special thanks are expressed to Drs. Marianne Barabasz, Dennis Warner, and Carol Wyatt. The study could not have been completed without their involvement.

The project was supported in part by the Washington State University Office of Grant and Research Development, and by grants to the second investigator.

Thanks also are expressed to REST Technologies Corporation of Huntington, New York.

24

Effects of Wet and Dry Flotation REST on Blood Pressure and Plasma Cortisol

John Turner, Jr., William Gerard, John Hyland, Pamela Nieland and Thomas Fine

Flotation Restricted Environmental Stimulation Therapy (F-REST) has been used successfully in the treatment of several stress-related disorders (Fine & Turner, 1982, 1985a; Rzewnicki et al., 1990; Koula et al., 1990). In F-REST (henceforth, REST) an individual lies supinely in thermoneutral buoyant fluid with minimal photic, auditory and tactile stimulation (Lilly, 1977). Deep relaxation reportedly accompanies REST (A. Barabasz, M. Barabasz, Dyer & Rather, 1990; Turner & Fine, 1983; Suedfeld, Ballard & Murphy, 1983). Relaxation has been shown to be associated with decreased activity of the adrenal axis (Davidson et al., 1979; Michaels, Huber & McCann, 1979; Jevning, Wilson & Davidson, 1978; McGrady et al., 1981). Plasma cortisol can be measured as an indicator of this axis, and levels have been shown to decrease during REST (Turner & Fine 1983; McGrady et al., 1987). In addition, a decrease in blood pressure has been a common finding in previous REST studies (Jacobs, Heilbronner & Stanley, 1985; Fine & Turner, 1982; Kristeller, Schwartz & Black, 1982; Suedfeld, Roy & Landon,

1982), indicating that, along with plasma cortisol, blood pressure can be a reliable index of the REST effect.

Despite the encouraging findings of physiological responses to REST, little is known regarding the mechanisms underlying REST effects. For example, which aspects of sensory restriction are necessary for the relaxation response to occur? In one study, Turner et al. (1989) found no differences in the blood pressure and cortisol response to REST whether light was present or absent in the REST environment, raising the possibility that absence of light is not a critical aspect of REST. How important are tactile stimulation, quiet, buoyancy and thermoneutrality? In order to begin addressing these questions, the present study compares blood pressure and plasma cortisol responses in standard flotation REST and in a modified version of REST in which the floater is separated from the fluid by a pliable plastic polymer membrane.

Materials and Methods

Nineteen healthy volunteers, ages 22-34 years, were recruited from a class of medical students. Twelve subjects were male, and seven were female. None of the subjects had experienced relaxation training previously. The subjects were on summer vacation, and no major stresses were reported during the study. All subjects were told they were participating in a study of physiological changes associated with relaxation. Subjects were randomly assigned to a REST-Wet or REST-Dry group. REST-Wet was an ovoid fiberglass chamber (Enrichment Enterprises Inc., Huntington, New York) 2.5 m long, 1.8 m wide and 1.1. m high. Subjects floated in a saturated epsom salt solution, specific gravity 1.28. The tank temperature was maintained at 34.5 ± 0.3° C. The chamber was completely enclosed, eliminating light. Subjects floated nude in a supine position. In this position the ears were submerged, resulting in a marked reduction of sound perception.

The REST-Dry environment was a rectangular chamber (Relaxation Dynamics, Inc., Boulder, Colorado) similar in dimensions and conditions to REST-Wet with several exceptions. First, a pliable, 15 mm. plastic polymer membrane separated the floater from the fluid, a $MgSO_4$ solution at 1.20 sp. gr. This condition was associated with tactile stimulation and low humidity. Second, subjects wore underclothing in the chamber. Third, thermoneutrality (comfort, with no perspiring) was approximately 29.5° C in this environment. Fourthly, although the sound level in the air was <20 db, the ears were exposed to the air, i.e., hearing was not attenuated by submersion.

The repeated-measures experimental design compared baseline vs. end-of-treatment (henceforth, treatment) in the REST-Wet (n = 10) and REST-Dry (n = 9) groups. The study period was five weeks, with two weeks of baseline and three weeks of treatment. Each subject experienced eight REST sessions, 40 min. each. Sessions were every third day during treatment. Baseline consisted of four visits, three days apart, in which blood pressure was measured and blood samples were taken. This procedure was also done during the treatment phase on non-session days between the last four sessions.

Systolic and diastolic blood pressure was measured five minutes after arrival while sitting quietly. Each reported value is the average of three measurements, taken two minutes apart, and calculated as mean arterial pressure (MAP = 1/3 (S-D) + D). Blood sampling consisted of two venous samples per visit, taken 20 minutes apart, after blood pressure. Samples were taken from the forearm via heparinized vacationer. They were iced and centrifuged, and the plasma was frozen until assay for cortisol, using a radioimmunoassay kit (Code COD2, Diagnostic Products, Los Angeles, California). Assessment of anxiety was made in each subject before and after REST sessions 1 and 8 using the Spielberger State Anxiety Scale (STA Form XI).

Data were subjected to two levels of analysis. Two-way repeated-measures ANOVA was used to determine differences across sessions. Specific differences were determined by Tukey test and F-test (Zar, 1984).

Results

Mean Arterial Pressure

In both REST-Wet and REST-Dry groups ANOVA established no differences among sessions within baseline or within treatment. In other words, MAP did not change during baseline or during the portion of treatment which was monitored. Therefore, across subject averages were pooled for sessions 1-4 and for sessions 5-8. MAP results are presented in Table 24-1. There were no differences in MAP between baseline REST-Wet (83.05 ± 0.97 mm Hg) and REST-Dry (82.50 ± 0.77 mm Hg). MAP in treatment was significantly lower than in baseline in both groups ($p < 0.05$ Tukey test). MAP values in treatment averaged 77.5 ± 1.52 for REST-Wet and 74.83 ± 1.42 for REST-Dry.

Table 24-1

Effect of Brief, Repeated Flotation REST on Mean Arterial Pressure

		Mean Arterial Pressure (mm Hg)	
CONDITION	n	BASELINE[a]	TREATMENT[a]
REST-Wet	10	83.05 ± 0.97[a]	77.05 ± 1.52[b]
REST-Dry	9	82.50 ± 0.77[a]	74.83 ± 1.42[c]

[a] Pooled values across visits 1-4 (baseline) or 5-8 (treatment).
[b] Different from baseline, repeated measures ANOVA ($p < 0.05$, Tukey test).
[c] Different from baseline, repeated measures ANOVA ($p < 0.01$, Tukey test).

Plasma Cortisol

ANOVA established no differences among sessions within baseline or within treatment for either REST-Wet or REST-Dry. In other words cortisol did not change during baseline or during the portion of treatment which was monitored in either group. Therefore across-subject averages were pooled for sessions 1-4 (baseline) and pooled for sessions 5-8 (treatment) in each group. Plasma Cortisol data are presented in Table 24-2.

There were no differences in plasma cortisol levels between REST-Wet and REST-Dry in baseline. There was no difference between baseline and treatment levels of plasma cortisol in the REST-Dry group. However, plasma cortisol was significantly ($p < 0.05$, Tukey test) lower in treatment than in baseline in the REST-Wet group.

Initial levels (before session 1) of state anxiety (SA) were greater in REST-Wet (ave. score = 43.1) than in REST-Dry (ave. score = 34.2) (Table 24-3). SA decreased within sessions for all sessions, with changes

Table 24-2

Effect of Brief, Repeated Flotation REST on Plasma Cortisol

		Mean Arterial Pressure (mm Hg)	
CONDITION	n	BASELINE[a]	TREATMENT[a]
REST-Wet	10	17.00 ± 0.06[a]	14.29 ± 0.54[b]
REST-Dry	9	16.70 ± 0.78	17.55 ± 1.26

[a] Pooled A and B samples averaged across sampling sessions 1-4 (baseline) or 5-8 (treatment).

[b] Different from baseline, repeated measures ANOVA ($p < 0.05$, Tukey test).

Table 24-3

Effect of Flotation REST on State Anxiety

Condition	n	STATE ANXIETY SCORE[a]					
		SESSION 1			SESSION 8		
		PRE	POST	Δ	PRE	POST	Δ
REST-Wet	10	43.1	28.0	-15.1	35.7	24.4	-11.3
REST-Dry	9	34.2	28.5	- 5.6	32.3	31.7	- 0.7

[a] Spielberger STA-XI state anxiety scale scores.

being greater in REST-Wet than in REST-Dry and greater in session 1 than session 8 for both groups. Comparison of presession SA revealed no significant differences between sessions 1 and 8 in either REST-Wet or REST-Dry. However, both groups showed a numerically lower SA score in presession 8 than in presession 1 and the change was larger in REST-Wet than in REST-Dry. Subjective reports indicated that both REST-Wet and REST-Dry were relaxing. Falling asleep was reported more frequently in REST-Dry (19% of sessions) than in REST-Wet (8% of sessions).

Discussion

Brief, repeated REST-Wet and REST-Dry sessions were associated with decreased MAP, while plasma cortisol was decreased only in REST-Wet. These results confirm previous reports of REST-Wet effects on MAP and cortisol (Turner & Fine 1991; Turner et al., 1989; Fine &

Turner, 1982). The similarity in MAP responses may reflect the occurrence of a relaxation response in both Wet and Dry REST. This is supported by subjective report and state anxiety data for both conditions of REST.

However, there were many differences between Wet and Dry REST which may be reflective of the differential cortisol response in the two groups. The difficulty lies in establishing a causative link between one or several of these differences and the cortisol difference. The present study does not permit this determination. Nonetheless, it may be useful to describe similarities and differences between REST-Wet and REST-Dry in the context of the observed effects on MAP and cortisol.

One of the first considerations is whether the different MAP and cortisol responses in REST-Wet and Dry are a matter of degree or type. For example, if MAP responds more readily to relaxation than cortisol, it is possible that REST-Wet was simply a stronger mediator of relaxation, passing the threshold for both responses. Alternatively, REST-Wet and Dry may be mechanistically different, tapping different aspects of the relaxation response, and thus affecting cortisol differently. The anxiety scale results tend to support the former possibility, since anxiety reduction was greater in REST-Wet than REST-Dry. This is potentially complicated, however, by the fact that anxiety was greater in REST-Wet at the outset i.e., before session 1. It has been our experience over numerous studies that a majority of subjects have at least mild anxiety prior to their first experience of REST-Wet, since it is an unknown to them. With few exceptions this did not persist beyond session 1.

The possibility that REST-Wet and REST-Dry act via different mechanisms is suggested by the EEG study reported elsewhere in this book by Fine, Mills and Turner. Both EEG amplitude and percent of time in alpha and theta frequencies were different during REST-Wet than during REST-Dry. Such differences in EEG could reflect differential influences of Wet and Dry conditions on regulation of MAP and cortisol. A further potentially complicating aspect of the EEG issue, however, is that sleeping occurred in a percentage of REST sessions. Normal nocturnal sleep in man has been associated with decreases in both MAP (Lydic, 1987) and cortisol (Weitzman et al., 1971). The cortisol response is probably too slow to have reacted by the end of the REST session. The MAP response may have been rapid enough that the REST decrease could be due to sleep in those subjects who slept. Examination of MAP responses in individual REST sessions, however, showed no difference between sessions with and without sleeping.

There were several physical-sensory differences between REST-Wet and REST-Dry, with the former unquestionably being associated with greater sensory restriction. Although the sound level was potentially greater in REST-Dry, both conditions were very quiet. The occurrence of sleep more than twice as often in REST-Dry as compared to REST-Wet would suggest that sound was not a major limitation to relaxation in REST-Dry.

Although the actual REST-Dry temperature was approximately 4° C cooler than in REST-Wet, the subjects reported feeling thermoneutral in both conditions. In other words the physical conditions dictated the temperature difference, but the temperature experience was similar in Wet and Dry. There remains the issue of the air-fluid interface, however. In REST-Wet the sensation of such an interface disappears when the temperature of the 100% humidity air and water are equal. The interface feeling between the 50% humidity air and the pliable membrane does not disappear. This provides some thermal input and probably contributes information for spatial orientation.

Perhaps the greatest single difference between sensory input in REST-Wet and REST-Dry is the contact with the fluid in the former and its absence in the latter. Floating in the fluid with its associated distribution of pressure equally to all points and the loss of sense of lying on a surface results in a marked attenuation of proprioceptive, kinesthetic and spatial information. Floating on a pliable membrane does not attenuate this information to nearly as great a degree.

The results of the present study do not permit firm conclusions as to why subjects in both REST-Wet and REST-Dry showed decreased MAP, and only those in REST-Wet showed decreased cortisol. We hypothesize that the response difference is more likely a matter of degree for several reasons. First, previous studies have shown that MAP and cortisol changes in response to REST-Wet were significantly correlated (Turner et al., 1990). Secondly, REST-Wet clearly provides greater reduction in sensory input than does REST-Dry. Thirdly, in a study comparing effectiveness of REST-Wet and biofeedback-assisted relaxation (a method completely different from REST that involves active learning) in decreasing MAP and hormones in hypertensives, both reduced MAP and only REST reduced the plasma cortisol, renin activity and aldosterone. It was suggested that REST was associated with deeper relaxation than biofeedback. While the simplest explanation for the findings of the present study is that REST-Wet is a more powerful relaxation tool than REST-Dry, with the response differences being a matter of degree, further studies will be required to test this hypothesis.

Acknowledgment

Partial funding of this study was provided by Needmor, Inc., Boulder, Colorado.

25

Relaxed and Alert: Patterns of T-Wave Amplitude and Heart Rate in a REST Environment

Gary Steel

One of the more constant areas of Restricted Environmental Stimulation Technique (REST) research has been psychophysiology. Perhaps the initial use of the psychophysiological approach was a consequence of D. O. Hebb's (1955a) theories regarding the concept of drive and its relationship to nervous system activity; more likely is that the fascination with psychophysiological measures was a natural outcome of the interest in the strange effects reported by subjects (e.g., odd visual sensations, changes in body perception) that issued from the first sensory deprivation laboratories (Heron, 1957, 1961). Whatever reasons may exist, the continued presence of psychophysiology in the REST research field is certainly due, in part, to the fact that its measures offer easily-quantifiable indicators of that nebulous construct of "arousal", a touchstone that has been a perennial favourite of REST theorists (Schultz, 1965) work on "sensoristasis", and Zuckerman's (1969a) ideas regarding "optimal level of stimulation".

Despite the early evidence of bizarre effects of reduced stimulation, recent studies have reported that such environments have relaxing effects (A. Barabasz, M. Barabasz, Dyer & Rather, 1990). Pre- and post-measures of heart rate and muscle tone after either flotation tank or water immersion experiences support the production of relation (Forgays & Belinson, 1986; Forgays & McClure, 1974; Lilly, 1977; Suedfeld, Ballard & Murphy, 1983). This apparent contradiction is likely due to differential expectations of the floater. It has been found that such expectations mediate responses to REST (M. Barabasz, A. Barabasz & O'Neill, 1991; Orne, 1986; Suedfeld, 1980; Zuckerman, 1969b).

The effect of cognitive set has even been shown to have some bearing on basic physiological functions; it has been found in prior sensory restriction studies that various autonomic nervous system (ANS) and central nervous system (CNS) related measures may be affected by expectations (A. Barabasz & M. Barabasz, 1986; Shepherd, Zubek & Saunders, 1967; Zubek, 1964; Zubek, Welch & Saunders, 1962; Zuckerman & Cohen, 1964). It is possible that two specific expectancy sets may have a significant influence on trends of psychophysiological arousal: 1) the amount of physical demand placed upon the body by an environment; and 2) the amount of time one has to prepare for these physical demands. It was hypothesized in this study that the time spent in preparation is based on the expected similarity of features of the first and second environments, and the duration one is to be in the first environment.

With respect to flotation research, it was thought that it should be possible to predict the order of the time points at which the lowest level of physiological arousal will occur, based only on the subject's beliefs about the float duration and the physical features of the environment that will follow the float. For example, subjects expecting a relatively short float and dissimilar conditions afterward would arrive at their lowest point in the shortest amount of time. Subjects expecting a long float and similar conditions will take the longest to reach their lowest point. Finally, if subjects are expecting either a long duration and dissimilar environment, or a short duration and a similar environment, then the low points should occur between the two points mentioned above.

Three indices of peripheral nervous system activity were chosen to test these hypotheses; two that represent the autonomic nervous system and one that represents somatic activity. It was felt that two cardiac measures, heart rate (HR) and T-wave amplitude (TWA), were necessary to properly index autonomic nervous system (ANS) activity. Although HR alone has been a standard dependent variable in psychophysiology, the Laceys (Lacey, 1967; Lacey & Lacey, 1970) have shown that, by itself, it can be an unstable or misleading indicator of autonomic nervous system activity.

Specific information about ANS activity, particularly about the separate contributions of the sympathetic and parasympathetic nervous systems, can be gained by examining HR and TWA together (Heslegrave & Furedy, 1979). Heart rate is influenced by both the parasympathetic and sympathetic nervous system (Larsen, Schneiderman & DeCarlo-Pasin, 1986), while it has been suggested that TWA, associated with the repolarization of the ventricular mass, is influenced solely by the sympathetic nervous system (Furedy, 1987; Furedy & Heslegrave, 1983; Matyas, 1976; Matyas & King, 1976; Scher, Hartman, Furedy & Heslegrave, 1986; cf. Bunnell, 1980; Schwartz & Weiss, 1983). Specifically, decreases in TWA indicate an increase in sympathetic activity.

T-wave amplitude has one other benefit as a measure: although measures of the cognitive effort expended by a floater are difficult to gather while he or she is in the tank, TWA may be one variable that permits access to this information (Furedy, 1987; Furedy, Heslegrave & Scher, 1984). Attenuation of TWA has been found to be positively related to cognitive effort in solving a mathematical task (Heslegrave & Furedy, 1979).

To give a more complete description of peripheral nervous system activity, it was felt that it was necessary to take some measure of the arousal of the somatic nervous system. Traditionally, REST researchers have used the electromyogram (EMG) as an index of somatic arousal. Therefore, EMG was chosen for the third variable.

Method

Design

Because the hypotheses in this study are temporal in nature, a repeated measures design was employed, utilizing mean HR, TWA, and EMG activity at five contiguous intervals as dependent variables. To test the effect of expectations, a between-subjects component was included, in which a subject's expectations were manipulated regarding float duration and the physical features of the tank immediately following his or her float. The resulting multivariate design was a 2 (short/long float) by 2 (similar/dissimilar environment), with three repeated measures.

Subjects

Fifty-four subjects were drawn from a list of flotation tank volunteers, which is compiled on an on-going basis in the lab of Dr. Peter Suedfeld at the University of British Columbia (UBC). All subjects were "novice" floaters (i.e., subjects having no prior experience in a float tank). Individuals were dropped as potential subjects if they met any of the following criteria: 1) taking psychoactive medication; 2) had a contagious or infectious condition; 3) were epileptic or had a history of fainting spells; 4) currently had hemorrhoids, cold sores, or a rash; 5) had ever been diagnosed as having abnormal heart activity; 6) had any allergies that may be activated by the tank environment; 7) were pregnant; 8) were asthmatic; 9) had been treated by a doctor for a serious medical condition in the last three months. Only one person did not meet the medical criteria. This person was taking prescribed tranquilizers.

Of the 53 subjects who passed the initial screening, 17 had to be dropped after an immediate post-float examination of their data indicated the presence of excessive artifact. Consequently, 36 subjects (18 men and 18 women) were included in the final analyses. The age of these subjects ranged from 18 to 40 years (mean = 24 yrs., mode =

21 yrs.). Because the volunteer list is compiled primarily through responses to posters displayed around campus, 81% of the individuals accepted as subjects were university students, many of whom were taking at least one psychology course. However, nearly one-fifth of the subjects were employed in a wide variety of non-academic occupations.

Procedure

During the initial telephone contact, the subject was asked to abstain from drinking any beverage that may contain any caffeine (i.e., coffee, tea, hot chocolate, or cola soft drinks) during the period two hours prior to his or her participation in the study.

Upon arriving at the lab, subjects were given a brief orientation tour of the facilities. The general functions of each of the pieces of equipment with which they would come into contact (tank, tank/lab intercom, and psychophysiological instruments) were explained in a non-technical manner. The subjects were informed that an experimenter would be monitoring them via the intercom so that they needed only to speak up should they feel that they wished to communicate with the experimenter for any reason. Besides complying with ethical standards, such orientation procedures have been shown to reduce any apprehension the subject may have with regards to sensory "deprivation" (Suedfeld, 1980).

It was during the orientation tour that the subject was first informed of the experimental condition to which he or she had been randomly assigned. Subjects in Group 1 were told that they would float for 40 minutes, after which there would be a 10 minute question period regarding their float experience. During the question period, conditions would be exactly as they had been during their float (no lights, no sound, same water temperature). Subjects in Group 2 were also told they were to float for 40 minutes, but that during the question period the lights in the tank would come on, they might hear some movement from the main lab (ostensibly from "lab workers" now being free to go about their business), and that the water temperature could drop to room temperature as the heating system was shut down. Subjects in

Groups 3 and 4 were told the same information as those in Groups 1 and 2, respectively, save that the length of the float was to be 80 minutes. All subjects were told that they would hear some "mellow" music to signal the end of their float and the beginning of the question period.

The subject was then asked to shower, and do a careful self-inspection for any cuts or abrasions. All such injuries were to be covered with either a liquid bandage or petroleum jelly. After the shower, the subject donned a bathrobe and went to the electrode preparation room.

Four Ag/AgCl electrodes, with Redux gel as a conducting agent, were used in this study. Site placements were as follows: 1) EMG: 2.5 cm. above the nasion, and 2.5 cm. above the left eyebrow, directly above the center of the pupil as the subject looked forward; 2) ECG: (upper) 2.5 cm. below the top of the sternum, and (lower) 2.5 cm. above the bottom of the sternum; 3) ECG alternative sites: left and right chest, approximately in the middle of a line representing where the deltoid muscle joins the pectoralis major muscle. These sites were chosen because pilot trials had shown them to remain relatively dry during the course of a one hour float. In addition, the EMG sites are used widely in biofeedback research on relaxation and muscle tension reduction.

Electrode placement was made difficult by the wide variation among the subjects with respect to head shape, body fat, pectoral muscle development, chest hair, breast shape and breast size. If resistance across the two ECG sites exceeded a previously set level (10,000 ohms), then the alternative sites detailed above were used. These alternative sites were required for three of the subjects, two males and one female. Once the electrodes had been successfully attached to the subject, the leads were plugged into a small, portable telemetry transmitter and the experimenter ensured that both the transmitter and receiver were performing properly. Subjects were reminded at this point about the particular experimental condition they were to experience. After this, they proceeded to the tank and began their float.

Each subject floated for 60 minutes in an Ova Systems flotation tank. This is a lightproof, sound-attenuated enclosure, approximately

2.75m long by 1.82m wide by 1.52m high, and shaped much like an egg. The water in the tank is 25 cm deep, saturated with Epsom salts (47% by volume), and is heated to 34° ±.5° C. Subjects floated face up, breathing normally. Data were gathered using a unique telemetry system, designed by UFI Inc. (California) which allowed for transmission, reception, and initial analysis of psychophysiological signals.

At the end of the hour, the physiological recording equipment was shut off and music was played into the tank, in accordance with the subject's expectations. However, after the music had played for a few minutes, the subject was informed, via the intercom, that he or she could step out and have his or her second shower, as the experimenter would be conducting the question period in the main part of the lab.

The post-float question period was actually a debriefing and information-exchange session. Subjects were handed a typewritten paragraph that informed them of the true conditions of their float. They were then given the opportunity to ask any questions that they may have had, either specifically about the study or about floating in general.

Results

Data Scoring and Reduction

The analog ECG and EMG waveforms were digitized using a hybrid of UFI and Beckman modules. The sampling rate was set to 100 samples/second, with each epoch lasting five seconds. Epochs began on a randomly determined second of each minute. The signal was then digitally filtered using a lowpass filter of 20 Hz, which allowed the signals to be viewed with recognizable components and the least amount of noise. The digitized EMG and ECG waveforms were then visually inspected on a computer screen to judge their overall clarity. It was apparent that the noise artifact present in the obtained signal prohibited analysis of the EMG signal.

T-wave amplitude was scored using criteria similar to those developed by Matyas and King (1975), in which TWA is defined as the difference between the P-Q isoelectric interval and the peak of the T-wave. Each subject's TWA's were averaged across each five-second epoch; generally, this yielded 60 mean TWA's per subject. In a few cases, however, an entire epoch was rendered unscorable due to a surge in the noise level. In these cases, the missing datum was set to the subject's own grand mean TWA.

Inter-beat intervals were measured, then converted to heart rates. Heart rate data were treated in the same manner as the TWA data, including the substitution procedure for missing data. It was decided to standardize the measures within each subject before the 12 minute means were calculated. Changing the TWA's and HR's to Z-score form allowed a direct, "metric-free" comparison of the activity of the two dependent variables. Finally, the data were averaged across the 12 minute intervals, yielding five means that were used as the data points in the analyses described below. These means are presented in Table 25-1.

Data were submitted to a multivariate analysis of variance (MANOVA) statistical procedure. The benefits of using the MANOVA versus multiple univariate repeated-measures analyses have been detailed elsewhere (O'Brien & Kister-Kaiser, 1985), but two points are particularly relevant to this study. First, the methodological design was inherently multivariate. Second, the use of MANOVA avoids the sphericity assumptions necessary, but usually unattainable, in univariate analyses.

All multivariate effects, save one were not significant. The overall test for within-subject trends, (linear, quadratic, cubic, and quartic) showed an extremely strong effect (multivariate $F(8,25) = 14.517$, $p < .001$). It was decided to investigate which trend(s) accounted for the multivariate result by probing using univariate analyses, adopting a conservative significance level of $p < .005$.

The results of the univariate analyses can be found in Table 25-2. It was immediately apparent that no single trend or measure caused the significant multivariate result. The TWA measure showed a strong linear trend and, to a somewhat lesser extent, a cubic trend. The HR also indicated a strong linear component, but the pattern was also influenced by a quadratic trend. These trends are expressed graphically in Figure 25-1.

Table 25-1

Interval Means for Standardized T-Wave Amplitude and Heart Rate by Expected Duration and Environment

	Condition				
	40 Minute		80 Minute		Grand
	Similar	Dissimilar	Similar	Dissimilar	Means
TWA					
Interval					
1	.37	.21	-.12	.11	.14
2	.37	.30	.51	.49	.42
3	-.19	.24	.12	.10	.07
4	-.27	-.30	-.12	-.31	-.25
5	-.28	-.46	-.39	-.38	-.38
HR					
Interval					
1	.43	.73	.61	.78	.64
2	.04	.11	.20	.08	.11
3	-.17	-.24	-.05	-.21	-.17
4	-.21	-.33	-.47	-.38	-.35
5	-.09	-.28	-.29	-.26	-.25

Table 25-2

Single *df* Polynomial Contrasts for "Internals" Effect

Trend	F(1,32)	p <
TWA		
Linear	31.56	.001
Quadratic	5.44	*n.s.*
Cubic	19.26	.001
Quartic	1.22	*n.s.*
HR		
Linear	49.98	.001
Quadratic	29.66	*n.s.*
Cubic	0.06	.001
Quartic	1.81	*n.s.*

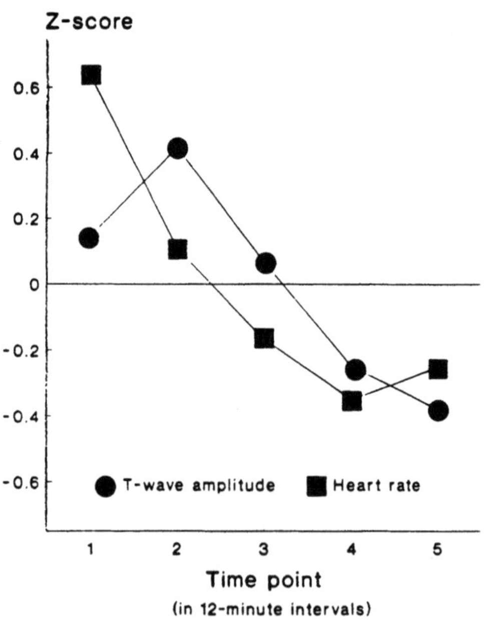

Figure 25-1. Trends of standardized (within-subject) T-wave amplitude and heart rate. Each interval represents 12 minutes.

Discussion

The results clearly offer no support for the influence of duration and following environment expectancy-sets, at least in respect to physiological functioning in the tank. Examining the significant trends in the data, the initial rise in TWA between Intervals 1 and 2 suggests that sympathetic nervous system activity is decreasing. One may suspect that autonomic nervous system arousal is generally decreasing, and this seems to be supported when one looks at the decrease in heart rate between these two points.

However, TWA begins to attenuate after Interval 2 and does not increase again, leading us to believe that sympathetic nervous system activity is increasing during all intervals but the first. When one turns to HR for corroboration of this increase of activity, it cannot be found. In fact, HR decreases from Interval 2 to Interval 4, rising slightly in Interval 5. This pattern is in opposition to the TWA trend, suggesting that the two measures are under the control of different systems.

With this in mind, one can see that as sympathetic nervous system activity increases (marked by TWA attenuation), a greater increase in parasympathetic nervous system activity must have accompanied it in order to bring about the decrease in HR. Rather than a general lowering of physiological arousal levels, the experience of floating is associated with a rise in activity of both sub-systems of the ANS.

Evidence from debriefing interviews indicates that the tank is perceived by a large number of novice floaters as an exploratory experience, as well as an environment in which one may mull over personal problems. If we consider that contemplative behavior requires cognitive effort, then the TWA pattern indicates that this behavior is on the increase 12 minutes after the subject enters the tank. Exploration and introspection are the orders of the day; after all, where else can one find so novel an environment, and one in which interruption of one's thoughts is so unlikely?

Alternatively, subjects may simply have been generating increasingly more complex images and thought patterns as their time in the tank wore on. It has been suggested that TWA attenuation is a potential marker of "a more selective and complexly organized set of cognitive processes, requiring higher levels of selective functioning or 'wakefulness'..." (Cacioppo, Petty & Morris, 1985, p. 381). Perhaps passing from one thought to the next brought about the chance to experience more interesting images; either by learning how to use the tank's unique environment for mental exploration, or through a lowering of mental blocks, the subject became more involved in the world of his or her mind. Consistent with Barabasz's (1982) hypothesis, it may not be that the level of internal stimulation increases. We may simply become better at detecting, and more interested in, the thoughts that are screened out by our interaction with the environment in everyday life.

Overall, the results of the two available measures indicate that the tank may be useful as a relatively rapid method of inducing deep relaxation. The key to using the tank most efficiently is in specifying what one wishes to derive from the experience. If physical relaxation is the goal, then a short stay of 30-40 minutes may suffice. If one wishes to experience the potential psychological benefits of tank-related cognitive activity, then a longer float session may be in order. Further research examining the temporal patterning of cardiovascular functioning and muscle activity of humans in the flotation tank is definitely in order.

26

A Method for Continuous Blood Sampling During Flotation REST

John Turner, Jr., Harmony Shroeder
and Thomas Fine

Flotation Restricted Environmental Stimulation Therapy (flotation REST) is a deep relaxation modality in which an individual lies supinely in a thermoneutral buoyant fluid with minimal photic, auditory and tactile stimulation (Lilly, 1977). Blood levels of several hormones, including aldosterone, renin activity, ACTH, LH, and cortisol, have been measured in association with flotation REST (henceforth, REST) and significant changes in the levels of several of these hormones have been reported (Turner & Fine 1983, 1991; Turner et al., 1989; McGrady et al., 1987). These studies have examined pre- to post-session and across-session changes in plasma levels of hormones. Although pre- to post-session decreases in plasma cortisol have been observed (Turner & Fine, 1983) in sessions as brief as 35 minutes, the characteristics and patterns of hormonal change during a REST session are unknown.

One of the difficulties faced in considering blood sampling during a REST session is the possible disruption of the REST experience in obtaining in-session samples. In the present repeated-measures study, a technique is demonstrated which uses an intravenous line to permit continuous blood sampling during the REST experience. Subject condition during REST was assessed via rating of physical and mental comfort and measurement of plasma cortisol.

Method

Subjects

Subjects were four healthy male medical student volunteers aged 22-30. The study was performed during summer vacation, and no major stresses were reported. Each subject experienced six sessions, 60 minutes each. Session 1 was baseline blood sampling in a Non-REST (waterbed) environment. The session consisted of reclining on a waterbed in a warm (85° F), dimly lit room. Sessions 2-5 were REST without blood sampling, and in the first three of these sessions the subject floated with the intravenous (i.v.) setup attached (no needle). Session 6 was continuous sampling in the REST environment.

Procedure

All blood sampling was done between 1100 and 1600 in consideration of diurnal cortisol release patterns (Weitzman et al., 1971).

Samples were taken via intravenous catheter using a 20 ga., 2.8 cm needle (Gelco Corp.) placed in the dorsal vein of the lower forearm. All i.v. operations were performed by a trained phlebotomist with extensive i.v. experience. The line was inserted into the forearm after the subject was in the REST chamber and extended his arm outside through a portal (see Figure 26-1). After i.v. placement, the subject drew his hand inside the chamber and rested it on a plastic foam slab 16 x 16 x 2 cm., which provided buoyancy to keep the i.v. site out of the fluid.

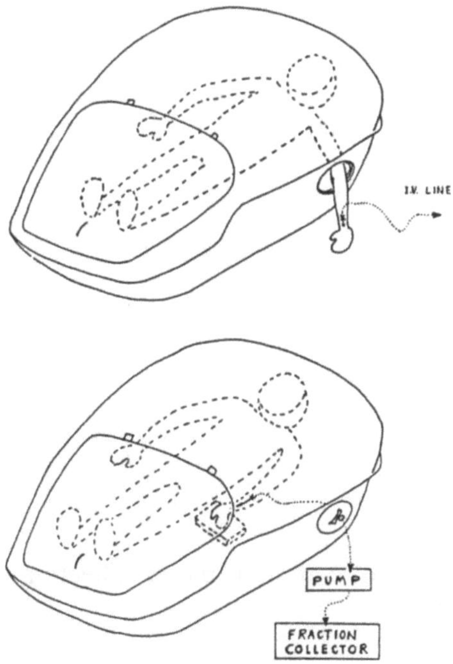

Figure 26-1. Diagram of subject in REST with intravenous monitoring system: a) subject with arm through portal to receive i.v. line, b) subject and i.v. system as it appears during collection.

Using a peristaltic pump, 70-90 ml of blood was withdrawn at a rate of 1.4 ml/minutes for 40-60 minutes. The blood was collected into heparinized tubes in 3 ml fractions. Silastic® tubing (16 ga.) was used throughout the collection system (see Figure 26-2). Total tubing length of the system from i.v. site to fraction tube was 1.9 m. Clotting within the system was prevented by continuous infusion of 51 mg heparin per minute in isotonic saline. The heparin line was inserted into the i.v. tubing approximately 1.0 cm distal to the i.v. site. Blood sample fractions were centrifuged at 3000 X g. for 20 minutes and plasma was decanted and frozen until assayed for cortisol. Plasma cortisol levels were determined by RIA kit (ICN Biomedical, Inc., Carson, California).

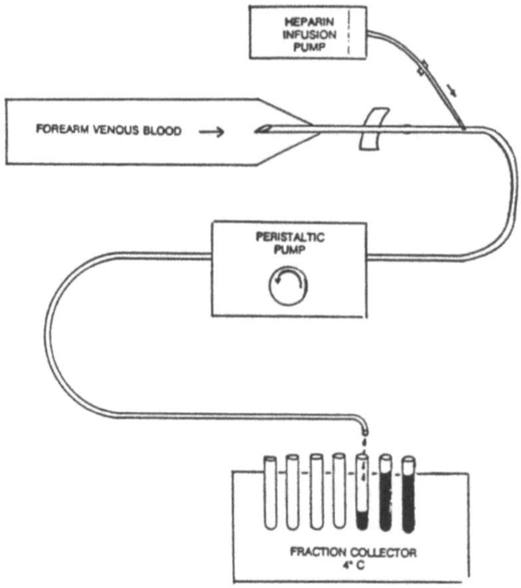

Figure 26-2. Diagram of continous blood collection system.

Each subject filled out a mental-physical comfort rating scale immediately after each session. Comfort was rated on a scale of 0 to 10, with 10 being consistent comfort and 0 being consistent discomfort. All subjects also gave a subjective report of each session's experience.

Results

Difficulties in blood collection were encountered initially due to clotting of blood in the i.v. system proximal to the heparin infusion site, and collection was not possible beyond 25 minutes. By soaking the hub and needle in heparin solution (100 mg/ml) and drying off the outside of the barrel prior to insertion, this problem was corrected. All sampling periods were at least 40 minutes, and four were 60 minutes. There were no differences in ratings of mental or physical comfort among the sessions (see Table 26-1).

Table 26-1

Mental and Physical Comfort Associated with Continuous Blood Sampling During Flotation REST

Condition	Comfort Rating ± S.E.	
	Mental Comfort[a]	Physical Comfort[a]
Non-REST with Blood Sampling[b]	7.5 ± 1.2	7.9 ± 0.8
REST with Mock Blood Sampling[c]	8.3 ± 1.1	8.8 ± 0.5
REST alone	8.5 ± 0.6	9.0 ± 1.0
REST with Blood Sampling	8.2 ± 0.6	8.7 ± 0.9

[a] Comfort is rated on a scale of 0 to 10, with 10 being consistent comfort and 0 being consistent discomfort (n=4).

[b] Consisted of reclining on a waterbed in a warm (85° F.), dimly lit room.

[c] Consisted of sampling procedure and paraphernalia without venipuncture.

There was no infection and no unusual bruising, swelling or tissue discoloration associated with the i.v. use, and no clotting failure was observed. Subjective reports regarding the REST experience were consistently positive, despite one subject's expression of anxiety about being in REST, prior to the initial experience. Three subjects stated that they had no reservations about having an i.v. line. One subject expressed mild concern. All subjects said that they felt much more comfortable knowing that an experienced phlebotomist was doing the i.v. work.

Plasma cortisol levels varied across fractions, and patterns varied among subjects. No consistent change was observed within a given session, and there were no consistent differences between patterns in Session 1 and Sessions 6, although the average levels of cortisol were higher in Session 1 than in Session 6. Representative cortisol data are shown in Figure 26-3.

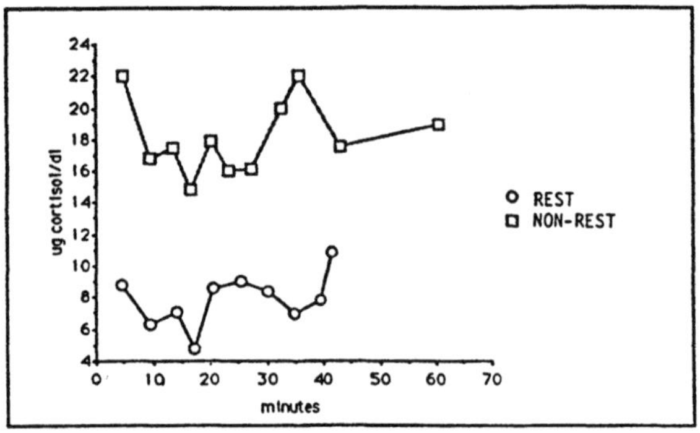

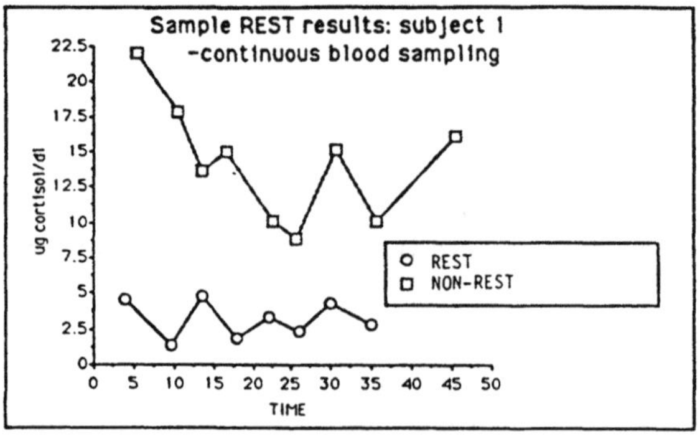

Figure 26-3. Plasma cortisol levels during a REST session and a Non-REST (waterbed) session: a) data from a single subject (D.D.), b) data averaged for all subjects.

Discussion

The results of this study demonstrate that blood may be collected continuously from subjects for up to 60 minutes during a REST experience. Heparinization of the i.v. needle and hub and continuous heparin infusion into the i.v. line distal to the i.v. placement site are necessary in this procedure to prevent clotting.

On the basis of the rating scales and subjective reports it appears that continuous blood withdrawal does not alter the subjects' perception of the REST experience. The cortisol data appear to be consistent with the subjective-rating data. Previous studies have shown that repeated, brief REST is deeply relaxing (A. Barabasz, M. Barabasz, Dyer & Rather, 1990; Turner & Fine, 1983; Suedfeld, Ballard, & Murphy, 1983) and is associated with decreased plasma cortisol (Turner & Fine, 1983, 1991; Turner et al., 1989). Since cortisol levels in the present study were lower in Session 6 than in baseline Session 1, it appears that in terms of the overall study, the presence of the i.v. line did not compromise the relaxation-REST response. On the other hand, the pre- to post-cortisol decrease (approximately 20%) in REST reported elsewhere (Turner & Fine, 1983) was not consistently observed in the present study. Two of the subjects showed a small decrease ($<12\%$) in cortisol during the monitored REST session, while one other subject showed no change and the fourth showed a slight increase.

The reason for this discrepancy is unknown. It may reflect a less relaxing experience in Session 6 associated with the presence of the i.v. line. This is, however, not consistent with the rating and report data. One possible explanation may be found in comparing the starting values in the two studies. The subjects in the present study showed beginning cortisol levels which averaged 40% lower than the starting values of the previous study and were even lower than the post session values of that study. Thus, it is possible that the cortisol values in the present study were already near minimum by Session 6 and could not decline further.

The results of this study are valuable and encouraging in providing a hitherto unavailable opportunity for continuous monitoring of blood-born substances during the REST experience.

27

REST as a Treatment for Children with Autism

John Harrison and Arreed Barabasz

Several studies suggest that average levels of stimulation may be too high for autistic children (C. Hutt, S. Hutt, Lee, & Ounsted, 1964; Margolies, 1977; Schechter, Shurley, Toussieng, & Maier, 1969; Suedfeld & Schwartz, 1983). Alternatively, others attribute the problem to a deprivation of sensory input (Moore & Shiek, 1971; Williams & Harper, 1974). Theories and evidence from clinical observations converge on a characterization of autism as an abnormal reaction to environmental stimuli or a dysfunction in the ability to adequately process average levels of stimuli (American Psychiatric Association, 1987; Fein, Waterhouse, Lucci, & Snyder, 1985; Ornitz & Ritvo, 1976; Wing & Gould, 1979). Bartak, Rutter, and Cox (1975) have shown that individuals with autism have limited or restricted interactions. Theories consistent with this evidence suggest that exposure to average levels of stimuli results in a cognitive processing breakdown and an abnormal (restrictive) response to the environment (e.g., Hermelin, 1976; Rutter, 1983; Shah & Wing, 1986). If these theories are correct, one would expect a reduction in the amount of stimuli these individuals are required to process to result in a reduction of autistic symptoms and a desire for stimulation. It is this theoretical perspective (Jones, 1969; Schechter et al., 1969; Suedfeld & Schwartz, 1983) that has encouraged the application of Restricted Environmental Stimulation Therapy (REST) to the treatment of children with autism.

Schechter et al. (1969) exposed three autistic boys (ages 5, 4.3, and 5.5) to an extended (68, 40, and 74 days, respectively) reduction in stimulation which resulted in the development of more satisfactory relationships, improved social and intellectual skills, and overall better adjustment to their environments. Suedfeld and Schwartz (1983) improved upon Schechter et al.'s (1969) methodological weaknesses by increasing the N to seven and instituting a control group which was matched for age with the experimental group. They employed pre- and post-test observational scales and standardized tests, whereas the Schechter et al. (1969) study relied primarily on clinical judgment and anecdotal reports. Suedfeld and Schwartz (1983) found significant increases in discrimination learning and social interaction, near significant increases on a measure of cognitive functioning, and near significant reductions in general autistic symptoms.

The present study extended the work of Suedfeld and Schwartz (1983). This included an increase in the number of subjects, the measurement of I.Q. to match subjects between REST and control conditions, the use of instruments which were less limited by ceiling effect, and research design improvements. A larger transdisciplinary research team was organized to make possible completely blind collection of data on the dependent variables. Finally, the present study responded to previous failures to adequately describe autistic samples (Kistner & Robbins, 1986).

On the basis of the REST and autism literature, the current study tested the hypotheses that REST would significantly: 1) increase autistic subjects' rate of discrimination learning on curriculum-based learning tasks; 2) increase cognitive performance on the Leiter International Performance Scale; 3) lower the frequency of autistic symptoms as measured on the Autism Behavior Checklist; 4) lower mean autistic social interaction on the Interaction Assessment; 5) increase the average length of verbal utterances and language age on a sample of vocal behavior; and 6) lower the frequency of autistic speech characteristics.

Method

Subjects

Subjects' parents volunteered for participation through an autism program and a special education program in two northwestern cities. Six males and six females ranging from 6.6 years to 20.5 years (mean age = 11.98 years; SD = 4.38 years), meeting the DSM III-R diagnostic criteria for autism (APA, 1987), were selected for participation in the study.

Volunteers were initially selected on the basis of information from medical/psychological records. Later, a screening procedure using the Autism Behavior Checklist (inter-rater reliability .95) (Krug, Arick, & Almond, 1980), was conducted for the final selection. Sixty-nine percent of the present sample received raw scores above the standardization sample mean while the remaining 31% received raw scores within one standard deviation below the mean.

Based on their performance on the Leiter International Performance Scale, 12 subjects were successfully matched and randomly assigned to experimental (mean I.Q. = 35.3; range = 8-72; SD = 28.14) and control groups (mean I.Q. = 39.0; range = 0-113; SD = 41.70). The experimental group mean age was 147.83 months (range = 81-209; SD = 65.90) compared to the control group mean age of 150.66 months (range = 88-201; SD = 44.38). There were no statistically significant pre-treatment differences between the experimental and control group on the intelligence test measure (Wilcoxon T = 8.50, Ns-R = 6, $p > .10$) or on the other pre-treatment test measures.

Treatment Setting

Three observation rooms in the Department of Clinical Psychology at Eastern Washington University, were used. The experimental room (REST condition) was about 4 x 7 meters. The room was dimly illuminated (approximately equivalent to that produced by six evenly distributed 4.5 watt night lights). Except for a mattress, a portable toilet behind a partition, and one ceiling camera monitor, there was no furniture. Forced air ventilation provided low level monotonous stimulation, and room temperature was maintained between 22.2-23.3° C. Behaviors were monitored from a central control room with visual (one-way mirrors), video, and audio capability.

The control condition setting was a larger (7 x 8 meters) fully illuminated room with four large windows and a wall mounted blackboard. The floor was covered with thick wall to wall carpet and the room was equipped with two mattresses, a variety of furniture, familiar age appropriate toys, and the parents' choice of a T.V. or radio. Meals were provided in the room and subjects were given access to bathroom facilities located several meters away from the control area. Behaviors were monitored from an observation room equipped with audio capability and a one-way window.

A nearby 5 x 4 meter stimulating play room was used for the pre- and post-treatment interaction assessment. The room was fully illuminated with natural and artificial light and was equipped with many gross and fine motor toys.

Procedure

Prior to commencement of the experiment, a general orientation session was conducted with the subjects' parents or legal guardians. Following the group orientation, each parent and child attended two pre-treatment orientations to the REST or control sites (as per Suedfeld, 1980, p.377).

Each child assigned to the experimental group wore pajamas and was told that he/she was going to have a good rest (Suedfeld & Schwartz, 1983). During the 34-hour treatment, interaction was limited to the presentation of meals, hygiene assistance and other health/safety requirements.

The control subjects were provided with opportunities for social contact with an experienced child caretaker. As per Suedfeld and Schwartz (1983), the control condition had normal lighting, free access to the entire room and its furnishings, meals, necessary health/safety provisions, and bathroom facilities. The condition was designed to control for potential novelty effects. It provided an experience where the child was relocated from familiar surroundings and placed in an environment where near typical levels of stimulation could be assured.

Assessment

The following baseline measures were conducted on all subjects approximately one month before the first of six successive treatment weekends during which the study was conducted. The Leiter International Performance Scale was administered by two clinical psychology graduate students. The Autism Behavior Checklist (ABC) was completed by each subject's classroom teacher. The Sample of Vocal Behavior was administered once to each subject by a graduate level communications disorders specialist with over 1,000 hours of supervised experience. The Interaction Assessment (IA) was administered to each subject twice a week for two weeks resulting in a mean IA baseline score. IA sessions were videotaped to allow for careful scoring and to maximize inter-rater reliability. The video tapes were scored by two research assistants trained to score the IA. Classroom teachers collected the curriculum-based discrimination learning baselines four times per week during the three weeks before each subjects's exposure to their respective treatment condition. Finally, one videotaped IA was conducted immediately before each experimental or control treatment. All classroom data were collected with an effort to avoid confounding variables which would likely influence subjects' performance. Raters and classroom teachers were blind to group assignment.

A research assistant and a parent/family member recorded the REST and control subject's behavior every 15 minutes throughout the treatment period. Both observers categorized the behavior on the basis of Suedfeld and Schwartz's (1983) observation of stress-and nonstress-related behaviors. The combination of parent and professional judgment served to validate the categorizations of these behaviors.

These research assistants had only a general knowledge of the hypotheses and were unaware of the alternative environments.

Immediately following treatment, each subject underwent another videotaped IA. IA data was also collected twice a week for two weeks following treatment. The Sample of Vocal Behavior was readministered two days after each treatment. The Leiter International Performance Scale and the ABC was readministered three weeks after each treatment. The discrimination learning measure was readministered four times a week for three weeks following each treatment. Finally, all parents were instructed to maintain a two-week follow-up log of behaviors which occurred outside of their child's typical range of behaviors at home.

Results

The behavioral logs, from the REST and control sessions, indicated low frequencies of observed stress in both groups. Children in the REST condition emitted 0.13 mean occurrences per hour, while children in the control condition emitted 0.10 mean occurrences per hour. Compared to the control group, the REST group emitted somewhat higher levels of stress in the initial hours, and somewhat lower levels in the latter hours. This trend is displayed in Figure 27-1.

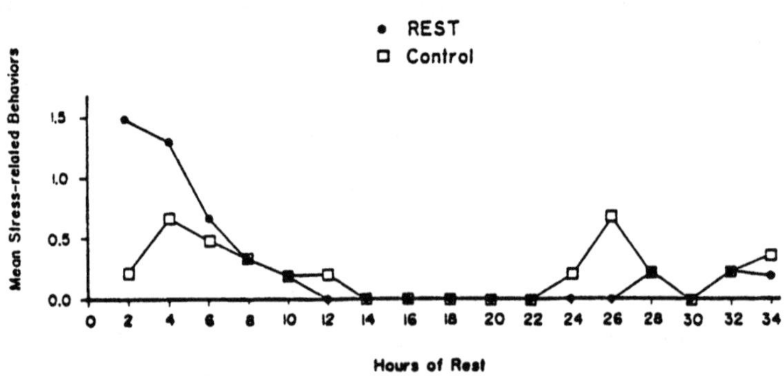

Figure 27-1. Mean occurrences of stress and nonstress-related behaviors in two hour intervals.

Behaviors displayed during REST included talking, giggling, feeling the walls, trying to observe their dim reflections in the one-way vision glass, attempting to open the door, and tantruming/crying episodes. All subjects completed the treatment. Following the 20-minute IA post-testing session, each child reunited with their parents. In an effort to detect the presence of negative feelings toward the REST experience, each child was allowed to briefly reenter the REST area. No reluctance or adverse reactions were observed. One child reentered the room with a notable positive facial expression and exploratory behavior. One REST subject approached the room saying, "Thanks for the weekend in the room." Upon reentering the room another subject immediately sat down on the mattress with no signs of stress. Another subject approached the room and smiled.

A Wilcoxon matched-pairs signed-ranks analyses suggested no positive effects of REST on intelligence test performance or vocal behavior (language age, average length, autistic speech characteristics). Point-by-point inter-rater reliability (Kazdin, 1982) ranged from .80 to 1.0 (mean = .90) on the Sample of Vocal Behavior throughout the data collection period.

The binomial expansion-split middle technique (Kazdin, 1982) and the rate of change (slope) analysis was used to compare the trend within and across the baseline and post-treatment phase for each of two curriculum based tasks per subject. No significant experimental or control group effects were found ($p > .10$, $z = 1.28$) (mcan point-by-point inter-rater reliability = .986; range = .83-1.0). Ceiling effects were observed on four tasks. Two tasks suggested false positive or false negative results related to steep pre-treatment trends in the data and excessive across trial variance.

Wilcoxon matched-pairs signed-ranks analyses revealed that both groups demonstrated lower post-treatment ABC scores as compared to pre-treatment ABC scores obtained at subject selection ($T = 0$, Ns-R = 6, $p < .01$) and just before treatment ($T = 1$, Ns-R = 6, $p < .03$). These results are shown in Table 27-1.

Table 27-1

Wilcoxon Matched-Pairs Signed-Ranks Test: Autism Behavior Checklist Results for Less Severe Subjects

Less severe symptom sample comparison	n	M Pretest (SD)	M Posttest (SD)	ES	Wilcoxon Ns-R	T	P<
S selection with post-treatment - exp	4	83.50 (16.9)	43.75 (12.1)	2.30	6	0	.06
S selection with post-treatment - con	4	79.75 (8.5)	62.75 (22.3)	1.56	6	2	.18
Pre-treatment with post-treatment - exp	4	68.75 (12.0)	43.75 (12.1)	4.51	6	0	.06
Pre-treatment with post-treatment - con	4	72.25 (15.1)	62.75 (22.3)	1.00	6	2	.18

(Alpha = .10)

Wilcoxon matched-pairs signed-ranks analyses were also conducted on IA scores obtained immediately pre- and post-treatment. The REST group demonstrated a trend toward significance showing greater ($p < .10$) within-group symptom reduction than the control group. However, older experimental subjects showed significant ($p < .05$) reductions not found in older controls ($p > .10$). Autistic social score reductions were noted in all older experimental subjects. These results appear in Table 27-2.

The two week follow-up data showed significant within-experimental ($T = 3$, Ns-R $= 6$, $p < .08$) and control ($T = 0$, Ns-R $= 6$, $p < .02$) group reductions. Initial mean point-by-point inter-rater reliability for the four IA subtests ranged from .80 to 1.0. Mean inter-rater reliabilities were maintained between .87 and 1.0 during data collection.

An analysis of parents' two-week follow-up anecdotal logs indicated that four of six (66%) experimental group parents reported improvements in their child's behavior during the first week post-

Table 27-2

Wilcoxon Matched-Pairs Signed-Ranks Tests: Interaction Assessment Immediately Pre- and Post-treatment

Group	n	M Pretest (SD)	M Posttest (SD)	ES	Wilcoxon Ns-R	T	P<
Exp	6	66.67 (10.6)	60.33 (8.2)	.36	6	7	.28
Con	6	53.83 (12.6)	53.83 (12.5)	.00	6	10	.50
Exp (older S)	4	68.50 (3.42)	59.25 (8.85)	3.19	4	0	.06
Con (older S)	4	48.75 (7.04)	48.50 (2.38)	.05	4	5	.56

(Alpha = .10).

treatment. Most reports indicated a deterioration during the second week post-treatment. One experimental group parent reported a variety of negative behaviors and symptoms and one parent's log could not be clearly categorized. Two of six control group parents reported negative post-treatment behaviors in their children. One reported improvement, and three reported no change. Two control group parents did not complete logs; but systematically obtained verbal reports revealed no atypical behaviors.

Discussion

The low frequencies of stress-related behaviors observed in this study were consistent with the Suedfeld and Schwartz (1983) observations. The careful and thorough pre-treatment orientation sessions appeared to facilitate subjects' adaptation to their respective environments.

Teachers' expectation for improvement on the ABC was a suspected confounding variable. This was supported by both groups' dramatic post-treatment reductions, despite teacher raters' blindness to subjects' group assignment. Despite these across group ABC reductions, significant within-REST group only reductions were found for subjects with less severe pre-treatment ABC symptoms.

Schechter et al. (1969), and Suedfeld and Schwartz (1983) found some support for increased social interaction as a result of REST. In the current study, REST subjects displayed a clear trend in this direction, immediately post-treatment. However, older experimental subjects showed much stronger significant experimental effects than younger subjects, while controls showed no such effects. The strength of this finding lies in the objectivity of the data collection procedure, which included standardized assessment, use of blind raters, and high inter-rater reliability.

In summary, significant autistic symptom reductions were found in older subjects and subjects with less severe autistic symptomatology. There was a 63% subject overlap between these responder subgroups. In addition, their I.Q.'s fell within the upper 58% of the total study sample. This suggests that the trend exhibited was consistent with other findings suggesting a relationship between I.Q., chronological age, and less severe autistic symptomatology (Rutter, 1970; Schopler & Mesibov, 1983; Wing, 1983).

The positive findings of this study support its theoretical basis which suggests that typical levels of environmental stimulation are too high for individuals with autism (e.g., C. Hutt, S. Hutt, Lee, & Ounsted, 1964; Suedfeld & Schwartz, 1983), and that REST may provide these individuals with more optimal interactions with their environment (Lilly, 1960; Jones, 1969; Suedfeld, 1969a).

It must be emphasized that the current study was exploratory and that its small number of subjects may not be representative of the population of autistic children. Replication with larger numbers of subjects is still needed to further test the apparent positive effects of REST on social interaction and general autistic symptoms. Future studies should add more structured/objective home-based follow-up procedures. Some ceiling effects occurred on discrimination learning tasks because subjects were not advanced to the next level of difficulty upon mastery. More careful monitoring could have been achieved by assigning greater numbers of assessment personnel or by reducing the number of learning tasks to be measured. Steep pre-treatment discrimination learning baseline trends and the effects of excessive across trial variance may be minimized in future studies by adding data points, or selecting more stable learning tasks. These methodological and procedural limitations may have concealed potential significant changes. Therefore, discrimination learning may still be an appropriate variable for further testing. Finally, future studies should consider increasing reliability and statistical power by conducting more in-depth measures on fewer dependent variables.

There may be several worthwhile applications of REST for children with autism. REST appears to provide a rationale for reducing stimulus complexity in the home and school environments. It would be particularly interesting to test the effects of brief REST sessions throughout the day to promote classroom attending. This is an important prerequisite to learning. Periodic sessions in the home may facilitate an increased desire for interactions with family members and peers. Changes at these levels might significantly increase the productivity and quality of life for children with autism.

28

The Effects of Consecutive Floats and Their Timing on Premenstrual Syndrome

Walter Jessen

Dalton (1987) defines Premenstrual Syndrome (PMS) as "any symptoms or complaints which regularly come between ovulation and the early phase of menstruation, but are absent at other times of the cycle." These symptoms run the gamut of depression or irritability to asthma, epilepsy and homicide. Although no woman suffers from all of the symptoms, any symptom can be so severe and so debilitating as to warrant extreme medical and/or psychiatric measures, only to quietly end at menses. Dalton (1987) documented that PMS is due to a hormone dysfunction, i.e., progesterone is either not secreted in an abundant supply or not long enough starting at ovulation. This can throw the woman into internal chaos both mentally and physically. If there was a way to naturally alter this hormone dysfunction without having to be conscious of diet or take progesterone this could make a big difference. Goldstein and Jessen (1989) determined that flotation REST, during PMS, radically reduces reported symptoms. The study examined the effects of one float on one cycle. Turner and Fine (1985b) used flotation REST to examine its effects on hormones. They found that it has a normalizing effect on the body by significantly reducing the hormonal activity of the pituitary adrenal axis. Although not statistically significant, they did note an increase in the luteinizing hormone. Lastly, they found that consecutive floats stabilized hormonal functioning. What's important about this research is that not only can flotation normalize hormonal functioning, it can also enhance the production of a hormone that potentiates the secretion of progesterone, the luteinizing hormone. Knowing that a very small change in hormone output can have enormous effects on menstrual and premenstrual activity, it was hypothesized that flotation during the premenstrual cycle could create just enough change to make a major difference in PMS, and do it naturally. Further, it was reasoned that consecutive floats might create the hormonal stabilization necessary for the body to create a new homeostasis and thus ameliorate the problem.

Thus, the study was designed to pose three questions: 1) Does flotation decrease the frequency of PMS symptoms and/or the degree of debilitation? 2) Does the timing of the float during the PMS cycle result in differential reductions in frequency and severity of symptoms? 3) Do the effects of consecutive floats stabilize or further decrease the frequency and severity of symptoms?

Method

Subjects

Originally there were 15 women randomly assigned to three groups. Due to attrition, all groups were reduced to four per group. There was no significant difference in age among the groups; the age range was 27 to 45 years. Each subject volunteered for the study, was not paid for their participation, and reported their history of PMS symptoms and documented their claims to having PMS. No attempt was made to match groups at baseline as to the degree of symptoms.

Procedure

There were two experimental groups and a control group. Subjects in the experimental groups were told "our study is examining whether or not flotation done once a month for three consecutive months has a significant effect on PMS." All subjects were required to self administer the Daniel-Goldstein Premenstrual Symptom Checklist, a self report instrument that measures the frequency and severity of 61 PMS symptoms. This was administered to determine a baseline before the floats, and subsequent to each float one day past mid PMS for a total of four administrations per subject. The control group was told to monitor their symptoms at the same intervals as the experimental groups. All checklists were self administered away from the experimental setting, presumably at home, and returned by mail in a postage-paid envelope to the experimenter. All experimental group subjects floated in a Samadhi I tank at the Regeneration Institute and all were floated by the experimenter. One experimental group floated on the day of ovulation, while the other experimental group floated at mid PMS.

Results

An analysis of variance, repeated measures design was used to analyze the data. Table 28-1 and 28-2 show no significant group differences with respect to either frequency or severity of symptoms.

There were significant treatment effects ($p < .01$) showing that changes were reported at the administration of the checklist on both the frequency and severity of symptoms in all groups. And there were significant interactions among groups, symptom severity was significant at $p < .05$ while a higher level of significance $p < .01$ was demonstrated with symptom frequency.

Post hoc analysis of the interactions revealed the following (see Figures 28-1 and 28-2).

Table 28-1

Frequency of PMS Symptoms x Groups

Source	SS	df	MS	F
Between S's	92,979.22	11		
A	20,076.79	2	10,038.40	1.24
S's within	72,902.43	9	8,100.27	
Within S's	27,523.75	36		
B	11,073.06	3	3,691.02	16.32*
AB	10,342.88	6	1,723.81	7.62*
B x S's within	6,107.81	27	226.22	

* p <.01

Table 28-2

Severity of PMS Symptoms x Groups

Source	SS	df	MS	F
Between S's	70,013.50	11	6,364.86	
A	18,927.13	2	9,463.57	1.67
S's within	51,086.37	9	5,676.26	
Within S's	34,783.50	36	966.21	
B	8,773.83	3	2,924.61	4.63*
AB	8,949.04	6	1,491.51	2.36**
B x S's within	17,060.63	27	631.88	

* p <.01
** p <.05

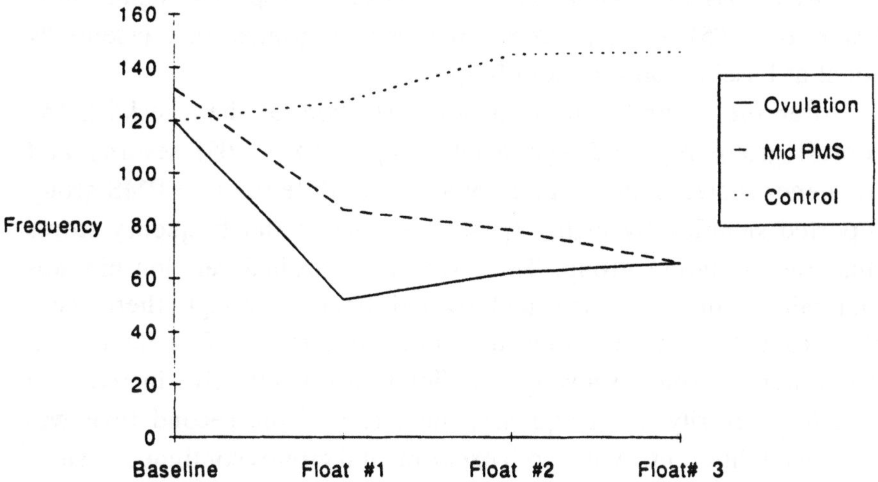

Figure 28-1. Symptoms frequency x group x float.

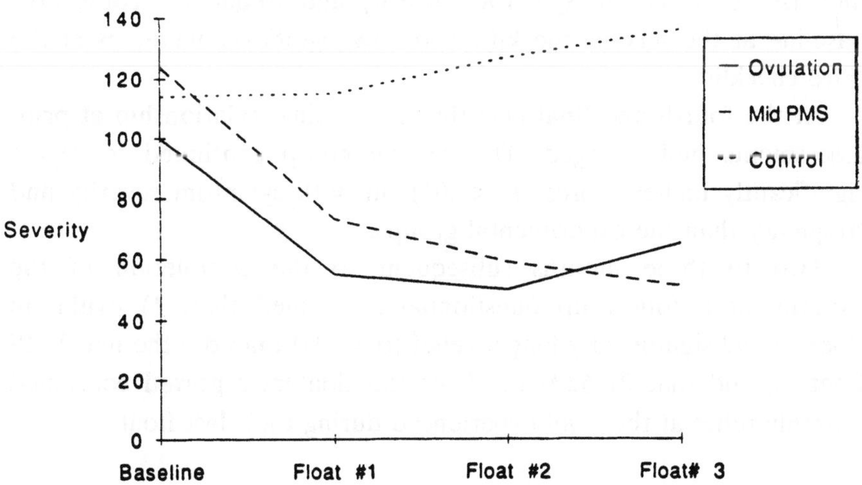

Figure 28-2. Symptom severity x group x float.

Control and mid PMS groups reported statistically equal symptom severity at baseline, while the ovulation group reported significantly lower ($p < .05$) severity scores. However, all groups were essentially equal at baseline on symptom frequency.

After the second and third administration of the checklist, the control group reported significantly higher ($p < .05$) severity and frequency scores than the mid PMS group, while the mid PMS group reported significantly higher ($p < .05$) severity and frequency scores than the ovulation group. Thus, the same ordinal relationship was maintained after the first and second float. Although there were significant decreases reported over baseline after the first float in all experimental groups showing that flotation was effective in reducing symptom severity and frequency, the effect of the second float was somewhat different. While both experimental groups continued to show more significant decreases in symptom severity after the second float, the ovulation group significantly increased ($p < .05$) symptom frequency at this point. Despite this increase, the ovulation group continued to report significantly lower frequency scores ($p < .05$), albeit less stable, than the mid PMS group. The control group reported a significant increase ($p < .05$) in symptom severity and frequency scores over baseline at the second checklist and now significant increases at the third checklist.

At the fourth and final checklist, the ordinal relationship at prior assessments had changed. The control group continued to report significantly higher scores ($p < .01$) on both symptom severity and frequency than the experimental groups.

Two to three months subsequent to the completion of the experiment a follow up questionnaire revealed that: 1) ovulation floaters had significantly longer relief ($p < .05$) than did the mid PMS floaters, and that 2) 62% of all of the floaters reported continued monthly relief at the level experienced during their last float.

Discussion

On both frequency and symptom severity scales, the mid PMS group showed a progressive and stable decrease in scores with significant decreases after the first and third floats. There was a linear relationship; as scores decreased on one scale they did the same on the other. The result may be due to the timing of the float. The float may deliver a powerful blow to the hormonal mechanisms active during PMS. Over floats the ovulation group reported more score variability on both scales than the mid PMS group. For example, the most obvious between group difference on the frequency scale was after the first float. The ovulation group reported a 67 point drop in symptom frequency from baseline and a 32 point difference below the mid PMS group scores after the first float; both differences are well beyond the .01 level of significance. After the next float the ovulation scores significantly increased over the first float. This suggests that floating at ovulation has a profound effect on how often a symptom will occur and that the effect may be unstable. Despite the fact that there is an obvious artifact, that the ovulation group reported these symptoms seven days after their float while the mid PMS group reported twenty four hours subsequent to floating, the post-experiment checklist revealed a startling observation.

The ovulation group reported significantly longer relief between floats than the mid PMS group. This suggests that floating at ovulation may be triggering a different mechanism than the mid PMS float--stimulating an increase of both the luteinizing and progesterone hormones versus the decrease of PMS hormones in the mid PMS group. These effects may be unstable but seemed to be longer lasting. Lastly, floating at ovulation resulted in significantly lower frequency and symptom severity scores than those reported by the mid PMS group. Even seven days after their float, the ovulation group still reported lower scores than the mid PMS group. Though consecutive monthly floats appeared to have the effect of progressively decreasing frequency and severity scores in the mid PMS group, the two consecutive floats followed by a third float two months later in the ovulation group served to increase scores on both scales. The artifact in the ovulation group, where 50% of this group on their third float, floated one month late, served to increase variability of responses. Perhaps the best consecutive float measure is to look at the post experimental results where 62% of the floaters reported continued relief at the same level or better than the last float. There was no difference due to timing of the float. However, this latter result can be criticized because memory over time may effect perception of symptoms. The anecdotal reports from husbands of these floaters are interesting. Husbands noted lasting results. They felt their stress levels decreased radically and domestic harmony returned.

29

Flotation REST, Physical Therapy and Psychological Intervention in the Treatment of Physical Disabilities

Roderick Borrie, James Dana, Sandra Perry and Martin Friedman

The use of flotation REST in the treatment of muscular disorders is relatively new. Until recently there existed only anecdotal reports of such application with a few individual patients. These suggested that flotation REST reduces muscle tone in patients with muscle hypertonicity.

The work of Sniffen et al. (1990), suggests that flotation may serve an important role in this respect as an adjunct to physical therapy. Although muscle tone reduction following flotation may be temporary, the functional gains that this affords in muscle retraining appear to be lasting.

This report presents an initial attempt to combine flotation REST with physical therapy and psychotherapy in the treatment of patients with disorders involving muscle tone. The four case studies presented here are cases in progress. While there are some shared variables, each case is representative of a different disability. All four cases involve disabilities resulting from neurological impairments. In three cases muscle hypertonicity was the dominate symptom; in one case ataxia was the main symptom. In two cases there is an emotional overlay of anger. Our data are based on reports from the involved physiatrist, physical therapists, occupational therapist, psychologist, parents, and the patients themselves.

Case One

Patient One is a 27-year-old male who, at age 17, suffered a basilar artery occlusion resulting in a stroke. The patient was comatose for one week. He remains quadraparetic with spasticity of upper and lower extremities; spasticity is most severe in his left arm. Through extensive stretching, matwork, and gait training, he had become able to ambulate with a rolling walker with forearm cuffs requiring stand-by assistance for distances up to 40 feet.

One and a half years ago this patient began a program of flotation REST. Flotation REST sessions were 60 to 90 minutes in length with specially prepared tape recorded messages containing guided images and mental rehearsals of targeted activities. In his physical therapy it was noted that after flotation he required less stretching prior to his functional activities. His muscle tone was consistently decreased after a flotation session. The carry-over enabled him to ambulate more frequently since less assistance was required. With improved balance and more even gait, he has now increased his walking distances up to three quarters of a mile. He walks and stands with a more erect posture. There has also been a marked improvement in his speech. Since he attends college courses this has been a noticeable advantage. He is now able to drink with a cup whereas before it was necessary to bend his head down to reach a straw.

Although the patient had no particular emotional problems, he described the effects of floating thus: "Before I started flotation, I had a fear of the unexpected. Like sitting in my chair without a seatbelt. What if I fell? Since I started floating I walk more because I have less fear. The relaxation physically has been tremendous. It's also helped me straighten out my life mentally. I can straighten out my thoughts and have less fear. I still have fear but I don't panic."

Case Two

Patient Two is a 23-year-old male who sustained traumatic brain injury (both cerebellar and brain stem) in a car accident six years ago. He remained comatose for 10 weeks. He was treated for a year and a half at another facility before beginning physical therapy at this facility. He presented with ataxia, poor balance and coordination (both static and dynamic), weakness on the left side, bilateral visual disturbances, short-term memory difficulties, mental concentration difficulties, and serious mood swings. Over the course of four years this patient made tremendous strides in functional capabilities. He remains ataxic but uses only a straight cane to walk. He completes a full Nautilus circuit independently and practices fine motor activities regularly. He was referred for flotation REST when he had reached a plateau in his gross motor recovery; his gait and dynamic balance had not improved in several months. He was also exhibiting tremendous anger, particularly with his family.

After several flotation sessions, it was noted that he appeared more relaxed and less shaky when at rest. When active, however, his gross motor capabilities may have suffered from the decrease in muscle tone that was attained. His high muscle tone may be necessary for controlling the effects of the ataxia. During the period he was floating, he was much calmer and in better control of his emotions. His family noted that his anger subsided. He was better able to deal with everyday stresses and to think more logically. He appeared better able to cope with the ramifications of his disability.

Case Three

Patient Three is an 8-year-old boy suffering from neurofibrotosis. Three years ago a partial resectioning of an astrocytoma of the left temporal lobe had no residual effect, however, a gross resectioning a year an a half later left him with right hemiparesis, spasticity of his right side and limbs. This patient came to our clinic for flotation REST only, since he received physical and occupational therapies elsewhere.

The first flotation session was only 15 minutes long since the patient was restless and splashed water in his eye. Nevertheless, pre and post float examination by a physiatrist showed reduced spasticity in the right leg, a loosening of the hamstrings, and bilateral loosening of the quadriceps. Gradually the patient was able to tolerate longer flotation sessions, working from the initial 15 minutes up to an hour by the seventh session. Each time he would float with either his mother or his father sitting at his head. By the eighth session he was able to float solo. All through this progress, the 8-year-old patient's restlessness was addressed by playing music and stories, and by talking to him over an intercom. For this purpose, tapes were specially prepared that contained his favorite story characters in situations that incorporated much imagery of physical movement--stretching, reaching, balancing, grabbing and the like.

A pre-evaluation before the eighth flotation session showed some carry-over in the reduced spasticity. After the float, he showed improved volitional elbow extension and flexion, reduction in right ankle clonus, improved range of motion in his right hip, and diminished abductor muscle tone.

His regular physical therapist was excited about the reduced tone and increased flexion in his right extremities and trunk. She noted that he was bearing more weight on his right foot and was beginning to increase the functional use of his right shoulder.

His occupational therapist reported that the improvement in his muscle tone meant that not as much preparation work was required to begin work on new motor movements. She found that two days after a flotation session he was using both sides in a more balanced way, with greater trunk rotation. However, by the sixth day following a flotation session, he again began to favor his right side and had a more spastic quality to his movement.

His mother reported that his gait and balance had improved after flotation. He was also able to stoop to pick things up and stand up again. He was more sure of his body, more coordinated, and less tactile defensive. He used to be hypersensitive to change in stimulation, but after floating he appeared less worried about getting hurt and thus moved around more confidently. Before he began floating his right leg was 1-1/4 inches shorter than his left, now it measures only a 1/2 inch shorter. The patient commented that the effects of flotation are that it makes him "loose as a goose".

Case Four

Patient Four is a 14-year-old male with a diagnosis of cerebral palsy since birth. He presented with right spastic hemiplegia. His right arm was weak and atrophied and had poor extension. Hypertonia was present in his right shoulder, elbow, and wrist. The right wrist also showed ulnar deviation. The patient's right achilles tendon and hamstrings were tight, requiring the use of a brace on his foot and ankle. He walked and ran independently, though, without full control of his right foot.

The emotional overlay was one of anger. He was particularly aggressive with the members of his family to the point that one of his episodes of destructiveness and aggression led to his hospitalization in a psychiatric unit. His self esteem was very low and he identified himself as a misfit to compensate. His mother had been overly protective of him and had accommodated his needs in deference to those of the rest of his family. The family presented as one in crisis dominated by a cycle of guilt, anger, resentment, and fear.

Physical therapy consisted of range of motion exercises and strength building exercises along with stretching of the right heel cord and hamstring. Following flotation the patient appeared more relaxed.

Stretching was easier and was maintained for longer periods.

During psychotherapy it became readily apparent that the patient was extremely manipulative and that apparent progress in therapy was not reflected in the situation at home where he continued to terrorize his family. The family was under such stress that it was decided to give flotation sessions to each family member. This strategy began to diffuse the crisis at home. The tone in the home changed as everyone reacted more slowly. As the mother puts it, "flotation slowed everyone's reaction times to the crisis. At first we needed the weekly fix (of flotation) but now even if we can't get a float the calmness stays. From the experience in flotation you learn to take the calm relaxed reaction with you". Flotation with the family members broke the guilt-anger cycle enough to allow some family therapy and behavior management strategies to be possible and to be effective in normalizing life at home.

At this point the patient continues with physical therapy and flotation with psychological intervention, however, the emphasis is now on building confidence, esteem, and physical capability.

Discussion

These four cases in progress demonstrate the interfacing of several therapies to meet the individual needs of patients in the rehabilitation process. It is impossible to extract the proportional effect of each therapeutic component. Nevertheless, the observations of all those involved suggest some distinct advantages of this integration.

Flotation consistently reduced muscle tone and increased range of motion. With problems of hypertonicity and spasticity this is an obvious advantage. It frees the physical and occupational therapists' time from the task of muscle loosening to the work of developing new movements and increasing function. With the problem of ataxia where high tone may be necessary to control involuntary shaking, the flotation induced relaxation may temporarily hinder function. Even when the physical benefits of flotation are less readily apparent, accompanying changes in attitude and coping abilities can still greatly enhance therapy efforts.

The actual role flotation plays in creating muscle tone reduction remains a question. When neurological impairment results in spasticity, the cortex has lost its ability to inhibit certain reflex arcs. The affected reflex arcs keep their related muscles contracted. Flotation may effect the spasticity in a number of ways. The reduced stimulus input may affect the cortex, slowing it down as recent research suggests, and sending generalized inhibitory signals to the whole body. It is also possible that the absorption of magnesium from the flotation solution directly inhibits the contraction of the muscles. As a third possibility, there may be some alteration of the feedback system of the spinal cord to the reflex arc that results from magnesium absorption, signal from the cortex, or from feedback from the skin. Changes in stimulation to the skin, such as temperature, can strongly influence muscle tone. Any combination of these possibilities may be occurring. Only by systematically examining the various elements of flotation REST will we determine what produces muscle tone reduction.

These cases also point out the importance of addressing emotional variables that often accompany physical disability and of working with the patient in a family context. Two of these cases were dominated by anger. In other cases we have seen, particularly pain cases, the predominant emotion is depression. Tension, stress and fear are other common emotional factors. Flotation REST combined with psychotherapy may provide an effective, time efficient means of addressing emotional barriers in the rehabilitation process. The amount of effect that interventions like mental rehearsal and guided imagery have on patients' rehabilitation efforts needs more systematic, controlled investigation.

30

Effects of Flotation REST on Range of Motion, Grip Strength and Pain in Rheumatoid Arthritics

John Turner, Jr., Anna DeLeon, Cathy Gibson and Thomas Fine

Rheumatoid arthritis (RA) is a chronic, progressive inflammatory disease of unknown etiology. It is a leading cause of long term disability with approximately 60% of the patients becoming disabled within 10 years (Whisler & Rothsmich, 1985). This disease, which commonly shows onset in the 20-55 age range, involves a systemic inflammation of the synovial membranes of joints as well as joint capsules, tendons, and tendon sheaths (O'Sullivan, Cullen, & Schmitz, 1981). It appears that the synovial membrane undergoes a local autoimmune response causing increased vascular permeability and collection of cellular blood elements. The infiltration causes the synovial membrane to become thickened and multicellular. As the disease progresses, chronic synovitis develops and destruction of cartilage and subchondral bone occurs.

The RA patient demonstrates a variety of physical symptoms, including inflammation, redness, and local heat at the joints. These symptoms are associated with pain, decreased range of motion, and decreased strength, especially in the hands. Traditional treatment for arthritis symptoms is moist heat in the form of hot packs, paraffin, and warm whirlpools (Moll, 1983). Moist heat decreases joint stiffness and muscle spasms as well as decreasing pain. Hydrotherapy has reportedly been beneficial in the management of RA symptoms. Tindall (1976) stated that patients exhibiting decreased range of motion and pain benefitted from pool therapy. It has been hypothesized that these benefits accrue from muscle relaxation associated with warm water and decreased strain of gravity associated with buoyancy.

There is evidence that various physiological and psychological stresses can exacerbate RA symptoms (Gordon, 1985). Thus, relaxation training may be beneficial for individuals with RA. Hypothetically, relaxation training involving moist heat should provide maximum relief from RA symptoms. One relaxation modality utilizing moist heat in a relaxing environment is flotation Restricted Environmental Stimulation Therapy (REST) in which the patient floats supinely in a light-free, minimal sound chamber which contains a saturated epsom salts solution maintained at 34.5° C. Preliminary research has shown that the use of flotation REST (henceforth, REST) is associated with decreased aspirin intake and decreased subjective pain reports in rheumatoid arthritis patients (Mereday, Lehman, & Borrie, 1988).

The present study was undertaken to determine the effects of REST on specific symptoms of RA. The study was intended to determine within and across session effects of REST on range of arm motion, grip strength and reported pain.

Materials and Methods

Four subjects previously diagnosed as having Stage II RA with moderate symptoms but otherwise in good health participated in this study. Subjects ranged from 52 to 69 years in age. Daily use of acetylsalicylic acid was <2 g. Two different REST environments were used in the study. The first, REST-Wet consisted of an ovid fiberglass chamber (Floatarium, Inc., Huntington, New York), 2.5 x 1.3 x 1.1 m., filled to 25 cm. depth with a saturated epsom salt ($MgSO_4$) solution having an approximate specific gravity of 1.28 and temperature maintained at 34.5 ± 0.3° C. The chamber was light-free and the sound level inside was <30db, with further attenuation due to submergence of the ears in the solution. The second environment, labelled REST-Dry, was a rectangular chamber similar in dimensions and conditions to REST-Wet with the exception that a pliable plastic polymer membrane separated the supinely floating subject from the buoyant fluid (Relaxation Dynamics, Inc., Boulder, Colorado).

Parameters

The physical parameters measured were the Range of Motion (ROM in degrees) of left and right shoulders and wrists and the grip strength (GS in Kg. force) of the hands. ROM was measured using a goniometer and GS was measured using a hand dynamometer. Subjective pain (SP) was assessed via the McGill Pain Questionnaire.

Protocol A

Two of the subjects experienced two REST-Wet sessions per week (three days apart) for five weeks, with each session lasting 45 minutes. ROM, GS, and SP were determined before and after sessions 1, 2, 9, and 10. For each session the procedure consisted of the following sequence: SP, ROM, GS measures, brief shower; REST; brief shower; SP, ROM, GS measures.

Protocol B

The remaining two subjects experienced biweekly (three days apart) REST-Wet sessions for two weeks followed by one week without sessions and then biweekly (three days apart) REST-Dry sessions for two weeks. Session length, within session procedure and parameters measured were identical to the first protocol. Pre- and post-measurements were taken in the first and last REST-Wet and in the first and last REST-Dry sessions.

Results

Protocol A

Each ROM value reported is based on the average of all ROM measurements taken at a given time, i.e., left shoulder and wrist and right shoulder and wrist. Initial shoulder ROM averaged for all subjects and conditions was 168° of 190° possible, and wrist ROM was 62° of 90° possible. Each GS value reported is based on left and right hand average. Initial GS averaged for all subjects and conditions was 10.3 Kg force.

Data from sessions 1 and 2 were pooled and data from Sessions 9 and 10 were pooled. ROM and GS data were normalized as percentages of the presession averaged for the initial two sessions. These percentages for ROM were be calculated as:

$$\frac{\text{complete ROM - initial observed ROM}}{\text{complete ROM - subsequent observed ROM}} \quad \text{x } 100$$

where complete ROM = 270°, i.e., complete shoulder (180°) and complete wrist (90°). These percentages for GS were calculated as (GS subsequent/GS initial) X 100. SP is reported as values ranging from 0 to 10 on a pain rating scale where 0 is no pain and 10 is extreme pain.

Both subjects showed increased ROM and GS and decreased SP within sessions and across sessions (see Figure 30-1). ROM and GS increased 15.4% and 16.8%, respectively, within sessions in the initial sessions. A pre-post increase of 8.8% for ROM and 21.2% for GS was observed in the final sessions. Reported pain decreased 57.4% within sessions in the initial sessions and decreased 15.5% within sessions in the final sessions. Across session changes were determined as average percent change from presession value for initial sessions to presession value for final sessions. ROM and GS increased 35.2% and 40.9%, respectively, across sessions, while SP decreased 53.0%.

Protocol B

Data processing and analysis was similar to Protocol A with the exception that the initial (baseline) values were based on session 1 only,

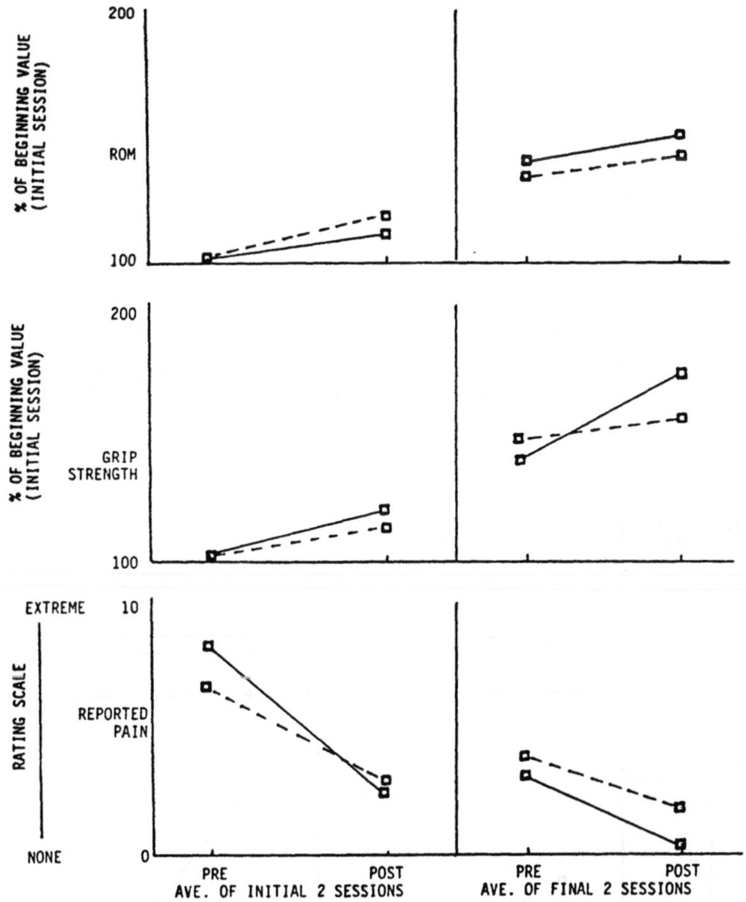

Figure 30-1. Within and across-session effects of brief; repeated REST-Wet on symptoms of rheumatoid arthritis. ROM = range of motion (mean for left and right at shoulder, forearm and wrist), GS = grip strength (mean for left and right), RP = reported pain from McGill Pain Questionnaire.

in REST-Wet and in REST-Dry. In the initial session of REST-Wet (see Figure 30-2) both subjects showed moderate within session increases in ROM (average 13.7% increase) and GS (average 18.5% decrease) and marked decreases in RP (average 67.5%). The within session pattern was similar in REST-Wet final sessions, but the response was not as great (see Figure 30-3). In REST-Dry ROM and

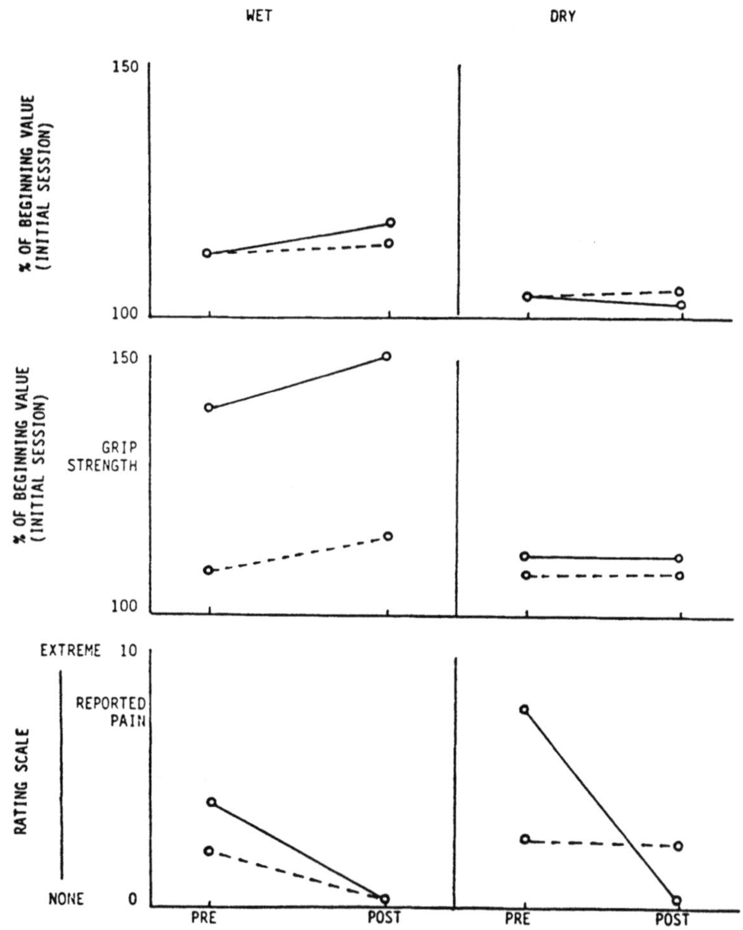

Figure 30-2. Session 1 results, Protocol B

GS increased 5.8% and 9.5%, respectively, and SP decreased 69.1% within initial sessions. With the exception of a 66.7% decrease in RP in one subject, no within session change was observed in final sessions.

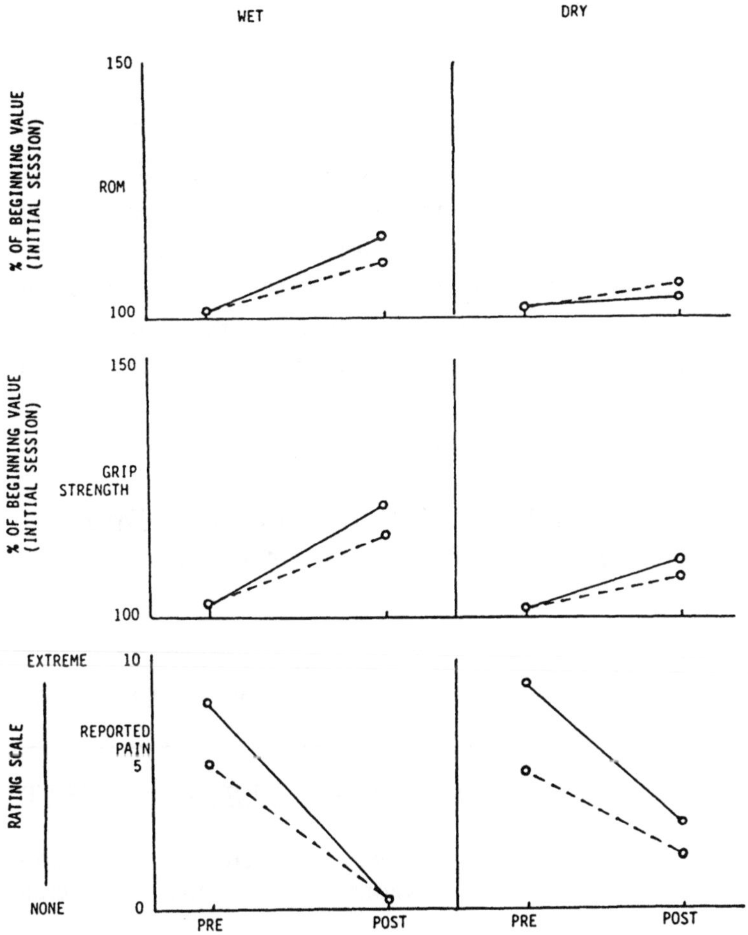

Figure 30-3. Within session effects of brief, repeated REST-Wet or REST-Dry on symptoms of rheumatoid arthritis: a) mean of initial two sessions and b) mean of final two sessions. ROM = range of motion (mean for left and right at shoulder, forearm and wrist), GS = grip strength (mean for left and right), RP = reported pain from McGill Pain Questionnaire.

Both subjects showed across-session increases in ROM and GS and decreases in SP in both REST-Wet and REST-Dry, with responses being 32-55% as great in REST-Dry as in REST-Wet (see Table 30-1).

Discussion

REST-Wet was consistently associated with improved ROM and GS and decreased pain both within and across sessions in all subjects, with all but one subject reporting no pain post session in several instances. Responses in REST-Dry were generally less consistent and less vigorous than in REST-Wet, both within and across sessions. The reasons for this are not known. Several factors may have been contributory. A major difference between the two conditions was the absence of contact with

Table 30-1

Effect of Brief, Repeated REST-Wet or REST-Dry on Symptoms of Rheumatoid Arthritis

Parameter	Across-Sessions Change (%)		
	REST-Wet across 4 sessions	REST-Wet across 8 sessions	REST-Dry across 4 sessions
Range of Motion	↑ 12.8	↑ 35.2	↑ 4.1
Grip Strength	↑ 24.5	↑ 40.9	↑ 10.2
Reported Pain	↓ 39.6	↓ 53.00	↓ 22.8

the fluid in REST-Dry. Since RA symptoms are reportedly relieved by moist heat, the presence of moisture and humidity in REST-Wet may have been more beneficial. However, the membrane in REST-Dry is also associated with differences in degree of auditory stimulation (ears are not submerged), temperature, kinesthesis, and spatial orientation. In other words REST-Wet and REST-Dry provide quite different experiences, making it impossible to attribute the difference in response to any single factor.

Another possible basis for the less vigorous responses in REST-Dry may be the protocol sequence. The REST-Wet sessions were experienced before the REST-Dry session by both subjects. Thus, it was possible that a significant portion of the total response was already achieved in REST-Wet, limiting the further response to REST-Dry. Alternatively, part of the vigor of the REST-Wet response may have been an "expectation" or placebo effect, exaggerating the difference between Wet and Dry. It seems unlikely that the former possibility was true, since the actual starting values for the parameters measured were similar for REST-Wet and REST-Dry. This fact would also suggest that there was little long-term carryover effect of the four REST-Wet sessions. This may be due to the small number of sessions, since studies using a larger number of REST-Wet sessions demonstrated significant carryover of across-session changes in blood pressure (Fine & Turner, 1982) and plasma cortisol (Turner & Fine, 1991) in some subjects. In this regard, both subjects experiencing eight REST-Wet sessions subjectively reported pain relief for 24-48 hours after a given session. However, even short-term (session to session) carryover seemed limited in the present study for ROM and GS, since the starting values for each REST-Wet session were usually closer to the previous pre-session value than to the post-session value.

The placebo issue cannot be resolved in the context of the present study, since there was no control condition. However, within session improvements continued to occur throughout the REST-Wet protocols in all four subjects, regardless of the number of sessions. Studies of placebo effects in biobehavioral treatment of hypertension have indicated that such effects show regression toward the mean after two or three sessions (Weiner, 1979). This would suggest that in the present study the placebo effect, if present, was not a major contributor to the outcome.

Despite the small number of subjects in this study, the responses in REST-Wet were substantial and consistent both within and among the parameters measured. The results suggest that the possible use of REST in the treatment of RA symptoms deserves further investigation.

Acknowledgment

The study was funded in part by Needmor, Inc., Boulder, Colorado.

References

Abramowicz, M. (Ed.). (1975). Antidepressant drugs. *The Medical Letter on Drugs and Therapeutics, 17*, 1-3.

Abramowicz, M. (Ed.). (1981). Choice of benzodiazepines. *The Medical Letter on Drugs and Therapeutics, 23*(9), 41-43 (b).

Abramowicz, M. (Ed.). (1981). Drugs that cause psychiatric symptoms. *The Medical Letter on Drugs and Therapeutics, 23*(3), 9-12 (a).

Achterberg, J. (1985). *Imagery in healing: Shamanism and modern medicine*. Boston: New Science Library.

Adams, H. B. (1964). Therapeutic potentialities of sensory deprivation procedures. *International Mental Health Research Newsletter, 6*(4), 7-9.

Adams, H. B. (1987). *Studies in REST: Arousability and the nature of alcohol and substance abuse.* Report for the U.S. Department of Health and Human Service.

Adams, H. B. (1988). Studies in REST III. REST, arousability, and the nature of alcohol and substance abuse. *Journal of Substance Abuse Treatment, 5*, 77-81.

Adams, H. B., Cooper, G. D., & Carrera, R. N. (1972). Individual differences in behavioral reactions of psychiatric patients to brief partial sensory deprivation. *Perceptual and Motor Skills, 34*, 199-217.

Adams, H. B., Cooper, G. D., Scott, J. C. (1987). Rest and reduced alcohol consumption. In J. W. Turner, Jr., & T. H. Fine (Eds.), *Proceedings of 2nd International Conference on REST.* Toledo: IRIS Publications.

Adams, H. B., Robertson, M. H., & Cooper, G. D. (1963). *Facilitating therapeutic personality change in patients by sensory deprivation.* Paper presented at the International Congress of Psychology.

Ader, R. (Ed.). (1981). *Psychoneuroimmunology*. New York: Academic Press.

Adler, T. (1990, January). Some negative feelings can fuel abuse of drugs. *APA Monitor* (pp. 6-7).

Altman, K., Grahs, C., & Friman, P. C. (1982). Treatment of unobserved trichotillomania by attention reflection and punishment of an apparent covariant. *Journal of Behavior Therapy and Experimental Psychiatry, 13*, 337-341.

American alliance for health, physical education, recreation, and dance. (1984). *Basketball Skills Test.* Reston: Author.

American Psychiatric Association. (1987). *Diagnostic and statistical manual of mental disorders* (3rd ed., revised). Washington, DC: Author.

Appley, M. H., & Trumball, R. (1967). *Psychological stress*. New York: Appleton-Century-Crofts.

Armitage, R., Hoffman, R., Loewy, D., & Moffitt, A. (1988). Interhemispheric EEG during REM and NREM sleep. *Sleep Research, 17*, 93.

Associated Press. (1989a, September 3). Theories abound about Bakker's nervous breakdown. *Courrier-Post.*

Associated Press. (1989b, October 15). Acquitted doctor plans suit: He blames drug for causing his violent behavior. *Asbury Park Press.*

Association of Sleep Disorders Centers. (1979). Diagnostic classification of sleep and arousal disorders (1st ed.), prepared by the Sleep Disorders Classification Committee, H. P. Roffwarg (Chairman), *Sleep, 2*, 1-137.

Atkinson, R. (1991, October). *Individual differences in afterimage persistence during waking and hypnosis: Effects of hypnotizability and visuospatial skills.* Paper presented at the scientific meeting of The Society for Clinical and Experimental Hypnosis. New Orleans, LA.

Ayd, F. J., & Blackwell, B. (Eds.). (1970). *Discoveries in biological psychiatry.* Philadelphia: J. B. Lippincott.

Azima, H., & Cramer, F. J. (1956). Effects of partial perceptual isolation in mentally disturbed individuals. *Diseases of the Nervous System, 17,* 117-122.

Azima, H., & Cramer-Azima, F. J. (1957). Studies on perceptual isolation. *Diseases of the Nervous System, 18,* 80-85.

Azima, H., Vispo, R. H., & Cramer-Azima, F. J. (1961). Observations on anaclitic therapy during sensory deprivation. In Solomon et al. (Eds.), *Sensory deprivation* (pp. 143-160). Cambridge: Harvard University Press.

Azima, H., & Wittkower, E. D. (1956). Gratification of basic needs in treatment of schizophrenia. *Psychiatry, 19,* 121.

Azima, H., Wittkower, E. D., & Latendresse, J. (1958). Object relations therapy of schizophrenic states. *American Journal of Psychiatry, 115,* 60.

Azrin, N. H., & Nunn, R. G. (1973). Habit reversal: A method of eliminating nervous habits and tics. *Behavior Research and Therapy, 11,* 619-628.

Azrin, N. H., & Nunn, R. G. (1978). *Habit control in a day.* New York: Simon & Schuster.

Azrin, N. H., Nunn, R. G., & Frantz, S. L. (1980). Treatment of hairpulling: A comparative study of habit reversal and negative practice training. *Journal of Behavior Therapy and Experimental Psychiatry, 11,* 13-20.

Bandura, A. (1977). Self-efficacy: Toward a unifying theory of behavioral change. *Psychological Review, 84(2),* 191-215.

Banquet, J. P. (1973). Spectral analysis of the EEG in meditation. *Electroencephalography and Clinical Neurophysiology, 35,* 143-151.

Banyai, E., Meszaros, I., & Csokay, L. (1985). Interaction between hypnotist and subject: A social psychophysiological approach (preliminary report). In D. Waxman, P. C. Mizra, M. Gibson, & M. A. Baker (Eds.), *Modern trends in hypnosis.* New York: Plenum Press.

Barabasz, A. (1977). *New techniques in behavior therapy and hypnosis.* Los Angeles, CA: Borden Publishers (second printing).

Barabasz, A. (1978). Electroencephalography, isolation and hypnotic capability at Scott Base, Antarctica. *New Zealand Antarctic Record, 1,* 35-42.

Barabasz, A. (1979). Isolation, EEG alpha and hypnotizability in Antarctica. In G. Burrows (Ed.), *Hypnosis 1979.* Amsterdam: Elsevier/North Holland Biomedica Press.

Barabasz, A. (1980a). EEG alpha, skin conductance and hypnotizability in Antarctica. *International Journal of Clinical and Experimental Hypnosis, 28,* 63-74.

Barabasz, A. (1980b). Effects of hypnosis and perceptual deprivation on vigilance in a simulated radar target detection task. *Perceptual and Motor Skills, 50,* 19-24.

Barabasz, A. (1980c, May). *Enhancement of hypnotic susceptibility following perceptual deprivation: Pain tolerance, electrodermal and EEG correlates.* Paper presented at the 2nd European Congress of Hypnosis, Dubrovnik, Yugoslavia.

Barabasz, A. (1982). Restricted environmental stimulation and the enhancement of hypnotizability: Pain, EEG alpha, skin conductance and temperature responses. *International Journal of Clinical and Experimental Hypnosis, 30,* 147-166.

Barabasz, A. (1983a). EEG alpha-hypnotizability correlations are not covariates of subject self-selection. *Biological Psychology, 17,* 169-173.

Barabasz, A. (1983b, March). *Effects of brief and long term REST on conformity of perception of figure inversion.* Paper presented at the 1st International

Conference on REST and Self Regulation, Denver, CO.
Barabasz, A. (1984a). Antarctic isolation and imaginative involvement. *International Journal of Clinical and Experimental Hypnosis, 32,* 296-300.
Barabasz, A. (1984b). Hilgard's neodissociation theory of hypnosis explains REST effects. *IRIS Bulletin, 2,* 2.
Barabasz, A. (1985, March). Enhancement of military pilot reliability by hypnosis and psychophysiological monitoring: In-flight and simulator data. *Aviation, Space and Environmental Medicine* (pp. 248-250).
Barabasz, A. (1990a). Effects of isolation on states of consciousness. In A. Harrison, Y. Clearwater & C. McKay (Eds.), *The human experience in Antarctica: Applications to life in space* (pp. 201-208). New York: Springer-Verlag.
Barabasz, A. (1990b, May). *Effects of sensory deprivation on EEG theta and skin conductance.* Paper presented at the 5th International Congress of Psychophysiology, Budapest, Hungary.
Barabasz, A. (1990c). Eingeschranke stimulation durch die Umwelt ruft spontane Hypnose fur die Schmerzkontrolle beim cold pressor test hervor. *Experimentelle und Klinishe Hypnose, 4,* Heft 2, 95-105.
Barabasz, A. (1990d). Flotation restricted environmental stimulation elicits spontaneous hypnosis. In R. Van Dyck, Ph.D., A. J. Spinhoven, W. Van der Does, Y. R. Van Rood, & W. DeMoor (Eds.), *Hypnosis: Current theory, research and practice* (pp. 113-120). Amsterdam: VU University Press.
Barabasz, A. (1990e, August). *Hypnotic responsiveness in flotation restricted environmental stimulation.* Paper presented at the 98th Annual Convention of the American Psychological Association, Boston.
Barabasz, A. (1990f). A review of Antarctic behavioral research. In A. Harrison, Y. Clearwater & C. McKay (Eds.), *The human experience in Antarctica: Applications to life in space* (pp. 21-30). New York: Springer-Verlag.
Barabasz, A. (1991a, October). *Clinical applications of restricted environmental stimulation: A conversation hour with Arreed Barabasz.* The 42nd Annual Meeting of the Society for Clinical and Experimental Hypnosis, New Orleans, LA.
Barabasz, A. (1991b, March). *Production of spontaneous hypnosis for pain control by REST.* Paper presented at 22nd Annual meeting of the Association for Applied Psychophysiology and Biofeedback, Dallas, TX.
Barabasz, A., Baer, L., Sheehan, D. V., & Barabasz, M. (1985). Effects of hypnosis and restricted environmental stimulation therapy (REST) on chronic smoking. In J. J. Sanchez-Sosa (Ed.), *Health and clinical psychology* (pp. 237-250). New York: Elsevier Science Publishers.
Barabasz, A., Baer, L., Sheehan, D. V., & Barabasz, M. (1986). A three year follow-up of hypnosis and restricted environmental stimulation therapy for smoking. *International Journal of Clinical and Experimental Hypnosis, 34,* 169-181.
Barabasz, A., & Barabasz, M. (1985). Effects of restricted environmental stimulation: Skin conductance, EEG alpha and temperature responses. *Environment and Behavior, 17,* 239-253.
Barabasz, A., & Barabasz, M. (1986). Antarctic isolation and inversion perception: Regression phenomena. *Environment and Behavior, 18(2),* 285-292.
Barabasz, A., & Barabasz, M. (1989). Effects of restricted environmental stimulation: Enhancement of hypnotizability for experimental and chronic pain control. *International Journal of Clinical and Experimental Hypnosis, 37,* 217-231.

Barabasz, A., & Barabasz, M. (1990). The effects of chamber REST on hypnotizability and chronic pain. In P. Suedfeld (Ed.), *Restricted environmental stimulation: Theoretical and empirical developments.* Springer-Verlag.

Barabasz, A., & Barabasz, M. (1992). Research Designs and Considerations, In E. Fromm & M. Nash (Eds.), *Contemporary Perspectives in Hypnosis Research.* New York: Guilford Press.

Barabasz, A., & Gregson, R. A. M. (1978). Effects of wintering-over on the perception of odorants at Scott Base. *New Zealand Antarctic Record, 1,* 14-23.

Barabasz, A., & Gregson, R. A. M. (1979). Antarctic wintering-over, suggestion and transient olfactory stimulation: EEG evoked potential and electrodermal responses. *Biological Psychology, 9,* 285-295.

Barabasz, A., Gregson, R. A. M., & Mullin, C. S. (1984). Questionable chronometry: Does Antarctic isolation produce cognitive slowing? *New Zealand Journal of Psychology, 13,* 71-78.

Barabasz, A., & Kaplan, G. M. (1989). Effects of restricted environmental stimulation (REST) on hypnotizability: A test of alternative techniques. In D. Waxman, D. Pedersen, I. Wilke, & P. Mellett (Eds.), *Hypnosis: The 4th European Congress at Oxford* (pp. 139-145). London:Whurr.

Barabasz, A., & Lonsdale, C. (1983). Effects of Hypnosis on P300 olfactory evoked potential amplitudes. *Journal of Abnormal Psychology, 92,* 520-525.

Barabasz, M. (1987a). *Imaginative involvement in Antarctica: Applications to life in space.* Paper presented at the NASA/NSF Conference. "The human experience in Antaractica: Applications to life in space". Sunnyvale, CA.

Barabasz, M. (1987b). Trichotillomania: A new treatment. *International Journal of Clinical and Experimental Hypnosis, 35,* 146-154.

Barabasz, M. (1989). Hypnotizability and weight loss in obese subjects. *International Journal of Eating Disorders, 8,* 335-341.

Barabasz, M. (1990a). Imaginative involvement in Antarctica: Applications to life in space. In A. Harrison, Y. Clearwater, & C. McKay (Eds.) *The human experience in Antarctica: Applications to life in space.* New York: Springer-Verlag.

Barabasz, M. (1990b). Treatment of bulimia with hypnosis involving awareness and control in clients with high dissociative capacity. *International Journal of Psychosomatics, 37,* 53-56.

Barabasz, M. (1991). Effects of aerobic exercise on transient mood state. *Perceptual and Motor Skills, 73,* 657-658.

Barabasz, M. (1991). Hypnotizability in bulimia. *International Journal of Eating Disorders, 10,* 117-120.

Barabasz, M., & Barabasz, A. (1987). Controlling experimental and situational demand variables in restricted environmental stimulation research. *Proceedings of the 2nd International Conference on Restricted Environmental Stimulation Research* (pp. 110-121). Toledo: IRIS Publications.

Barabasz, M., Barabasz, A., & Dyer, R. (1990, August). *Effects of restricted environmental stimulation therapy (REST) on alcohol consumption.* Paper presented at the 98th Annual Convention of the American Psychological Association, Boston, MA.

Barabasz, M., Barabasz, A., & Mullin, C. S. (1983). Effects of brief Antarctic isolation on absorption and hypnotic susceptibility. *International Journal of Clinical and Experimental Hypnosis, 31,* 235-238.

Barabasz, M., Barabasz, A., & O'Neill, M. (1991). Effects of experimental context, demand characteristics and situational cues: New data. *Perceptual and Motor Skills, 73,* 83-92.

Barber, T. X. (1969). *Hypnosis: A scientific approach.* New York: Van Nostrand Reinhold.

Bargmann, E., Wolfe, S. M., & Levin, J. (1982). *Stopping Valium: and Ativan, Centrax, Dalmane, Librium, Paxipam, Restoril, Serax, Tranxene, Xanax.* Washington, DC: Public Citizen's Health Research Group.

Barnard, G. W. (1987). Personal communication (letter).

Barrett, D. (1979). The hypnotic dream: Its relation to nocturnal dreams and waking fantasies. *Journal of Abnormal Psychology, 88,* 584-591.

Bartak, L., Rutter, M., & Cox, A. (1975). A comparative study of infantile autism and specific developmental receptive language disorder: I. The children. *British Journal of Psychiatry, 126,* 127-145.

Batten, D. E. (1961). *The effects of sensory deprivation on auditory and visual sensitivity.* Unpublished doctoral dissertation, Washington State University, Pullman, WA.

Battig, W. F. (1979). Are the important "individual differences" between or within individuals? *Journal of Research in Personality, 13,* 546-558.

Beaumont, J. G., Young, A. W., & McManus, I. C. (1984). Hemisphericity: A critical review. *Cognitive Neuropsychology, 1,* 191-212.

Bechtel, R. (1987, August). The third-quarter phenomenon. In A. A. Harrison & M. M. Connors (Chairs). *The human experience in Antarctica: Application to life in space.* Symposium conducted in San Jose.

Beck, A. (1976). *A cognitive therapy and emotional disorders.* New York: Universities Press.

Becton-Dickinson. (1986). *Simultaneous two color enumeration of human T and B cells in peripheral blood.* Becton-Dickinson Immunocytometry Systems, Mountain View, CA.

Bednar, R. L., Wells, M. G., & Peterson, S. R. (1989). *Self-esteem: Paradoxes and innovations in clinical theory and practice.* Maryland: American Psychological Association Press.

Beecher, H. K. (1959). *Measurement of subjective responses: Quantitative effect of drugs.* New York: Oxford University Press.

Belinson, M. J., & Forgays, D. G. (1985). *Flotation isolation as a relaxation environment.* In J. J. Sanchez-Sosa (Ed.), *Health and clinical psychology* (pp. 467-477). New York, NY: Elsevier Science.

Best, J. A., Owen, L. E., & Trentadue, R. L. (1978). Comparison of satiation and rapid smoking in self-managed smoking cessation. *Addictive Behaviors, 3,* 71-78.

Best, J. A., & Suedfeld, P. (1982). Restricted environmental stimulation therapy and behavioral self-management in smoking cessation. *Journal of Applied Social Psychology, 12,* 408-419.

Bexton, W. H. (1953). *Some effects of perceptual isolation on human subjects.* Unpublished doctoral dissertation. McGill University, Montreal.

Bexton, W. H., Heron, W., & Scott, T. H. (1954). Effects of decreased variation in the environment. *Canadian Journal of Psychology, 8,* 70-76.

Biderman, A. D., & Zimmer, H. (Eds.). (1961). *The manipulation of human behavior.* New York: Wiley.

Bigelow, G., Cohen, M., Liebson, I., & Faillace, L. A. (1972). Abstinence or moderation? Choice by alcoholics. *Behavior Research and Therapy, 10,* 209-214.

Bixler, E. O., Kales, A., Soldatos, C. R., Kales, J. D., & Healy, S. (1979). Prevalence of sleep disorders in the Los Angeles metropolitan area. *American Journal of Psychiatry, 136*, 1257-1262.

Blanc, G., Hervé, D., Simon, H., Lisoprawski, A., Glowinski, J., & Tassin, J. P. (1980). Response to stress of mesocortico-frontal dopaminergic neurons in rats after long-term isolation. *Nature, 284*, 265-267.

Blanchard, E., McCoy, G., Musso, A., Acerra, M., Pallmeyer, T., Gerardi, R., Cotch, P., Siracusa, & Andrasik, F. (1986). A controlled comparison of thermal biofeedback and relaxation training in the treatment of essential hypertension: Short-term and long-term outcome. *Biofeedback and Self-Regulation, 11*, 52.

Blanchard, E., Appelbaum, K., Guarnieri, P., Neff, D., Andrasik, F., Jaccard, J., & Barron, K. (1988). Two studies of the long-term follow-up of minimal therapist contact treatments of vascular and tension headache. *Journal of Consulting and Clinical Psychology, 56*, 427-432.

Bootzin, R. R. (1972). Stimulus control treatment for insomnia. *Proceedings of the 80th Annual Convention of the American Psychological Association, 7*, 593-601.

Borkovec, T. D. (1982). Insomnia. *Journal of Consulting and Clinical Psychology, 50*, 880-895.

Borkovec, T. D., & Hennings, B. L. (1978). The role of physiological attention-focusing in the relaxation treatment of sleep disturbance, general tension, and specific stress reaction. *Behaviour Research and Therapy, 16*, 7-19.

Bornstein, P. H., & Rychtarik, R. G. (1978). Multi-component behavioral treatment of trichotillomania: A case study. *Behavior Research and Therapy, 16*, 217-220.

Borrie, R. A., & Suedfeld, P. (1980). Restricted environmental stimulation therapy in a weight reduction program. *Journal of Behavioral Medicine, 3*, 147-161.

Bowen, R. C. (1978). The effect of diazepam on the recovery of endogenously depressed patients. *Journal of Clinical Pharmacology, 18*, 280-284.

Bowers, P. G., & Bowers, K. S. (1979). Hypnosis and creativity: A theoretical and empirical rapprochement. In E. Fromm & R. E. Shor (Eds.), *Hypnosis: developments in research and new perspectives*. New York: Aldine.

Brownell, K. D. (1980). Obesity: Understanding and treating a serious, prevalent, and refractory disorder. *Journal of Consulting and Clinical Psychology, 50*, 820-840.

Brownell, K. D., Marlatt, G. A., Lichtenstein, E., & Wilson, G. T. (1986). Understanding and preventing relapse. *The American Psychologist, 41*, 767-782.

Brownfield, C. A. (1964a). Deterioration and facilitation hypotheses in sensory deprivation research. *Psychological Bulletin, 61*, 304-313(a).

Brownfield, C. A. (1964b). Sensory deprivation: A comprehensive survey. *Psychologia, 7*, 63-93.

Brownfield, C. A. (1965). *Isolation: Clinical and experimental approaches*. New York: Random House.

Brownfield, C. A. (1981, May 9). *Reduced environmental stimulation therapy (REST)*. Paper read, in part, at the Maryland Psychological Association Symposium on Environmental Therapies in the Treatment of Alcoholism, Behavior Disorder and Substance Abuse. Towson State University, Towson, Maryland.

Budzynski, T. (1974). Relaxation training program: Arms and legs, heavy and warm. Bio-Feedback Systems, Inc. New York: BMA Audio Cassettes.

Budzynski, T. H. (1976). Biofeedback and the twilight states of consciousness. In: G. E. Schwartz & D. Shapiro (Eds.), *Consciousness and Self-Regulation. Vol. 1*. New York: Plenum.

Budzynski, T. H. (1990). Hemispheric asymmetry and REST. In P. Suedfeld, J. W. Turner, Jr., & T. H. Fine (Eds.), *Restricted environmental stimulation: Theoretical and empirical developments in flotation REST.* New York: Springer Verlag.

Bunnel, D. E. (1980). T-wave amplitude and P-Q interval: Relationships to non-invasive indices of myocardial performance. *Psychophysiology, 17(6),* 592-597.

Burns, N. M., Chambers, R. M., & Hendler, E. (Eds.). (1963). *Unusual environments and human behavior.* New York: Free Press of Glencoe.

Burns, R. B., & Dobson, C. B. (1984). *Introductory psychology* (pp. 106-109). MTP Press Limited, Lancester.

Cacioppo, J. T., Petty, R. E., & Morris, K. J. (1985). Semantic, evaluative, and self-referent processing: Memory, cognitive effort, and somatovisceral activity. *Psychophysiology, 22(4),* 371-384.

Cacioppo, J. T., & Tassinary, L. G. (1990). Inferring psychological significance from physiological signals. *American Psychologist, 45,* 16-28.

Carrington, P. (1977). *Freedom in meditation.* Garden City: Anchor Press/ Doubleday.

Cautela, J. R. (1967). Covert sensitization. *Psychological Reports, 20,* 459-468.

Chen, A. C. N., Dworkin, S. F., & Bloomquist, D. S. (1981). Cortical power spectrum analysis of hypnotic pain control in surgery. *International Journal of Neuroscience, 13,* 127-136.

Chertok, L. (1966). *Hypnosis.* Pergamon Press, Oxford.

Cohen, S. I., Silverman, A. J., & Shmavonian, B. M. (1962a). Neurophysiological, humoral, and personality factors in response to sensory deprivation. In R. A. Cleghorn (Ed.), *Proceedings of the Third World Congress of Psychiatry* (pp. 1004-1009). Toronto: University of Toronto Press.

Cohen, S. I., Silverman, A. J., & Shmavonian, B. M. (1962b). Psychophysiological studies in altered sensory environments. *Journal of Psychosomatic Research, 6,* 259-281.

Cole, C. W., & Goldstein, G. S. (1971). Consumption of ethanol as a function of sensory isolation. *Training and Motivation, 2,* 363-370.

Coleman, R. M., Roffwarg, H. P., Kennedy, S. J., Guilleminault, C., Cinque, J., Cohn, M. A., Karacan, I., Kupfer, D. J., Lemmi, H., Miles, L. E., Orr, W. C., Phillips, E. R., Roth, T., Sassin, J. F., Schmidt, H. S., Weitzman, E. D., & Dement, W. C. (1982). Sleep-wake disorders based on a polysomnographic diagnosis: A national cooperative study. *Journal of the American Medical Association, 247,* 997-1003.

Collins, R. L., Rothblum, E. D., & Wilson, G. T. (1986). The comparative efficacy of cognitive and behavioral approaches to the treatment of obesity. *Cognitive Therapy and Research, 10,* 299-318.

Colvin, R. H., & Olson, S. B. (1983). A descriptive analysis of treatments highly successful at maintaining weight loss. *Addictive Behaviors, 8,* 287-295.

Cooper, G. D., Adams, H. B., & Scott, J. C. (1988). Studies in REST I. Reduced environmental stimulation therapy (REST) and reduced alcohol consumption. *Journal of Substance Abuse Treatment, 5,* 61-68.

Cooper, G. D., McGraw, J., Pasternak, R., Paznak, R., & Adams, H. B. (1977). A new treatment for alcohol abuse: Preliminary report. Unpublished manuscript, George Mason University (pp. 7-8). Summarized in *Alcoholism and Alcohol Education,* July 27.

Cooper, J. (1980). Reducing fears and increasing assertiveness: The role of dissonance reduction. *Journal of Experimental Social Psychology, 16*, 199-213.
Cooper, L. F., & Erickson, M. H. (1954). *Time distortion in hypnosis.* Baltimore: The Williams & Wilkins Company.
Corby, J. C., Roth, W. T., Zarcone, V. P., & Kopell, B. S. (1978). Psychophysiological correlates of the practice of Tantric Yoga meditation. *Archives of General Psychiatry, 35*, 571-577.
Courtney, J., Davis, J. M., & Solomon, P. (1961). Sensory deprivation: The role of movement. *Perceptual and Motor Skills, 13*, 191-199.
Cowen Leib-Failacie, (1977)
Crawford, H. J. (1982). Hypnotizability, daydreaming styles, imagery vividness, and absorption: A multidimensional study. *Journal of Personality and Social Psychology, 42*, 915-926.
Crawford, H. J. (1989). Cognitive and physiological flexibility: Multiple pathways to hypnotic responsiveness. In V. Ghorghui, P. Netter, H. Eysenck, & R. Rosenthal (Eds.), *Suggestion and suggestibility: Theory and research.* Heidelberg and New York: Springer.
Crawford, H. J. (1990a, July). *Cold pressor pain with and without suggested analgesia: EEG correlates as moderated by hypnotic susceptibility level.* Paper presented at the 5th International Congress of Psychophysiology, Budapest, Hungary.
Crawford, H. J. (1990b). Cognitive and psychophysiological correlates of hypnotic responsiveness and hypnosis. In M. L. Fass & D. Brown (Eds.), *Creative mastery in hypnosis and hypnoanalysis: A festschrift for Erika Fromm* (pp. 47-54). Hillsdale, New Jersey: Lawrence Erlbaum.
Crawford, H. (1990c, March). *Delving deeply into the tank: Implications for psychophysiological research.* Invited address, 4th International Conference on REST, Washington, D.C.
Crawford, H. (1990d, December.). Personal communication.
Crawford, H. J. (1991). *Psychophysiological correlates of hypnosis.* Chapter in preparation.
Crawford, H. J., & Allen, S. N. (1983). Enhanced visual memory during hypnosis as mediated by hypnotic responsiveness and cognitive strategies. *Journal of Experimental Psychology: General, 112*, 662-685.
Crawford, H. J., & Barabasz, A. (in press). Treatment of phobias and intense fears by hypnosis and REST. In J. W. Rhue, S. J. Lynn, & I. Kirsch (Eds.), *Handbook of Clinical Hypnosis.* Washington, DC: American Psychological Association.
Crawford, H. J., Brown, A. M., & Moon, C. E. (1991). *Sustained attentional abilities: Differences between low and high hypnotizables.* Manuscript under editorial review.
Crawford, H. J., Clarke, S. N., Kitner-Triolo, M., & Olesko, B. (1989, August.). *EEG correlates of emotions: Moderated by hypnosis and hypnotic level.* Paper presented at the American Psychological Association annual meeting, New Orleans, Louisiana.
Crawford, H. J., Gur, R., Skolnick, B., Gur, R., & Benson, D. (1986, July). *Regional cerebral blood flow and hypnosis: Differences between low and high hypnotizables.* Paper presented at 3rd International Conference of the International Organization of Psychophysiology, Vienna, Austria.
Crawford, H. J., Nomura, K., & Slater, H. (1983). Spatial memory processing: Enhancement during hypnosis. In J. E. Shorr, J. Conella, G. Sobel, & L. Robin (Eds.), *Imagery: Theoretical aspects and applications.* New York: Plenum.

Crawford, H. J., Wallace, B., Nomura, K., & Slater, H. (1986). Eidetic-like imagery in hypnosis: Rare but there. *American Journal of Psychology, 99,* 527-546.

Crocket, R., Sandison, R., and Walk, A. (Eds.). (1963). *Hallucinogenic drugs and their therapeutic use.* London: J.Q. Lewis.

Dalton, K. (1987). *Once a month.* California: Hunters House.

Daniel, A. (1985). Uses of REST in a private practice, utilizing a flotation tank. In T. H. Fine & J. W. Turner (Eds.), *Proceedings of the 1st international conference on REST and self-regulation* (pp. 198-200). Toledo, OH: Medical College of Ohio.

Davidson, D. M., Winchester, M. A., Taylor, C. B., Alderman, E. A., & Ingles, N. B. (1979). Effects of relaxation therapy on cardiac performance and sympathetic activity in patients with organic heart disease. *Psychosomatic Medicine, 41,* 303-309.

Davis, J. M., McCourt, W. F., & Solomon, P. (1960). The effect of visual stimulation on hallucinations and other mental experiences during sensory deprivation. *American Journal of Psychiatry, 116,* 889-892.

DeBenedittis, G., Panerai, A. A., & Villamira, M. A. (1989). Effects of hypnotic analgesia and hypnotizability on experimental ischemic pain. *International Journal of Clinical and Experimental Hypnosis, 37(1),* 55-69.

Deikman, A. J. (1966). Deautomatization and the mystic experience. *Psychiatry, 29,* 324-338.

DePascalis, V., & Palumbo, G. (1986). EEG alpha asymmetry: Task difficulty and hypnotizability. *Perceptual and Motor Skills, 62,* 139-150.

DePascalis, V., Silveri, A., & Palumbo, G. (1988). EEG asymmetry during covert mental activity and its relationship with hypnotizability. *International Journal of Clinical and Experimental Hypnosis, 36,* 38-52.

Derogatis, L. R. (1977). *SCL-90-R (Revised Version Manual-I).* Baltimore, MD.

Dershewitz, R. A., & Christophersen, E. R. (1984). Childhood household safety: An overview. *American Journal of Diseases in Children, 138,* 85-88.

Doane, B. K. (1955). *Changes in visual function with perceptual isolation.* Unpublished doctoral dissertation, McGill University, Montreal.

Doane, B., Mahatoo, W., Heron, W., & Scott, T. (1959). Changes in perceptual function after isolation. *Canadian Journal of Psychology, 13,* 210-219.

Dumas, R. A., & Spitzer, S. E. (1978). Influences of subject self-selection on the EEG alpha-hypnotizability correlation. *Psychophysiology, 15(6),* 606-608.

Dunn, O. J. (1961). Multiple comparisons among means. *Journal of the American Statistical Association, 56,* 52-64.

Dyer, R. A. (19__). *Effects of restricted environmental stimulation therapy on the creation of specific food aversions in overweight females.* Unpublished doctoral dissertation, Washington State University, Pullman, WA.

Dyer, R., Barabasz, A., & Barabasz, M. (1990, March). Effects of REST on body fat reduction and food aversion. Paper presented at the 4th International Conference on REST, Washington, DC.

Edmonston, W. E., Jr. (1979). The effects of neutral hypnosis on conditioned responses: Implications for hypnosis as relaxation. In E. Fromm & R.E. Shor (Eds.), *Hypnosis: Developments in research and new perspectives.* New York: Aldine.

Edwards, R. A., & Medlicott, R. W. (1980). Advantages and disadvantages of benzodiazepine prescription. *New Zealand Medical Journal, 92,* 357-359.

Ellis, A. (1962). *Reason and emotion in psychotherapy.* New York: Lyle Stuart.
Engs, R. C. (1977). Drinking patterns and drinking problems of college students. *Journal of Studies on Alcohol, 38,* 2144-2156.
Engstrom, D. R. (1976). Hypnotic susceptibility, EEG-alpha and self-regulation. In G. E. Schwartz & D. Shapiro (Eds.), *Consciousness and self regulation.* New York: Plenum Press.
Epstein, L. H., & Peterson, G. L. (1973). The control of undesired behavior by self-imposed contingencies. *Behavior Therapy, 4,* 91-95.
Erickson, M. H. (1980). *The collected papers of Milton H. Erickson on hypnosis, Vol. I.* Rossi, E. L. (Ed.). Irvington, New York.
Evans, F. J. (1967). Suggestibility in the normal waking state. *Psychological Bulletin, 67,* 114-129.
Evans, F. J. (1974). The placebo response in pain reduction. In J. J. Bonica (Ed.), *Advances in Neurology, 4, Pain.* New York: Raven Press.
Evans, F. J. (1979). Hypnosis and sleep: Techniques for exploring cognitive activity during sleep. In E. Fromm & R. E. Shor (Eds.), *Hypnosis: Developments in research and new perspectives* (pp. 139-183). New York: Aldine.
Ewer, T. C., & Stewart, D. E. (1986). Improvement in bronchial hyper-responsiveness in patients with moderate asthma after treatment with a hypnotic technique: A randomized controlled trial. *British Medical Journal, 293,* 1129-1132.
Eysenck, H. J., & Furneaux, W. D. (1945). Primary and secondary suggestibility: An experimental and statistical study. *Journal of Experimental Psychology, 35,* 485-503.
Farah, M. J. (1988). The neuropsychology of mental imagery: Converging evidence from brain-damaged and normal subjects. In J. Stiles-Davis, M. Kritchevsky, & U. Bellugi (Eds.), *Spatial cognition: Brain bases and development.* Hillsdale, New Jersey: Erlbaum.
Fehr, F. S., & Stern, J. A. (1967). The effect of hypnosis on attention to relevant and irrelevant stimuli. *International Journal of Clinical and Experimental Hypnosis, 15,* 134-143.
Fein, D., Waterhouse, L., Lucci, D., & Snyder, D. (1985). Cognitive subtypes in developmentally disabled children: A pilot study. *Journal of Autism and Developmental Disorders, 15,* 77-95.
Feldman, M. D. (1986). Paradoxical effects of benzodiazepines. *North Carolina Medical Journal, 47(6),* 311-312.
Fine, T. H., & Turner, J. W., Jr. (1982). The effect of brief restricted environmental stimulation therapy in the treatment of essential hypertension. *Behaviour Research and Therapy, 20,* 567-570.
Fine, T. H., & Turner, J. W., Jr. (1987). The effect of REST on EMG biofeedback and plasma cortisol. In J. W. Turner, Jr. & T. H. Fine (Eds.), *2nd International Conference on Restricted Environmental Stimulation Proceedings* (pp. 148-155). Toledo, OH: Iris Publication #1392822406-1.
Fisher, S., & Greenberg, R. P. (Eds.). (1989). *The limits of biological treatments for psychological distress: Comparisons with psychotherapy and placebo.* Hillsdale, NJ: Erlbaum.
Fiske, D. W., & Maddi, S. R. (Eds.). (1961). *Functions of varied experience.* Homewood, Ill.: Dorsey Press.
Fogel, S., & Hoffer, A. (1962). The use of hypnosis to interrupt and reproduce an LSD-25 experience. *Journal of Clinical and Experimental Psychopathology, 23,* 11-

16.

Forgays, D. G., & Belinson, M. J. (1986). Is flotation isolation a relaxing environment? *Journal of Environmental Psychology, 6,* 19-34.

Forgays, D. G., & McClure, G. N. (1974). A direct comparison of the effects of the quiet room and water immersion isolation techniques. *Psychophysiology, 11(3),* 346-349.

Frank, J. D. (1965). *Persuasion and healing.* Baltimore: The John Hopkins Press.

Freedman, S. J., & Greenblatt, M. (1959). *Studies in human isolation* (WADC Tech. Rep., Contract No. 59-266). Wright-Patterson AFB, OH: Aero-Medical Laboratory, Wright Air Development Center.

Freedman, S. J., & Held, R. (1960). Sensory deprivation and perceptual lag. *Perceptual and Motor Skills, 11,* 277-280.

Fretz, B. R. (1982). Perspectives and definition. *The Counseling Psychologist, 10,* 15-19.

Fromm, E. (1981). How to write a clinical paper. *International Journal of Clinical and Experimental Hypnosis, 29,* 5-9.

Furedy, J. J. (1987). Beyond heart rate in the cardiac psychophysiological assessment of mental effort: The T-wave amplitude component of the electrocardiogram. *Human Factors, 29(2),* 183-194.

Furedy, J. J., & Heslegrave, R. J. (1983). Consideration of recent criticisms of the T-wave amplitude index of myocardial sympathetic activity. *Psychophysiology, 20(2),* 204-211.

Furedy, J. J, Heslegrave, R. J., & Scher, H. (1984). Psychophysiological and physiological aspects of T-wave amplitude in the objective study of behavior. *Pavlovian Journal of Biological Science, 19(4),* 182-194.

Gabrielli, W. F., Jr., Volavka, J., Pollock, V. E., Schulsinger, F., & Itil, T. M. (1982). Electroencephalograms in children of alcoholic fathers. *Psychophysiology, 19,* 404-407.

Galbraith, G. C., London, P., Leibovitz, M. P., Cooper, L. M., & Hart, J. T. (1970). EEG and hypnotic susceptibility. *Journal of Comparative and Physiological Psychology, 72,* 125-131.

Galski, T. S. (1981). The adjunctive use of hypnosis in the teatment of trichotillomania: A case report. *American Journal of Clinical Hypnosis, 23,* 198-201.

Garver, R. B. (1977). The enhancement of human performance with hypnosis through neuromotor facilitation and control of arousal level. *American Journal of Clinical Hypnosis, 19,* 177-181.

Geiser, D. S. (1989). Psychosocial influences on human immunity. *Clinical Psychology Review, 9,* 689-715.

Gill, M. M., & Brenman, M. (1959). *Hypnosis and related states.* New York: International Universities Press.

Glowinski, J., Tassin, J. P., & Thierry, A. M. (1984). The mesocortico-prefrontal dopaminergic neurons. *TINS, 7,* 415-418.

Goldberger, L., & Holt, R. R. (1958). Experimental interference with reality contact (perceptual isolation): Method and group results. *Journal of Nervous and Mental Disorders, 127,* 99-112.

Golding, L. (Ed.). (1982). *Y's way to physical fitness* (rev.). Champaign, IL: Human Kinetics.

Goldstein, A. P. (1962). *Therapist-patient expectancies in psychotherapy.* New York:

Pergamon Press.
Goldstein, D., & Jessen, W. (1990). Flotation Effect on Premenstrual Syndrome in J. W. Turner, Jr. & T. H. Fine (Eds.), *Restricted environmental stimulation: Research and commentary* (pp. 260-266). Toledo: MCO.
Goldstein, L., Sugarman, A. A., Marjerrison, G., & Stoltzfus, N. (1973, October). *The EEG and differential hemispheric functions.* Paper presented at the Conference on Aspects of Transformation of Consciousness, Montreal. R. M. Bucke Memorial Society. cit. Cohen, H. D., Rosen, R. C., and Goldstein, L. (1976). *Archives of Sexual Behavior, 5,* 186-199.
Gollwitzer, P. M., Earle, W. B., & Stephan, W. G. (1982). Affect as a determinant of egotism: Residual excitation and performance attributions. *Journal of Personality and Social Psychology, 43,* 702-709.
Gordon, D. A. (1985). *Rheumatoid arthritis.* New York, NY: Elsevier Science Publishing Company, Inc.
Greenberg, H. R., & Sarner, C. A. (1965). Trichotillomania. *Archives of General Psychiatry, 12,* 482-489.
Greenberg, R. P., & Fisher, S. (1990). To prescribe or not to prescribe. Register Report: *Newsletter for Psychologist Health Service Providers, 16(No.1), 5,* 10-11.
Greenblatt, D. J., Shader, R. I., Divoll, M., & Harmatz, J. S. (1984). Adverse reactions to triazolam, flurazepam, and placebo in controlled clinical trials. *Journal of Clinical Psychiatry, 45(5),* 192-195.
Griffiths, R. R., Bigelow, G. E. T., & Liebson, I. (1973, August). *Alcohol self-administration and social interaction in alcoholics.* Paper presented at the meeting of the American Psychological Association, Montreal.
Gruzelier, J. (1987). The neuropsychology of hypnosis. In M. Heap (Ed.), *Hypnosis: Current clinical, experimental and forensic practices.* London: Croom Helm.
Gruzelier, J. (1990, July). *Shifts in cerebral asymmetry during hypnosis.* Paper presented at the 5th International Congress of Psychophysiology, Budapest, Hungary.
Gruzelier, J., Brow, T., Perry, A., Rhonder, J., & Thomas, M. (1984). Hypnotic susceptibility: A lateral predisposition and altered cerebral asymmetry under hypnosis. *International Journal of Psychophysiology, 2,* 131-139.
Gruzelier, J., Thomas, M., Brow, T., Conway, A., Golds, J., Jutai, J., Liddiard, D., McCormack, K, Perry, A., & Rhonder, J. (1987). Involvement of the left hemisphere in hypnotic induction. In B. Taneli, C. Perris, & D. Kemali (Eds.), *Neurophysiological correlates of relaxation and psychopathology* (pp. 6-17). *Advances in Biological Psychiatry, 16,* 1-5,
Guilleman, R., Vargo, T., Rossier, J., Minich, S., Long, N., Rivier, C., Vale, W., & Bloom, F. (1977). β-Endorphin and adrenocorticotropin are secreted concomitantly by the pituitary gland. *Science, 197,* 1367-1370.
Gunderson, E. K. E. (1973). Individual behavior in confined and isolated groups. In J. E. Rasmussen (Ed.), *Man in isolation and confinement.* Chicago: Aldine.
Gurdjieff, G. I. (1973). *Views from the real world.* New York: Dutton Press.
Haberman, M. A. (1987). Spontaneous trance as a possible cause for persistent symptoms of the medically ill. *American Journal of Clinical Hypnosis, 29,* 171-176.
Hales, D. (1981). *The complete book of sleep: How your nights affect your days.* Don Mills, Ontario: Addison-Wesley.
Hall, E. G., & Erffmeyer, E. S. (1983). The effects of visuo-motor behavior rehearsal with videotaped modeling on free throw accuracy of intercollegiate

female basketball players. *Journal of Sport Psychology, 5,* 343-346.

Hall, H. R. (1983). Hypnosis and the immune system: A review with implications for cancer and the psychology of healing. *American Journal of Clinical Hypnosis, 25*(2-3), 92-103.

Hall, H. R. (1989). Research in the area of voluntary immunomodulation: Complexities, consistencies and future research considerations. *International Journal of Neuroscience, 47*(1-2), 81-89.

Halldin, J. (1985). Alcohol consumption and alcoholism in an urban population in Sweden. *Acta Psychiatrica Scandinavica, 71,* 128-140.

Harmon, L. (1982). Scientific affairs-The next decade. *The Counseling Psychologist, 10,* 31-37.

Harrison, J., & Barabasz, A. (1990, March). *REST as a treatment for children with autism.* Presented at the 4th International Conference on REST, Washington, DC.

Harrison, J., & Barabasz, A. (1991). Effects of REST in the treatment of children with autism. *Child Study Journal, 21,* 153-166.

Hartley, J. T., Birnbaum, I. M., & Parker, E. S. (1978). Alcohol and storage deficits: Kinds of processing. *Journal of Verbal Learning and Verbal Behavior, 17,* 635-647.

Hartz, A. J., Kalkhoff, R. K., Rimm, A. A., & McCall, R. J. (1979). A study of factors associated with the ability to maintain weight loss. *Preventive Medicine, 8,* 471-483.

Hebb, D. O. (1949). *The organization of behavior.* New York: Wiley.

Hebb, D. O. (1955a). Drives and the C.N.S. (conceptual nervous system). *Psychological Review, 62,* 243-254.

Hebb, D. O. (1955b). The mammal and his environment. *American Journal of Psychology, 111,* 826-831.

Hebb, D. O. (1958). The motivating effects of exteroceptive stimulation. *American Psychologist, 13,* 109.

Hebb, D. O. (1966). *A Textbook of Psychology.* Philadelphia: W.B. Saers.

Hebb, D. O., Heath, E. S., & Stuart, E. A. (1954). Experimental deafness. *Canadian Journal of Psychology, 8,* 152-156.

Hebert, R., & Lehmann, D. (1979). Theta bursts: An EEG pattern in normal subjects practicing the transmeditational technique. *EEG and Clinical Neurophysiology, 42,* 397-405.

Helzer, J. E. (1987). Epidemiology of alcoholism. *Journal of Consulting and Clinical Psychology, 55,* 284-292.

Hermelin, B. (1976). Coding and the sense modalities. In L. Wing (Ed.), *Early Childhood Autism* (pp. 135-168). New York: Pergamon.

Heron, W. (1957). The pathology of boredom. *Scientific American, 196,* 52-56.

Heron, W. (1961). Cognitive and physiological effects of perceptual isolation. In P. Solomon, P. Kubzansky, P. Liederman, J. Mendelson, T. Trumbull, & D. Wexler, (Eds.), *Sensory deprivation* (pp. 6-33). Cambridge: Harvard University Press.

Heron, W., Bexton, W. H., & Hebb, D. O. (1953). Cognitive effects of decreased variation in the sensory environment. *American Psychologist, 8,* 1-28.

Heron, W., Doane, B., & Scott, T. (1956). Visual disturbances after prolonged perceptual isolation. *Canadian Journal of Psychology, 10,* 13-18.

Heslegrave, R. J., & Furedy, J. J. (1979). Sensitivities of HR and T-wave amplitude

for detecting cognitive and anticipatory stress. *Physiology and Behavior, 22*(1), 17-23.
Hilgard, E. R. (1965). *Hypnotic susceptibility.* New York: Harcourt, Brace & World.
Hilgard, E. R. (1974a). Imaginative involvement: Some characteristics of the highly hypnotizable and non hypnotizable. *International Journal of Clinical and Experimental Hypnosis, 22*(2), 138-156.
Hilgard, E. R. (1974b). Toward a neo-dissociation theory of multiple cognitive controls in human functioning. *Perspectives in Biology and Medicine, 17,* 301-316.
Hilgard, E. R. (1977a). *Divided consciousness: Multiple controls in human thought and action.* New York: Wiley.
Hilgard, E. R. (1977b). The problem of divided consciousness: A neodissociation interpretation. *Annals of the New York Academy of Sciences, 296,* 48-59.
Hilgard, E. R. (1989, in preparation). A neodissociation theory of divided consciousness.
Hilgard, E. R., & Hilgard, J. R. (1975). *Hypnosis in the relief of pain.* Los Altos, CA: Kaufmann.
Hilgard, J. R. (1974). Imaginative involvement: Some characteristics of the highly hypnotizable and the non-hypnotizable. *International Journal of Clinical and Experimental Hypnosis, 22,* 138-156.
Hilgard, J. R. (1979). *Personality and hypnosis: A study of imaginative involvement,* (2nd ed.). Chicago: University of Chicago Press.
Hilgard, J. R., & Lebaron, S. (1983). *Hypnotherapy of pain in children with cancer.* Los Altos, Calif: William Kaufman Inc.
Hilgard, J. R., & Morgan, A. (1975). Standard hypnotic clinical scale. In E. R. Hilgard & J. R. Hilgard (Eds.), *Hypnosis in the relief of pain.* Palo Alto: Kaufman.
Hoffer, A. (1965). LSD: A review of its present status. *Clinical Pharmacological Therapy, 183,* 49-57.
Hollister, L. E. (1978). Treatment of depression with drugs. *Annals of Internal Medicine, 89(1),* 78-84.
Hull, J. G. (1981). A self-awareness model of the causes and effects of alcohol consumption. *Journal of Abnormal Psychology, 90,* 586-600.
Hull, J. G., & Young, R. D. (1983). The self-awareness reducing effects of alcohol: Evidence and implications. In J. Suls & A. Greenwald (Eds.), *Psychological Perspectives on the Self, 2,* 159-190.
Hutchinson, M. (1984a, November). One man, one float. *Esquire,* 329-30.
Hutchinson, M. (1984b). *The book of floating: Exploring the private sea* (pp. 13-14). New York: Quill. William Morrow.
Hutt, C., Hutt, S. J., Lee, D., & Ounsted, C. (1964). Arousal and childhood autism. *Nature, 204*(4961), 908-909.
Huxley, A. (1954). *The doors of perception.* New York: Harper and Row.
Huxley, A. (1958). *Brave new world revisited.* New York: Harper and Brothers.
Israel, A. C., Silverman, W. K., & Solotar, L. C. (1986). An investigation of family influences on initial weight status, attrition, and treatment outcome in a childhood obesity program. *Behavior Therapy, 17,* 131-143.
Jackson, A. L., & Warner, N. L. (1986). Preparation, staining and analysis by flow cytometry of peripheral blood leukocytes. In N. R. Rose, H. Friedman, & H. L. Fahey (Eds.), *Manual of clinical laboratory immunology (3rd ed.),* (pp. 226-235), Washington, DC: American Society for Microbiology.
Jacobs, G. D., Heilbronner, R. L., & Stanley, J. M. (1985). The Effects of Short

Term Floatation REST on Relaxation: A Controlled Study. In J. W. Turner, Jr., & T. H. Fine, (Eds.) *REST and self-regulation: Proceedings of the 1st International Conference* (pp. 179-185). Denver, CO., IRIS Publ., Toledo, OH.

Jacobson, E. (1970). *Modern Treatments of Tense Patients.* Springfield, IL: Charles Thomas.

Jacobson, G. R. (1971). *Sensory deprivation and field dependence in alcoholics.* Unpublished doctoral dissertation, Illinois of Technology.

Janoski, M. L., & Kugler, J. (1987). Relaxation, imagery and neuroimmunomodulation. *Annals of the New York Academy of Sciences, 496,* 772-730.

Jevning, R., Wilson, A., & Davidson, J. M. (1978). Adrenocortical activity during meditation. *Hormones and Behavior, 10,* 54-60.

Jones, A. (1969). Stimulus-seeking behavior. In J. P. Zubek (Ed.), *Sensory deprivation: Fifteen years of research* (pp. 167-206). New York: Appleton-Century-Crofts.

Jones, F. W., & Holmes, D. S. (1976). Alcoholism, alpha production and biofeedback. *Journal of Consulting and Clinical Psychology, 44,* 224-228.

Kammerman, M. (Ed.). (1977). *Sensory isolation and personality change.* Springfield: Charles C. Thomas.

Kaplin, G. M., & Barabasz, A. F. (1988). Enhancing hypnotizability: Differential effects of flotation restricted environmental stimulation technique and progressive muscle relaxation. *Australian Journal of Clinical and Experimental Hypnosis, 16,* 39-51.

Karlin, R., Cohen, A., & Goldstein, L. (1982). *A shift to the right: Electroencephalographic changes from rest to hypnotic induction.* Unpublished manuscript.

Karlin, R., Goldstein, L., Cohen, A., & Morgan, D. (1980). *Quantitated EEG, hypnosis and hypnotizability.* Paper presented at the annual meeting of the American Psychological Association.

Kasamatsu, A., & Hirai, T. (1966). An electroencephalographic study on the Zen meditation. *Folia Psychiatrica et Neurologia Japonica, 20,* 315-336.

Kazdin, A. C., & Wilcoxin, L. A. (1976). Systematic desensitization and non-specific treatment effects: A methodological evaluation. *Psychological Bulletin, 83(5),* 729-758.

Kazdin, A. E. (1982). *Single-Case Research Designs.* New York: Oxford.

Kihlstrom, J. F. (1987). The cognitive unconscious. *Science, 237(4821),* 1445-1452.

Kiloh, I. G., & Osselton, J. W. (1961). *Clinical Electroencephalography.* London: Butterworths.

Kirkendall, D. R., Gruber, J. J., & Johnson, R. E. (1987). *Measurement and evaluation for physical educators.* Champaign: Human Kinetics.

Kissen, A. T., Reifler, C. B., & Thaler, V. H. (1964). Modification of thermoregulatory responses to cold by hypnosis. *Journal of Applied Psychology, 19,* 1043-1050.

Kistner, J., & Robbins, F. (1986). Brief report: Characteristics of methods of subject selection and description in research on autism. *Journal of Autism and Developmental Disorders, 16(1),* 77-82.

Klein, K. B., & Spiegel, D. (1989). Modulation of gastric acid secretion by hypnosis. *Gastroenterology, 96,* 1383-1387.

Knox, N. (1989, December 10). Mass murderer link. *The Shotgun News* (p. 3).

Koslin, B. L., Pargament, B., & Suedfeld, P. (1971). An uncertainty model of opinion change. In P. Suedfeld (Ed.), *Attitude change: The competing views.* Chicago: Aldine-Atherton.

Koula, G. M., Kemp, J. C., Keane, K. M., & Belden, A. D. (1990). Replication of a clinical outcome study on a hospital-based stress management and behavioral medicine program utilizing flotation REST and biofeedback. In P. Suedfeld, J. W. Turner Jr., & T. H. Fine (Eds.), *Restricted environmental stimulation: Theoretical and empirical developments in flotation REST* (pp. 202-209). New York, NY: Springer-Verlag.

Krantz, D. S. (1979). A naturalistic study of social influences on meal size among moderately obese and non-obese subjects. *Psychosomatic Medicine, 41,* 19-26.

Kris, E. (1951). On preconscious mental processes. In D. Rapaport (Ed.), *Organization and pathology of thought.* New York: Columbia University Press.

Kristeller, J., Schwartz, G. E., & Black, H. (1982). The use of restricted environmental stimulation therapy in treatment of essential hypertension: Two case studies. *Behaviour Research and Therapy, 20,* 561-566.

Kroger, W. S., & Fezler, W. D. (1976). *Hypnosis and behavior modification: Imagery conditioning.* Philadelphia: J. B. Lippincott.

Krug, D. A., Arick, J. R., & Almond, P. (1980). *Autism screening instrument for educational planning.* Oregon: ASIEP Ed. Co.

Kubie, L. S., & Margolin, S. (1944). The process of hypnotism and the nature of the hypnotic state. *American Journal Psychiatry, 100,* 611-622.

LaBriola, F., Karlin, R., & Goldstein, L. (1987). EEG laterality changes from prehypnotic to hypnotic periods. In B. Taneli, C. Perris, & D. Kemali (Eds.), *Neurophysiological correlates of relaxation and psychopathology: Advances in Biological Psychiatry, 16,* 1-5.

Lacey, J. I. (1967). Somatic response patterning and stress: Some revisions of activation theory. In M. H. Appley, & R. Trumbull (Eds.), *Psychological stress: Issues in research* (pp. 14-44). New York: Appleton-Century-Crofts.

Lacey, J. I., & Lacey, B. C. (1970). Some autonomic-central nervous system interrelationships. In P. Black (Ed.), *Physiological correlates of human emotion* (pp. 205-227). New York: Academic Press.

Larbig, W. et al. (1982). EEG and slow brain potentials during anticipation and control of painful stimulation. *EEG Clinical Neurophysiology, 53,* 298-309.

Larsen, P. B., Schneiderman, N., & DeCarlo Pasin, R. (1986). Physiological bases of cardiovascular psychophysiology. In M. G. H. Coles, E. Donchin, & S. W. Porges (Eds.). *Psychophysiology: Systems, processes, and applications.* New York: Guilford.

Lazarus, R. S. (1966). *Psychological stress and the coping process.* New York: McGraw-Hill.

Lazarus, R. S., & Folkman, S. (1984). *Stress, appraisal and coping.* New York: Springer.

Lee, A. B., & Hewitt, J. (1987). Using visual imagery in a flotation tank to improve gymnastic performance and reduce physical symptoms. *International Journal of Sport Psychology, 18,* 223-230.

Lennie, B. A. (1976). Treatment of trichotillomania by covert sensitization. *Journal of Behavior Therapy and Experimental Psychiatry, 7,* 75-76.

Leuner, H. (1969). Guided affective imagery (GAI): A method of intensive psychotherapy. *American Journal of Psychotherapy, 23,* 4-22.

Levitt, E. E., Brady, J. P., Ottinger, D. R., & Hinesley, R. (1962). Effects of sensory restriction on hypnotizability. *Archives of General Psychiatry, 7,* 343-344.

Lickey, M., & Gordon, B. (1983). *Drugs for mental illness: A revolution in psychiatry.* New York: W.H. Freeman.

Lilly, J. C. (1956). Mental effects of reduction in ordinary levels of physical stimuli on intact healthy persons. *Psychiatric Research Reports, 5,* 1-28. Washington, DC: American Psychiatric Association.

Lilly, J. C. (1960). Discussion of paper by J. T. Shurley. *American Journal of Psychiatry, 117,* 544-545.

Lilly, J. C. (1965). Mental effects of reduction of ordinary levels of physical stimuli on intact, healthy persons. *Psychiatric Research Reports (Whole No. 5).*

Lilly, J. C. (1975). *The deep self: Profound relaxation and the tank isolation technique.* New York: Simon and Schuster.

Lilly, J. C. (1977). *The deep self* (p. 118). New York: Simon & Schuster.

Lilly, J. C. (1981). *The deep self: Profound relaxation and the tank isolation technique* (rev. ed.). New York: Warner Books.

Lilly, J. (1985, March). The science of isolation. Presented at the 2nd International Conference on REST, New Orleans.

Lilly, J. C., & Shurley, J. T. (1961). Experiments in solitude, in maximum achievable isolation with water suspension, of intact, healthy persons. In *Psychophysiological aspects of space flight* (pp. 238-247). New York: Columbia University Press.

Lindsley, D. B. (1957). Psychophysiology and motivation. In M. R. Jones (Ed.), *Nebraska symposium on motivation* (pp. 44-105). Lincoln: University of Nebraska Press.

Lindsley, D. B. (1961). Common factors in sensory deprivation, sensory distortion, and sensory overload. In P. Solomon, P. E. Kubzansky, P. H. Leiderman, J. H. Mendelson, R. Trumbull, & D. Wexler (Eds.), *Sensory deprivation* (pp. 174-194). Cambridge, MA: Harvard.

Lobb, L. G., & Schaefer, H. H. (1971). Successful treatment of anorexia nervosa through isolation. *Psychological Reports, 30,* 245-246.

Loor, M., Daston, P., & Smith, I. R. (1967). An analysis of mood states. *Educational and Psychological Measurement, 27,* 89-96.

Lowe, M. R., & Fisher, E. B., Jr. (1983). Emotional reactivity, emotional eating, and obesity: A naturalistic study. *Journal of Behavioral Medicine, 6,* 135-149.

Lydic, R. (1987). State-dependent aspects of regulatory physiology. *FASEB Journal, 1,* 6-15.

Lynn, D. J. (1985). I am now talking with your right hemisphere: A critical evaluation of the lateralization hypothesis. In K. Zeig (Ed.), *Ericksonian Psychotherapy Vol. I Structures* (pp. 448-458). New York: Brunner/Mazel.

MacAndrew, C. (1981). What the MAC scale tells us about men alcoholics. *Journal of Studies on Alcohol, 42,* 604-625.

MacLeod-Morgan, C. (1979). Hypnotic susceptibility, EEG theta and alpha waves, and hemispheric specificity. In G. D. Burrows, D. R. Collison, & L. Dennerstein (Eds.), *Hypnosis 1979.* Amsterdam: Elsevier-North Holland.

MacLeod-Morgan, C. (1982). EEG lateralization in hypnosis: A preliminary report. *Australian Journal of Clinical and Experimental Hypnosis, 10,* 99-102.

MacLeod-Morgan, C. (1985). Hemispheric specificity and hypnotizability: An overview of ongoing EEG research in South Australia. In D. Waxman, P. C. Misra, M. G. Gibson, & M. A. Basker (Eds.), *Modern trends in hypnosis.* Plenum Press, New York.

MacLeod-Morgan, C., & Lack, L. (1982). Hemispheric specificity: A physiological concomitant. *Psychophysiology, 19,* 687-690.

MacNeil, J., & Thomas, M. R. (1976). The treatment of obsessive compulsive hair pulling by behavioral and cognitive contingency manipulation. *Journal of Behavior Therapy and Experimental Psychiatry, 7,* 391-392.

MacNeill, M., & Zubek, J. P. (1967). Effects of prolonged visual deprivation (dark-rearing) on the weight of the sensory cortex of the rat. *Canadian Journal of Psychology, 21,* 177-183.

Margolies, P. (1977). Behavioral approaches to the treatment of early infantile autism: A review. *Psychological Bulletin, 84,* 249-264.

Markus, H. (1977). Self-schemata and processing information about the self. *Journal of Personality and Social Psychology, 35,* 63-78.

Massong, S. R., Edwards, R. P., Range-Sitton, L., & Hailey, B. J. (1980). A case of trichotillomania in a three-year-old treated by response prevention. *Journal of Behavior Therapy and Experimental Psychiatry, 11,* 223-225.

Mastellone, M. (1974). Aversion therapy: A new use for the old rubber band. *Journal of Behavior Therapy and Experimental Psychiatry, 5,* 311-312.

Matyas, T. A. (1976). T-wave amplitude stability during sinus arrhythmia in the resting man. *Physiology and Behavior, 16,* 115-117.

Matyas, T. A., & King, M. G. (1976). Stable T-wave effects during improvement in heart rate control with biofeedback. *Physiology and Behavior, 16,* 15-20.

McAleney, P. J., Barabasz, A., & Barabasz, M. (1990). Effects of flotation restricted environmental stimulation on intercollegiate tennis performance. *Perceptual and Motor Skills, 71,* 1023-1028.

McGlashan, T., Evans, F., & Orne, M. (1969). The nature of hypnotic analgesia and placebo response to experimental pain. *Psychosomatic Medicine, 31,* 227-246.

McGrady, A. V., Tan, S. V., Crane, R., Fine, T., & Yonker, R. (1979). Biochemical correlates of biofeedback in essential hypertension. *Biofeedback and Self-Regulation, 4,* 258.

McGrady, A. V., Turner, J. W., Jr., Fine, T. H., & Higgins, J. T. (1987). Effects of biobehaviorally-assisted relaxation training on blood pressure, plasma renin, cortisol, and aldosterone levels in borderline essential hypertension. *Clinical Biofeedback & Health, 10(1),* 16-25.

McGrady, A. V., Yonker, R., Tan, S. Y., Fine, T., & Woerner, M. (1981). The effect of biofeedback-assisted relaxation training on blood pressure and selected biochemical parameters in patients with essential hypertension. *Biofeedback and Self-Regulation, 6(3),* 343-353.

McKirnan, D. J., & Peterson, P. L. (1988). Stress, expectancies, and vulnerability to substance abuse: A test of a model among homosexual men. *Journal of Abnormal Psychology, 97,* 461-466.

McNair, D. M., Loor, M. (1964). An analysis of mood in ceurotics. *Journal of Abnormal and Social Psychology, 69,* 620-627.

McNair, D. M., Loor, M., & Droppleman, L. F. (1981). *Profile of mood state manual.* San Diego, CA: Educational and Industrial Testing Service.

Meerloo, J. A. M. (1955). Medication into submission: The danger of therapeutic coercion. *Journal of Nervous and Mental Disorders, 122,* 353-360.

Meerloo, J. A. M. (1956). *The rape of the mind.* Cleveland: World Publishing.

Melchiori, L. G., & Barabasz, A. (1990). Effects of flotation REST on simulated instrument flight performance. In J. Turner, & T. Fine (Eds.), *Restricted environmental stimulation: Research and commentary* (pp. 196-203). Toledo:

MCO Press.
Mellinger, G. D., Balter, M. B., & Uhlenhuth, E. H. (1985). Insomnia and its treatment: Prevalence and correlates. *Archives of General Psychiatry, 42,* 225-232.
Melville, A., & Johnson, C. (1983). *Cured to death: The effects of prescription drugs.* New York: Stein & Day.
Melzack, R. (1954). The genesis of emotional behavior. *Journal of Comparative and Physiological Psychology, 47,* 166-168.
Melzack, R., & Perry, C. (1975). Self-regulation of pain, use of alpha feedback and hypnotic training for the control of chronic pain. *Experimental Neurology, 46,* 452-469.
Melzack, R., & Scott, T. H. (1957). The effects of early experience on the response to pain. *Journal of Comparative and Physiological Psychology, 50,* 155.
Mereday, C., Lehman, C., & Borrie, R. (1990). Flotation for the management of rheumatoid arthritis. In P. Suedfeld, J. W. Turner, Jr., & T. H. Fine (Eds.), *Restricted environmental stimulation: Theoretical and empirical developments in flotation REST* (pp. 169-173). New York, NY: Springer-Verlag.
Meszaros, I., Banyai, E. I., & Greguss, A. C. (1985). Evoked potential correlates of verbal versus imagery coding in hypnosis. In D. Waxman, P. C. Misra, M. Gibson, & M. A. Basker (Eds.), *Modern trends in hypnosis.* New York and London: Plenum Press.
Meszaros, I., Banyai, E. I., & Greguss, A. C. (1986). *Enhanced right hemisphere activation during hypnosis: EEG and behavioral task performance evidence.* Paper presented at the 3rd international conference of the International Organization of Psychophysiology, Vienna, Austria.
Meszaros, I., Crawford, H. J., Szabo, Cs., Nagy-Kovacs, A., & Revesz, M. A. (1989). Hypnotic susceptibility and cerebral hemisphere preponderance. In V. Ghorghui, P. Netter, H. Eysenck, & R. Rosenthal (Eds.), *Suggestion and suggestibility: Theory and research.* Heidelberg and New York: Springer.
Metropolitan Life Insurance Company. (1984, Jan-Mar). *Statistical Bulletin, 64,* 21.
Michaels, R. R., Huber, M. J., & McCann, D. S. (1976). Evaluation of transcendental meditation as a method of reducing stress. *Science, 192,* 1242-1244.
Migály, P. (1987a, July). *Integrated approach of hypnotic theories and hallucinatory states, Part 1, Electrophysiological similarities of hallucinatory states.* Paper presented at the 4th European Congress of Hypnosis in Psychotherapy and Psychosomatic Medicine, Oxford.
Migály, P. (1987b, July). *Integrated approach of hypnotic theories and hallucinatory states, Part 2, Neurotransmitter model of hypnotic phenomena.* Paper presented at the 4th European Congress of Hypnosis in Psychotherapy and Psychosomatic Medicine, Oxford.
Migály, P. (1987c, July). *Integrated approach of hypnotic theories and hallucinatory states, Part 3, Psychological considerations.* Paper presented at the 4th European Congress of Hypnosis in Psychotherapy and Psychosomatic Medicine, Oxford.
Migály, P. (1988, March). *Sensory deprivation and the hypnotic phenomena: Some similarities.* Paper presented at The American Society of Clinical Hypnosis 30th Annual Scientific Meeting. Chicago, IL.
Migály, P. (1991, April). *Hallucinogenic drugs and treatment opportunities with hypnosis.* Paper presented at The American Society of Clinical Hypnosis 33rd Annual Scientific Meeting, St. Louis, MO.

Migály, P., & Jakab, T. (1986). Psychomimetic side effect of ketamine anaesthesia and the mechanism of action of drugs reducing these effects. Hallucination and neurotramsmitters: A review. (Hun.) *Orvosi Hetilap, 127,* 1201-1206.

Migály, P., Jakab, T., & Károvits, J. (1987). A consideration of ketamine-dreams. *Neuroscience, 22,* Supplement, S66.

Miller, G. A. (1956). The magical number seven, plus or minus two: Some limits on our capacity for processing information. *Psychological Review, 63,* 81-97.

Miller, M., Barabasz, A. F., & Barabasz, M. (1991). Effects of active alert and relaxation hypnotic inductions on cold pressor pain. *Journal of Abnormal Psychology, 100,* 223-226.

Miller, M. F., & Barabasz, M. (1987). *Effects of REST on the perception of abstract figure pairs.* Presented at the 3rd International Conference on REST. New York, NY.

Miller, M. F., & Barabasz, M. (1989). Effects of REST on the perception of abstract figure pairs. In T. Fine & J. Turner (Eds.), *REST 1989.* Toledo: MCOT.

Mills, M. J., & Eth, S. (1987). Consent and liability: Special problems with anxiolytics. *Journal of Clinical Psychiatry, 48(12),* 29-32.

Mogar, R. E. (1969). Current status and future trends in psychedelic (LSD) research. In C. Tart (Ed.), *Altered states of consciousness.* New York: Wiley.

Moll, J. M. (1983). *Management of rheumatic disorders.* New York, NY: Raven Press.

Moore, D. J., & Shiek, D. (1971). Toward a theory of early infantile autism. *Psychological Review, 78(5),* 451-456.

Morgan, A. H., & Hilgard, J. R. (1975). Stanford hypnotic clinical scale (SHCS). In E. R. Hilgard & J. R. Hilgard (Eds.), *Hypnosis in the relief of pain* (pp. 209-221, Appendix A.). Los Altos, CA: Kaufmann.

Muller, E. E., & Genazzani, A. R. (1984). *Central and peripheral endorphins basic and clinical aspects.* New York, NY: Raven Press.

Murphy, A. L., Karlin, R., Hochron, S., Lehrer, P. M., Swartzman, L., & McCann, B. (1989). Hypnotic susceptibility and its relationship to outcome in the behavioral treatment of asthma: Some preliminary data. *Psychological Reports, 65,* 691-698.

Naranjo, C., & Ornstein, R. E. (1977). *On the psychology of meditation.* Baltimore: Penguin Books.

Nicassio, P., & Bootzin, R. (1974). A comparison of progressive relaxation and autogenic training as treatments for insomnia. *Journal of Abnormal Psychology, 83,* 253-260.

Nicholas, P., & Dwyer, J. (1986). Diets for weight reduction: Nutritional considerations. In K. D. Brownell & J. P. Foreyt (Eds.), *Handbook of eating disorders* (pp. 122-144). New York: Basic Books.

O'Brien, R. G., & Kister Kaiser, M. (1985). MANOVA method for analyzing repeated measures designs: An extensive primer. *Psychological Bulletin, 97(2),* 316-333.

O'Sullivan, S., Cullen, K., & Schmitz, T. (1983). *Physical rehabilitation: Evaluation and treatment procedures.* Philadelphia, PA: F. A. Davis Company.

Olness, K. N. (1988, December). Personal communication.

O'Neil, M. (1989). Physical self concept and psychologicalmood state: Their relationship to aerobic exercies. Unpublished doctoral dissertation, Washington State University, Pullman, WA.

Orne, M. T. (1979). On the simulating subject as a quasi-control group in hypnosis research: What, why and how. In E. Fromm & R. E. Shor (Eds.), *Hypnosis: Research: Developments and new perspectives* (2nd ed., pp. 432-565). Chicago: Aldine.

Orne, M. T. (1986, August). *Demand characteristics in REST and health psychology.* Paper presented at the 3rd annual meeting of the International REST Investigators Society, New York, New York.

Orne, M. T., & Scheibe, K. E. (1964). The contribution of non-deprivation factors in the production of sensory deprivation effects: The psychology of the panic button. *Journal of Abnormal Psychology, 68,* 3-12.

Ornitz, E. M., & Ritvo, E. (1976). The syndrome of autism: A critical review. *American Journal of Psychiatry, 133,* 609-618.

Ornstein, R. E. (1977). *The psychology of consciousness* (2nd ed.). New York: Harcourt, Brace, Jovanovich.

Pena, F. (1963). *Perceptual isolation and hypnotic susceptibility.* Unpublished doctoral dissertation, Washington State University, Pullman, WA.

Peniston, E. G., & Kulkosky, P. J. (1989). Alpha-theta brainwave training and beta-endorphin levels in alcoholics. *Alcoholism: Clinical and Experimental Research, 13,* 271-279.

Perry, G. (1985). The personal nature of the REST experience. In T. Fine & J. Turner, Jr. (Ed.s). *The First International Conference on REST and Self-Regulation: Proceedings* (pp. 194-198). Toledo, OH: IRIS Publications.

Pollak, C. (1979). *The sleep log. Homer, New York:* Metrodesign Associates.

Price, V. (1978). Disorders of the hair in children. *Pediatric Clinics of North America, 25,* 305-321.

Propping, P. (1977). Genetic control of ethanol action on the central nervous system: An EEG study in twins. *Human Genetics, 35,* 309-334.

Radtke, H. L., Spanos, N. P., Armstrong, L. A., Dillman, N., & Biosvenue, M. E. (1983). Effects of electromyographic feedback and progressive relaxation training on hypnotic susceptibility: Disconfirming results. *The International Journal of Clinical and Experimental Hypnosis, 31(2),* 98-106.

Rank, D., & Suedfeld, P. (1978). Positive reactions of alcoholic men to sensory deprivation. *International Journal of Addiction, 13,* 805-813.

Raphael, Sally Jessy (Host). (1989, October 3). Peeping Tom Murders [television show]. Transcript from New York: Journal Graphics, Incorporated (Show No. 1013, Transcript No. 290).

Rasmussen, J. (Ed.) (1973). *Man in isolation and confinement.* Chicago: Aldine.

Reyher, J. (1964). Brain mechanisms, intrapsychic processes and behavior: A theory of hypnosis and psychopathology. *American Journal of Clinical Hypnosis, 7,* 107-119.

Robertson, M. H. (1961a). Sensory deprivation and some therapeutic considerations. *Psychological Record, 11,* 343-347.

Robertson, M. H. (1961b). Theoretical implication of sensory deprivation. *Psychological Record, 11,* (4)33-42.

Roffwarg, H. P., Herman, J. H., Bowe-Anders, C., & Tauber, E. S. (1978). The effects of sustained alterations of waking visual input on dream content: A preliminary report. In A. M. Arkin, J. S. Anrtobus, & S. J. Ellman (Eds.), *The mind in sleep: Psychology and psychophysiology,* Hillsdale, NJ: Lawrence Erlbaum.

Rolin, J. (1956). *Police drugs.* Translated by L. J. Bendit. New York: Philosophical Library.

Rossier, J., French, E. D., River, C., Ling, N., Guillemin, R., & Bloom, F. E. (1977). Foot-shock induced stress increases β-endorphin levels in blood but not brain. *Nature, 270,* 618-620.

Rowen, R. (1981). Hypnotic age regression in the treatment of trichotillomania. *American Journal of Clinical Hypnosis, 23,* 195-197.

Russell, J. A. (1980). A circumplex model of affect. *Journal of Personality and Social Psychology, 3,* 1161-1178.

Russell, J. A., & Snodgrass, J. (1986). Plans and the environment. In D. Stokols & I. Altman (Eds.), *Handbook of Environmental Psychology.* New York: Wiley.

Rutter, M. (1970). Autistic children: Infancy to adulthood. *Seminars in Psychiatry, 2,* 435-450.

Rutter, M. (1983). Cognitive deficits in the pathogenesis of autism. *Journal of Child Psychology and Psychiatry, 24,* 513-531.

Ruzyla-Smith, P., & Barabasz, A. (1990, March). *Effects of flotation REST on the immune response: T- and B-cells, helper and suppressor T-cells.* Paper presented at the 4th International Conference on REST, Washington, DC.

Ruzyla-Smith, P., Barabasz, A., Barabasz, M., & Warner, D. (In preparation). Effects of hypnosis on the immune response in high and low hypnotizable subjects.

Ryan, H. F., Merrill, F. B., Scott, G. E., Krebs, R., & Thompson, B. L. (1968). Increase in suicidal thoughts and tendencies: Association with diazepam therapy. *Journal of the American Medical Association, 203(13),* 135-137.

Rzewnicki, R., Wallbaum, A. B. C., Steele, H., & Suedfeld, P. (1990). REST for muscle contraction headaches: A comparison of two REST environments combined with progressive muscle relaxation training. In P. Suedfeld, J. W. Turner, Jr. & T. H. Fine (Eds.), *Restricted environmental stimulation: Theoretical and empirical developments in flotation REST* (pp. 174-183). New York, NY: Springer-Verlag.

Sabourin, M. E. (1982). Hypnosis and brain function: EEG correlates of state-trait differences. *Research Communications in Psychology, Psychiatry and Behavior, 7,* 149-168.

Sabourin, M. E., Cutcomb, S. D., Crawford, H. J., & Pribram, K. (1990). EEG correlates of hypnotic susceptibility and hypnotic trance: Spectral analysis and coherence. *International Journal of Psychophysiology, 10,* 125-142.

Saletu, B. (1987). Brain function during hypnosis, acupuncture and transcendental meditation. In B. Taneli, C. Perris, & D. Kemali (Eds.), *Neurophysiological correlates of relaxation and psychopathology: Advances in Biological Psychiatry, 16,* 18-40.

Sanders, R. S. (1967). The utilization of sensory deprivation procedures for increasing hypnotic susceptibility. Unpublished doctoral dissertation, Michigan State University.

Sanders, R. S., & Reyher, J. (1969). Sensory deprivation and the enhancement of hypnotic susceptibility. *Journal of Abnormal Psychology, 74,* 375-381.

Sanderson, K. V., & Hall-Smith, P. (1970). Tonsure trichotillomania. *British Journal of Dermatology, 82,* 343-350.

Saper, B. (1971). A report on behavior therapy with outpatient clinic patients. *Psychiatric Quarterly, 45,* 209-215.

Sarbin, T. R., & Sable, R. (1979). Hypnosis and psychophysiological outcomes. In

E. Fromm & R. E. Shor (Eds.), *Hypnosis: Developments in research and new perspectives* (2nd ed.). New York: Aldine.

Schachtel, E. G. (1959). Perception as creative experience: Critique of the concept of regression in the service of the ego. *Metamorphosis.* New York: Basic Books.

Schachter, S. (1964). The interaction of cognitive and physiological determinants of emotional state. In L. Berkowitz (Ed.), *Advances in experimental social psychology* (Vol. 1, pp. 49-80). New York: Academic Press.

Schacter, D. L. (1977). EEG theta waves and psychological phenomena: A review and analysis. *Biological Psychology, 5,* 47-82.

Schechter, M. D., Shurley, J. T., Toussieng, P. W., & Maier, W. J. (1969). Sensory isolation therapy of autistic children: A preliminary report. *Journal of Pediatrics, 74,* 564-569.

Schopler, E., & Mesibov, G. B. (Eds.). (1983). *Autism in adolescents and adults.* New York: Plenum Press.

Schowalter, J. E. (1989). Psychodynamics and medication. *Journal of the American Academy of Child & Adolescent Psychiatry, 28,* 681-684.

Schultz, D. (1965). *Sensory restriction: Effects on behavior.* New York: Academic Press.

Schultz, J. H., & Luthe, W. (1959). *Autogenic Training.* New York: Grune and Stratton.

Schwartz, G. E. (1983). Disregulation theory and disease: Applications to the repression/cerebral disconnection/cardiovascular disorder hypothesis. *International Review of Applied Psychology, 32,* 95-118.

Schwartz, P. J., & Weiss, T. (1983). T-wave amplitude as an index of cardiac sympathetic activity: A misleading concept. *Psychophysiology, 20(6),* 696-701.

Scott, T. H. (1954). *Intellectual effects of perceptual isolation.* Unpublished doctoral dissertation, McGill University, Montreal.

Scott, T. H., Bexton, W. H., Heron, W., & Doane, B. K. (1959). Cognitive effects of perceptual isolation. *Canadian Journal of Psychology, 13,* 200-209.

Selzer, M. L. (1980). Alcoholism and alcoholic psychosis (3rd ed.). In H. J. Kaplan, et al. (Eds.), *Comprehensive Textbook of Psychiatry, 2* (pp. 1629-1645). Baltimore: Williams & Wilkins.

Shah, A., & Wing, L. (1986). Cognitive impairments affecting social behavior in autism. In E. Schopler & G. Mesibov (Eds.), *Social behavior in autism* (p. 88). New York & London: Plenum.

Shapiro, A. (1971). Placebo effects in medicine, psychotherapy and psychoanalysis. In A. Bergin & S. Garfield (Eds.), *Handbook of psychotherapy and behavior change.* New York: Wiley.

Sheehan, P. W. (1979). Hypnosis and the processes of imagination. In E. Fromm and R. Shor (Eds.), *Hypnosis: Developments in research and new perspectives.* New York: Aldine.

Sheehan, P. W., & McConkey, K. M. (1982). *Hypnosis and experience.* N.J.: Earlbaum.

Shepherd, J. M., Zubek, J., & Saers, M. G. (1967). EEG changes during sensory and perceptual deprivation studies. *Electroencephalography and Clinical Neurophysiology, 22,* 191.

Sher, H., Hartman, L. M., Furedy, J. J., & Heslegrave, R. J. (1986). Electrocardiographic T-wave changes are more pronounced in Type A than in Type B men during mental work. *Psychosomatic Medicine, 48(3-4),* 159-166.

Siegel, S., & Castellan, Jr., N. J. (1988). *Nonparametric statistics for the behavioral sciences.* New York: McGraw-Hill.

Sifford, D. (1990, January 28). When one drug treats many psychiatric illnesses. *The Philadelphia Inquirer.*

Sigelman, D. W. (1989, November). Halcion: Waking up to the dangers of a sleeping pill. *Trial,* 38-43.

Siler, W. A. (1979). *Death by prescription.* Nashville: Sherbourne Press, Inc.

Smith, S., & Lewty, W. (1959). Perceptual isolation using a silent room. *Lancet, 2,* 342-345.

Sniffen, J., DeTurk, W., Mereday, C., & Lehmann, C. (1990). *Effects of flotation in magnesium sulfate on muscle tone in children with Cerebral Palsy.* A paper presented at the American Physical Therapy Association Conference, Anaheim, CA.

Soldatos, C. R., Kales, A., Bixler, E. O., & Vela-Bueno, A. (1985). Behavioral side effects of benzodiazepine hypnotics. *Clinical Neuropharmacology, 8,* S112-S117 (Supplement #1).

Soldatos, C. R., Sakkas, P. N., Bergiannaki, J. D., & Stefanis, C. N. (1986). Behavioral side effects of triazolam in psychiatric inpatients: A report of five cases. *Drug Intelligence and Clinical Pharmacy, 20,* 294-297.

Solomon, P., Kubzansky, P., Liederman, P., Mendelson, J., Trumbull, R., & Wexler, D. (Eds.). (1961). *Sensory deprivation: A symposium.* Cambridge, MA: Harvard University Press.

Sonstroem, R. J., & Bernardo, P. (1982). Intraindividual pregame state anxiety and basketball performance: A re-examination of the inverted-U curve. *Journal of Sport Psychology 4,* 235-245.

Spiegel, D., & Barabasz, A. (1988). Effects of hypnotic hallucination on P300 evoked potential amplitudes: Reconciling conflicting findings. *American Journal of Clinical Hypnosis, 331,* 11-17.

Spiegel, D., Bierre, P., & Rootenberg, J. (1988, May). *Hypnotic alteration of somatosensory perception.* Paper presented at the annual meeting of the American Psychiatric Association, Montreal, Canada.

Spiegel, D., Cutcomb, S., Ren, C., & Pribram, K. (1985). Hypnotic hallucination alters evoked potentials. *Journal of Abnormal Psychology, 13(3),* 249-255.

Spiegel, H., & Spiegel, D. (1978). *Trance and treatment: Clinical uses of hypnosis.* Washington, DC: American Psychiatric Press, Inc.

Stanley, J., Mahoney, M., & Reppert, S. (1987). REST and the enhancement of sports performance: A panel presentation and discussion. In J. W. Turner & T. H. Fine (Eds.), *Proceedings of the 2nd International Conference on Restricted Environmental Stimulation* (pp. 168-183). Toledo, OH: MCO Press.

Steck, W. D. (1979). The clinical evaluation of pathologic hair loss. *Cutis, 24,* 293-301.

Stern, G. (1980). Physiological and mood effects of salt water flotation. Unpublished manuscript, University of Colorado, Denver.

Striegel-Moore, R., & Rodin, J. (1986). The influence of psychological variables in obesity. In K. D. Brownell & J. P. Foreyt (Eds.), *Handbook of eating disorders* (pp. 99-121). New York: Basic Books.

Strupp, H., & Bergin, A. E. (1972). *Changing frontiers in the science of psychotherapy.* Chicago: Aldine.

Stuart, R. B. (1967). Behavioral control of overeating. *Behavior Research & Therapy, 5,* 357-365.

Stuart, R. B. (1971). A three-dimensional program for the treatment of obesity. *Behavior Research & Therapy, 9,* 177-186.

Stunkard, A. J. (1959). Eating patterns and obesity. *Psychiatric Quarterly, 33,* 284-292.

Stunkard, A. J. (1976). *The pain of obesity.* Palo Alto, CA: Bull Publishing Company.

Stunkard, A. J. (1986). The control of obesity: Social and community perspectives. In K. D. Brownell & J. P. Foreyt (Eds.), *Handbook of eating disorders* (pp. 213-228). New York: Basic Books.

Suedfeld, P. (1969a). Changes in intellectual performance and in susceptibility to influence. In J. P. Zubek (Ed.), *Sensory deprivation: Fifteen years of research* (pp. 126-166). New York: Appleton-Century-Crofts.

Suedfeld, P. (1969b). Theoretical formulations: II. In J. P. Zubek (Ed.), *Sensory deprivation: Fifteen years of research* (pp. 433-448). New York: Appleton-Century-Crofts.

Suedfeld, P. (1972). *Attitude manipulation in restricted environments: Theory and research.* Symposium paper read at the XXth International Congress of Psychology, Tokyo.

Suedfeld, P. (Ed.). (1977). Therapeutic uses of sensory deprivation and social isolation.

Suedfeld, P. (1980). *Restricted environmental stimulation: Research and clinical applications.* New York: Wiley.

Suedfeld, P. (1984). Restricted environmental stimulation therapy (REST). In J. D. Matarazzo, W. Weiss, J. A. Herd, N. E. Miller, & W. M. Weiss (Eds.). *Behavioral health: A handbook of health enhancement and disease prevention* (pp. 755-763). New York: Wiley.

Suedfeld, P. (1985, March). *Presidential address.* Presented at the 2nd International Conference on REST, New Orleans.

Suedfeld, P. (1987, August). *Presidential address.* Presented at the 3rd International Conference on REST, New York City.

Suedfeld, P., & Baker-Brown, G. (1987). Restricted environmental stimulation therapy of smoking: A parametric study. *Addictive Behaviors, 12,* 263-267.

Suedfeld, P., & Ballard, E. (1984, September). The uses of REST: Do we need procedural specificity? Presented at the International Congress of Psychology, Acapulco, Mexico.

Suedfeld, P., Ballard, E. J., & Murphy, M. (1983). Water immersion and flotation: From stress experiment to stress treatment. *Journal of Environmental Psychology, 3,* 147-155.

Suedfeld, P., Bernaldez, J. P., & Stossel, D. L. (1989). The Polar psychology project: A cross national investigation of polar adaptation. *Arctic Medical Research, 48,* 91-94.

Suedfeld, P., & Best, J. A. (1977). Satiation and sensory deprivation combined in smoking therapy: Some case studies and unexpected side-effects. *The International Journal of the Addictions, 12,* 337-359.

Suedfeld, P., & Bruno, T. (1990). Flotation REST and imagery in the improvement of athletic performance. *Journal of Sport and Exercise Psychology, 12,* 82-85.

Suedfeld, P., & Clarke, J. C. (1981). Specific food aversions acquired during restricted environmental stimulation. *Journal of Applied Social Psychology, 11,* 538-547.

Suedfeld, P., & Kristeller, J. L. (1982). Stimulus reduction as a technique in health psychology. *Health Psychology, 4,* 337-357.

Suedfeld, P., Roy, C., & Landon, P. B. (1982). Restricted environmental stimulation therapy in the treatment of essential hypertension. *Behaviour Research and Therapy, 20,* 553-559.

Suedfeld, P., & Schwartz, G. (1983). Restricted environmental stimulation therapy (REST) as a treatment for autistic children. *Developmental and Behavioral Pediatrics, 4(3)* 196-201.

Suinn, R. (1986). *Seven steps to peak performance: The mental training manual for athletes.* Toronto, Canada: H. Huber.

Szasz, T. S. (1960). The myth of mental illness. *American Psychologist, 15,* 113-118.

Szasz, T. S. (1961). *The myth of mental illness: Foundations of a theory of personal conduct.* New York: Hoerber-Harper.

Taneli, B., & Krahne, W. (1987). EEG changes of transcendental meditation practitioners. *Neurophysiological correlates of relaxation and psychopathology. Advances in Biological Psychiatry, 16,* 41-71.

Tart, C. T. (1966). Types of hypnotic dreams and their relation to hypnotic depth. *Journal of Abnormal Psychology, 71,* 377-382.

Taylor, J. G. (1963). A behavioral interpretation of obsessive compulsive neurosis. *Behavior Research and Therapy, 1,* 237-244.

Tebecis, A. K., Provins, K. A., Farnbach, R. W., & Pentony, P. (1975). Hypnosis and the EEG: A quantitative investigation. *Journal of Nervous and Mental Disease, 161,* 1-17.

Tellegen, A., & Atkinson, G. (1974). Openness to absorbing and self altering experiences ("absorption"), a trait related to hypnotic susceptibility. *Journal of Abnormal Psychology, 83,* 268-277.

Tellock, P. E., & Suedfeld, P. (1976). Inducing belief instability without a persuasive message: The roles of attitude centrality, individual cognitive differences, and sensory deprivation. *Canadian Journal of Behavioral Science, 8,* 324-333.

Tichalsky, F. (1984). *REST for smoking control.* Presented at the International Congress of Psychology. Acapulco, Mexico.

Tindall, A. (1976). *Exercise in water.* In M. H. Duffild (Ed.). Baltimore, MD: Williams and Wilkins.

Turner, J. W., Jr., & Fine, T. H. (1983). Effects of relaxation associated with brief restricted environmental stimulation therapy (REST) on plasma cortisol, ACTH, and LH. *Biofeedback and Self-Regulation, 9,* 115-126.

Turner, J. W., Jr., & Fine, T. H. (1985a). Effects of restricted environmental stimulation therapy (REST) on self-control of heart rate. In J. J. Sanchez-Soza (Ed.), *Health and Clinical Psychology* (pp. 477-490). New York, NY: Elsevier Science Publ.

Turner, J. W., Jr., & Fine, T. H. (1985b). Hormonal changes associated with restricted environmental stimulation therapy (REST). In T. H. Fine & J. W. Turner, Jr. (Eds.), *Proceedings of the 1st International Conference on REST and Self-Regulation* (pp. 17-39). Toledo, OH: IRIS.

Turner, J. W., Jr., & Fine, T. H. (1987). *Second International Conference on REST.* IRIS Publishing, Toledo, OH.

Turner, J. W., Jr., & Fine, T. H. (1990a). Hormonal changes associated with restricted environmental stimulation therapy. In P. Suedfeld, J. Turner, & T. Fine (Eds.), *Restricted environmental stimulation theoretical and empirical developments in flotation REST.* New York, NY: Springer-Verlag.

Turner, J. W., Jr., & Fine, T. H. (1990b). Restricted environmental stimulation influences plasma cortisol levels and their variability. In J. W. Turner, Jr., & T. H. Fine (Eds.), *Restricted environmental stimulation: Research and commentary* (pp. 71-78). Toledo, OH: Medical College of Ohio Press.

Turner, J. W., Jr., & Fine, T. H. (1991, in press). Restricting environmental stimulation influences variability and levels of plasma cortisol. *Journal of Applied Physiology.*

Turner, J. W., Jr., Fine, T., Ewy, G., Sershon P., & Frelich, T. (1989). The presence or absence of light during flotation restricted environmental stimulation: Effects on plasma cortisol, blood pressure and mood. *Biofeedback and Self-Regulation, 14,* 291-300.

Turner, J. W., Jr., Fine, T. H., McGrady, A., & Higgins, J. T. (1987). Effects of biobehavioraly assisted relaxation training on blood pressure and hormone levels and their variation in normotensives and essential hypertensives. In J. W. Turner, Jr., & T. H. Fine (Eds.), *Proceedings of the Second International Conference on REST* (pp. 87-109). Toledo, OH: IRIS.

Turner, J. W., Jr., Gerard, W., Hyland, J., Neilands, P., & Fine, T. H. (1991a, in press). Effects of wet and dry flotation REST on blood pressure and plasma cortisol. In A. Barabasz (Ed.), *Clinical and experimental restricted environmental stimulation: New developments and perspectives.* New York: Springer-Verlag.

Turner, J. W., Jr., Schroeder, H., & Fine, T. H. (1991b, in press). A method for continuous blood sampling during flotation REST. In A. Barabasz (Ed.), *Clinical and experimental restricted environmental stimulation: New developments and perspectives.* New York: Springer-Verlag.

Ulett, G. A., Akpinar, S., & Itil, T. M. (1972). Hypnosis: Physiological and pharmacological reality. *American Journal of Psychiatry, 128,* 799-805.

Van Itallie, T. B. (1985). Health implications of overweight and obesity in the United States. *Annals of Internal Medicine, 103,* 983-988.

Van Oot, P. H., Lane, T. W., & Borkovec, T. D. (1983). Sleep disturbances. In H. Adams & P. B. Sutker (Eds.), *Comprehensive handbook of psychopathology* (pp. 683-723). New York: Plenum Press.

van Wulfften Plathe, P. M. (1958). Sensory and motor deprivation as psychopathological stress. *Aeromedica Acta (Netherlands), 6,* 155-168.

van Wulfften Plathe, P. M. (1959). Sensory and motor deprivation as a psychopathological stress. *Folia Psych Neur Neurochirug (Netherlands), 62,* 407-421.

van Wulfften Plathe, P. M. (1962). Fluctuations in level of consciousness caused by reduced sensorial stimulation and by limited motility in solitary confinement. *Psychiat Neurol Neurochirug (Amsterdam), 65,* 377-401.

Vernon, J. A. (1964). *Inside the black room.* New York: Clarkson N. Potter.

Vogel, W., Broverman, D. M., & Klaiber, E. L. (1968). EEG and mental abilities. *Electroencephalography and Clinical Neurophysiology, 24,* 166-175.

Wagaman, J., & Barabasz, A. (1990). *Effects of flotation REST on collegiate athletic performance: Basketball.* Presented at the 4th International Conference on Restricted Environmental Stimulation, Washington, DC, March 22-23.

Wagaman, J., Barabasz, A., & Barabasz, M. (1991). Flotation REST and imagery in the improvement of collegiate basketball performance. *Perceptual and Motor Skills, 72,* 119-122.

Wallace, B. (1978). Restoration of eidetic imagery via hypnotic age regression:

More evidence. *Journal of Abnormal Psychology, 87,* 673-675.
Wallace, R. K., & Benson, H. (1972). The physiology of meditation. *Scientific American, 226*(2), 84-90.
Wanberg & Horn, (1987)
Watson, D., & Clark, L. A. (1984). Negative affectivity: The disposition to experience aversive emotional states. *Psychological Bulletin, 96,* 465-490.
Watson, D., & Tellegen, A. (1985). Toward a consensual structure of mood. *Psychological Bulletin, 98*(2), 219-235.
Weiner, H. (1979). *Psychobiology of essential hypertension.* New York, NY: Elsevier North Holland, Inc.
Weitzenhoffer, A. M., & Hilgard, E. R. (1962). *Stanford Hypnotic Susceptibility Scale, Form C.* Palo Alto, CA: Consulting Psychologists Press.
Weitzman, E. D., Fukushima, D., Nageire, C., Roffwarg, H., Gallagher, T. F., & Hellman, L. (1971). Twenty-four hour pattern of the episodic secretion of cortisol in normal subjects. *Journal of Clinical Endocrinology and Metabolism, 33,* 14-22.
Werch, C. E., & Gorman, D. R. (1988). Relationship between self control and alcohol consumption patterns and problems of college students. *Journal of Studies on Alcohol, 49,* 30-37.
West, L. J. (Ed.). (1962). *Hallucinations.* New York: Grune & Stratton.
Wexler, D., Mendelson, J., Leiderman, P. H., & Solomon, P. (1958). Sensory deprivation: A technique of studying psychiatric aspects of stress. *Archives of Neurology and Psychiatry, 79,* 225-233.
Whisler, R., & Rothsmich, N. (1985). *Rheumatoid arthritis.* New York, NY: Grune and Stratton, Inc.
Wickramasekera, I. (1969). The effects of sensory restriction on susceptibility to hypnosis: A hypothesis, some preliminary data, and theoretical speculation. *The International Journal of Clinical and Experimental Hypnosis, 17(4),* 217-224.
Wickramasekera, I. (1970). Effects of sensory restriction on susceptibility to hypnosis: A hypothesis and more preliminary data. *Journal of Abnormal Psychology, 76,* 69-75.
Wickramasekera, I. (1971). Effects of EMG feedback restriction on susceptibility to hypnosis: Preliminary observations. *Proceedings of the 79th Annual Convention of the American Psychological Association, 6(part 2),* 783-784.
Wickramasekera, I. (1973). Effects of electromyographic feedback on hypnotic susceptibility: More preliminary data. *Journal of Abnormal Psychology, 82(1),* 74-77.
Wickramasekera, I. (1976). *Biofeedback, behavior therapy and hypnosis.* Chicago: Nelson Hall.
Wickramasekera, I. (1977a). On attempts to modify hypnotic susceptibility: Some psycho-physiological procedures and promising directions. *Annals of the New York Academy of Sciences, 296,* 143-153.
Wickramasekera, I. (1977b). The placebo effect and biofeedback for headache pain. In *Proceedings of the San Diego Biomedical Symposium.* New York: Academic Press.
Wickramasekera, I. (1979). *A model of the patient at high risk for chronic stress related disorders: Do beliefs have biological consequences?* Paper presented at the Annual Convention of the Biofeedback Society of America, San Diego, CA.
Wickramasekera, I. (1980). A conditioned response model of the placebo effect: Predictions from the model. *Biofeedback and Self-Regulation, 5(1),* 5-18.

Wickramasekera, I. (1983). *A model of people at high risk.* Paper read at the International Stress and Tension Control Society, Brighton, England.
Wickramasekera, I. (1985). A conditioned response model of the placebo effect: Predictions from the model. In L. White, B. Tursky, & G.E. Schwartz (Eds.), *Placebo: Theory, research, and mechanisms.* New York: Guilford Press.
Wickramasekera, I. (1986). A model of people at high risk to develop chronic stress related somatic symptoms: Some predictions. *Professional Psychology: Research and Practice, 17*(5), 437-447.
Wickramasekera, I. (1988). *Clinical behavioral medicine: Some concepts and procedures.* New York: Plenum.
Wickramasekera, I. (1989). Enabling the somatizing patient to exit the somatic closet: A high-risk model. *Psychotherapy: Theory, Research, Practice, Training, 26*(4), 530-544.
Wickramasekera, I. (1990). *Psychophysiological monitoring as another royal road to the unconscious.* Paper presented at the annual meeting of the Association for Applied Psychophysiology and Biofeedback, Washington, DC.
Wickramasekera, I. (1991). *Psychophysiological monitoring: Another 'royal road' to the unconscious mind.* Paper presented at the annual meeting of the Association for Applied Psychophysiology and Biofeedback, Dallas, Texas.
Wilfrey, D., & Konce, J. (1986). Differential physical and psychological effects of exercise. *Journal of Counseling Psychology, 33,* 337-342.
Williams, S., & Harper, J. (1974). A study of etiological factors at critical periods of development in autistic children. *International Journal of Mental Health, 3*(1), 90-99.
Wing, L. (1983). Social and interpersonal needs. In E. Schopler & G. Mesibov (Eds.), *Autism in adolescents and adults* (pp. 337-354). New York: Plenum Press.
Wing, L., & Gould, J. (1979). Severe impairments of social interaction and associated abnormalities in children: Epidemiology and classification. *Journal of Autism and Developmental Disorders, 9*(1), 11-29.
Wojcikiewicz, A., & Orlick, T. (1987). The effects of post-hypnotic suggestion and relaxation with suggestion on competitive fencing anxiety and performance. *International Journal of Sport Psychology,* 18, 303-313.
Wolf, M. (1978). Social validity: The case for subjective measurement or how applied behavioral analysis is finding its heart. *Journal of Applied Behavioral Analysis, 11,* 203-214.
Wolfe, S. M. (Ed.). (1985). The risks of tranquility. *Health Letter, 1*(4), 5-6.
Wolfe, S. M. (Ed.). (1987). Drug-induced tranquility. *Health Letter, 3*(4), 6-8.
Wolfe, S. M. (Ed.). (1988). VERSED: Another dangerous drug slips through the DA's sieve. *Health Letter, 4*(3), 1-4.
Wolfe, S. M., Fugate, L., Hulstrand, E. P., & Kamimoto, L. E. (1988). *Worst pills, best pills: The older adults' guide to avoiding drug-induced death or illness.* Washington: Public Citizen's Health Research Group.
Woodburn, H. (1961). Cognitive and physiological effects of perceptual isolation. In P. Solomon, P. Kubzansky, P. H. Leiderman, J. Mendelson, R. Trumbull, & D. Wexler (Eds.), *Sensory Deprivation* (pp. 6-33). Cambridge, Mass: Harvard Univ. Press.
Woods, J. H., Katz, J. L., & Winger, G. (1987). Abuse liability of benzodiazepines. *Pharmacological Reviews, 39*(4), 251-419.
Woolfolk, R. L., Carr-Kaffashan, L., McNulty, T. F., & Lehrer, P. M. (1976).

Meditation training as a treatment for insomnia. *Behavior Therapy, 7,* 359-365.
Wolpe, J. (1973). *The practice of behavior therapy.* New York: Pergamon Press.
Wright, L., Schaefer, A. B., & Solomons, J. G. (1979). *Encyclopedia of Pediatric Psychology.* Baltimore: University Park Press.
Zar, J. H. (1984). *Biostatistical analysis.* Englewood Cliffs, NJ: Prentice-Hall.
Zawadaski, Z. (1971). A rare case of persistent trichotillomania in an adult. *Polish Medical Science and History,* 77-78.
Zeig, J. K. (1974). Hypnotherapy techniques with psychotic in-patients. *American Journal of Clinical Hypnosis, 17,* 56-59.
Zillmann, D. (1983). Transfer of excitation in emotional behavior. In J. Caccioppo & R. Petty (Eds.), *Social Psychophysiology.* New York: Guilford Press.
Zisook, S. (1990, February 5). Personal communication (letter).
Zisook, S., & DeVaul, R. A. (1977). Adverse behavioral effects of benzodiazepines. *Journal of Family Practice, 5(6),* 963-966.
Zubek, J. (1964). Behavioral and EEG changes after 14 days of perceptual deprivation. *Psychonomic Science, 1,* 57-58.
Zubek, J. P. (1969a). Physiological and biochemical effects. In J. P. Zubek (Ed.), *Sensory deprivation: Fifteen years of research* (pp. 254-288). New York: Appleton-Century-Crofts.
Zubek, J. P. (Ed.). (1969b). *Sensory deprivation: Fifteen years of research.* New York: Appleton-Century-Crofts.
Zubek, J. P. (1973). Behavioral and physiological effects of prolonged sensory and perceptual deprivation: A review. In J. E. Rasmussen (Ed.), *Man in isolation and confinement* (pp. 9-83). Chicago: Aldine.
Zubek, J., Welch, G., & Saers, M. G. (1962). Electroencephalographic changes after 14 days of perceptual deprivation. *Science, 139,* 490-492.
Zuckerman, M. (1969a). Theoretical formulations: I. In J. Zubek (Ed.), *Sensory deprivation: Fifteen years of research* (pp. 404-432). New York: Appleton-Century-Crofts.
Zuckerman, M. (1969b). Variables affecting deprivation results. In J. Zubek (Ed.), *Sensory deprivation: Fifteen years of research* (pp. 47-84). New York: Appleton-Century-Crofts.
Zuckerman, M. (1979). *Sensation seeking: Beyond the optimal level of arousal.* Hillside, NJ: Erlbaum.
Zuckerman, M., & Cohen, N. (1964). Is suggestion the source of reported visual sensations in perceptual isolation? *Journal of Abnormal and Social Psychology, 68,* 655-660.

Springer Nature Customer Service Center GmbH

Printed by Libri Plureos GmbH

in Hamburg, Germany

MIX
Papier aus verantwortungsvollen Quellen
Paper from responsible sources
FSC® C105338

If you have any concerns about our products,
you can contact us on
ProductSafety@springernature.com

In case Publisher is established outside the EU,
the EU authorized representative is:
Springer Nature Customer Service Center GmbH
Europaplatz 3, 69115 Heidelberg, Germany

Printed by Libri Plureos GmbH
in Hamburg, Germany